THE STRENGTH TRAINING BIBLE

FOR SENIORS

The Ultimate Fitness Guide
for the Rest of Your Life

Dr. Karl Knopf

VELO press

Portions of *The Strength Training Bible for Seniors* have been previously published in a different format.

Published by:

velopress®

an imprint of Ulysses Press
PO Box 3440
Berkeley, CA 94703
www.velopress.com

VeloPress is the leading publisher of books on sports for passionate and dedicated athletes around the world. Focused on cycling, triathlon, running, swimming, nutrition/diet, and more, VeloPress books help you achieve your goals and reach the top of your game.

ISBN: 978-1-64604-747-5
Library of Congress Control Number: 2024934522

Printed in United States
10 9 8 7 6 5 4 3 2 1

Project managers: Brian McLendon, Kierra Sondereker
Managing editor: Claire Chun
Editor: Mary Calvez
Proofreader: Renee Rutledge
Photographs: © Rapt Production and © Robert Holmes Photography
Front cover/interior design and layout: Jake Flaherty Design
Models: Grant Bennett, Fred Brevold, Vivian Gunderson, Rob Harrison, Jack Holleman, Karl Knopf, Michael O'Meara, Jeff Rankin, Phyllis Ritchie, Toni Silver, Kym Sterner

Please Note: This book has been written and published strictly for informational purposes, and in no way should be used as a substitute for consultation with health care professionals. You should not consider educational material herein to be the practice of medicine or to replace consultation with a physician or other medical practitioner. The author and publisher are providing you with information in this work so that you can have the knowledge and can choose, at your own risk, to act on that knowledge. The author and publisher also urge all readers to be aware of their health status and to consult health care professionals before beginning any health program. This book is independently authored and published and no sponsorship or endorsement of this book by, and no affiliation with, any trademarked events, brands, or other products mentioned or pictured within, is claimed or suggested. All trademarks that appear in this book belong to their respective owners and are used here for informational purposes only. The author and publisher encourage readers to patronize the events, brands, and other products mentioned and pictured in this book.

CONTENTS

PART 2: CORE STRENGTH   123

CORE-STRENGTHENING PROGRAMS **133**

EXERCISES FOR CORE STRENGTH **141**

PART 3: WEIGHT AND RESISTANCE TRAINING   211

WEIGHT AND RESISTANCE TRAINING EXERCISES 227

PART 4: KETTLEBELLS   287

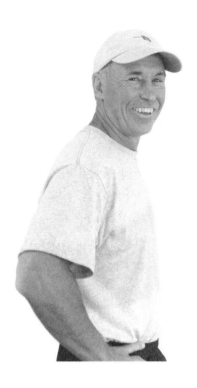

INTRODUCTION

Grow strong, not old.

The fountain of youth has been discovered! However, it's not in a bottle, an injection, or a pill. It's found in a daily dose of sensible physical activity. While many seniors—people 50 and older—understand the importance of aerobic exercise, many neglect a critical component to successful aging: maintaining strength and power. Specifically, a lack of strength and power in our legs, trunk, and arms reduces our ability to attend to basic activities of daily living. This weakness increases the risk of falling and reduces our independence.

Many people let their age exclude them from being the healthiest and fittest person they can be. Every day we have the ability to determine how we want to age. To a large extent how well we age has to do with how we eat, sleep, think, and move. Our attitude toward aging largely influences how we age. The decisions we make daily, such as choosing to eat well and engage in regular physical activity, are the foundation of successful living. If you view the process as a time of decline and frailty, you will be fighting each birthday rather than making every year the best year of your life. Also, if you allow advertisers to make you feel bad about living, then you will continue to deny aging rather than embrace it.

More and more research supports the conclusion that we can control our own aging, and recent scientific studies have exploded the myth that strength training isn't effective as we age. As a recent headline in the *Washington Post* proclaimed, "It's never too late to lift weights: Older bodies can still build muscle." This book will help you do that.

The people who live long and thrive often report that the success of their aging was largely influenced by their positive attitude, being physically active, eating healthily, moderating their consumption of alcohol, getting adequate rest and sleep, and staying socially engaged. If we want society to change its attitude about aging, we need to start bragging about our age rather than denying it. We also need to be proactive and take steps today to positively influence our health. A simple rule of thumb for healthy aging is the 80-20 rule: Do healthy, positive things at least 80 percent of the time.

Many scientists believe that with a healthy lifestyle, we may be able to turn back the biological clock 10 to 20 years or at least slow it down. A healthy, active person ages approximately half a percent a year, compared to an inactive person with poor health habits, who ages at approximately two percent a year. If you do the math, you can see how a healthy lifestyle can make a significant difference over a period of a lifetime. To maintain a fit lifestyle, engage in strength training two to three times a week, aim for 30 minutes of aerobic exercise five days a week, and stretch daily. When coupled with an aerobic exercise program, *The Strength Training Bible for Seniors* is designed to be a single resource to help you create your own personalized plan for getting and remaining strong and flexible.

This book is divided into four sections, each designed to give you the foundations you need to create a customizable full-body strength exercise plan to gain power, muscle, and flexibility so you can remain healthy and active throughout your senior years:

- **Stretching:** to ensure flexibility and prevent muscle strains and ligament injuries
- **Core Strength:** to build up the powerhouse of the body, from the tops of your legs to the shoulder area
- **Weights:** to strengthen muscles in your core, arms, and legs
- **Kettlebells:** to improve explosive muscle power

A quote from a former student: "I don't want to just survive, I want to thrive! Active aging is not a journey to the grave with the intention of arriving with regrets, but rather to skid in broadside, thoroughly totally worn out, and loudly proclaiming, WOW, what a ride! I hate exercise but I hate not being able to do what I want more." Another student once told me, "Age is just a number and mine is not listed." A 75-year-old student told me that she didn't care about her age because she feels better and more empowered than ever before. She went on to say that how you feel and act is more important than the number of candles on a cake and that being active every day makes her feel better than the day before.

The intent of this book is to assist you to train well and train smart, not hard. It does not have hard-and-fast rules. The only rule in this book is to learn to listen to your body and heed what it says. The aim of this book is to teach you to turn inward and feel what is best for you. Throughout this book, you'll also find answers to the frequently asked questions of stretching and strength training. No one knows your body better than you do! You are the captain of your ship, and everyone else is a member of your fitness crew. Never let anyone "should" you!

Remember that you hold the key to your wellness. Create the life you want. It is never too late to feel great! Too often as we age we think we are too old or too disabled to be active and physically fit. Both are wrong! The key to happy aging is to change what you can and accept what you cannot.

Try to remodel yourself daily; what you do today determines your tomorrows. With this mindset, you can grow well, not old!

"In the end we cannot become what we need to be by remaining what we are."

—Max De Pree

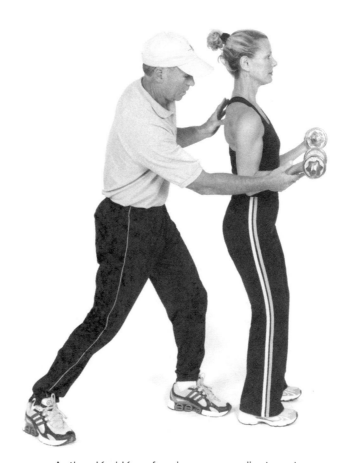

Author Karl Knopf makes some adjustments.

GETTING STARTED

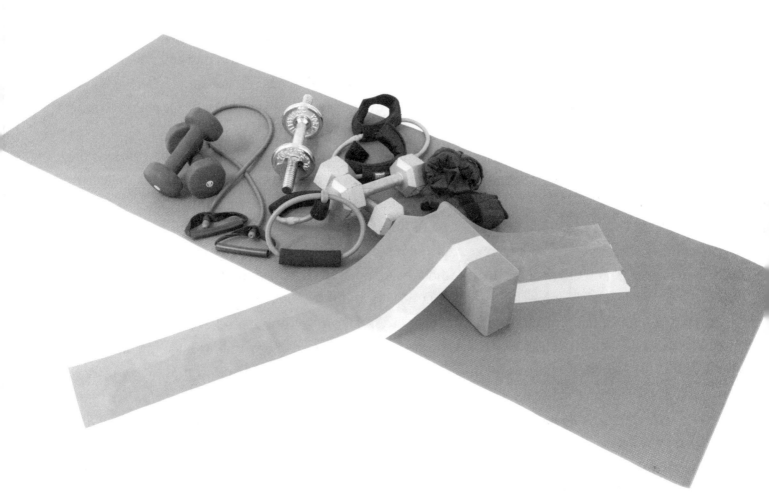

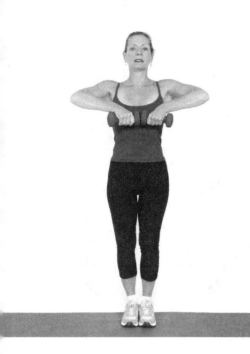

FIT FOR LIFE

Hippocrates said it so well more than 2000 years ago: "All parts of the body, which have function, if used in moderation and exercised to which each is accustomed, become thereby healthy and well developed and age slowly. But if left idle become liable to disease, defective in growth and age quickly." Mickey Mantle said the same thing, but in a simpler way: "If I knew I was going to live this long I would have taken better care of myself."

Strength training is the single most critical step you can take to retard aging. The human body has over 400 voluntary muscles—it's a machine that was designed for movement. Yet, in this technology-driven age, we consistently invest in products that reduce our need to move. Do you remember the days when you had to get out of the car to open the garage door? Or get up to adjust the thermostat instead of through your smartphone? Even these simple bouts of physical activity required muscular strength. Unfortunately, all these wonderful labor-saving devices that we use daily hasten the process of sarcopenia (age-related loss of muscle mass and strength). To keep our muscles from withering away from disuse, we must challenge them frequently.

Young people frequently exercise to look better. In middle age, people often exercise for the health of it. However, in order to age well and remain fully independent, we need to exercise for the function of it. Too often, older people find that many of the activities of daily living that they once found simple have become challenging. Many of my older students joined my classes because steps seemed higher than they used to be, chairs were harder to get out of, and even the act of lifting a bag of groceries caused strain. Much of the decline often associated with normal aging has more to do with a loss of muscular strength and function than the number of trips around the sun.

A great deal of strength is lost between the ages of 30 and 50. If a person participates in a regular strength-training routine, the loss of strength can be minimized. Fortunately, it is never too late to turn your fitness life around. Numerous studies have proven that both men and women in their 80s and 90s can regain their strength and function by engaging in sensible and regular strength training; in cases of arthritis, several studies have shown that when the muscles around an arthritic joint get stronger, the load placed on that joint decreases. I have personally witnessed a woman in my strength class lose about 30 pounds and dramatically improve her ability to get around; she no longer uses a walker and can pick things up off the floor easily, which she was unable to do a year ago. Today she has more energy and is having a lot more fun than she ever remembered. All these positive results can be derived by a slight reduction in calories to lose weight slowly and permanently, combined with a daily dose of strength training and aerobic exercise.

IF YOU REST, YOU RUST

People who do not engage in a regular strength-training routine throughout their lives will lose 40 to 50 percent of their muscle mass and 50 percent of their muscular strength by age 65. This loss is not without consequence—these people can become so weak that doing simple daily activities becomes very difficult. A recent study revealed just how much negative impact a sedentary lifestyle can have on aging. The study looked at adults aged 55 to 64 and found that 40 percent of women had a difficult time lifting and carrying 10 pounds; 20 percent of men within this age bracket found the same task difficult. This study also revealed that almost 25 percent of both men and women had a difficult time walking a quarter of a mile briskly. The saddest part of this report stated that by age 65, untrained individuals had lost as much as 80 percent of their strength.

The chart below gives you an idea of the percent of muscle loss in some major muscle groups.

MUSCLE GROUP	% OF STRENGTH LOSS
Back & arms	30–40%
Legs	47%
Hand & grip strength	42%

This decline can be responsible for loss of independent living skills and can exacerbate existing disabilities. While this information is both alarming and discouraging, the good news is that it is never too late to feel great and recapture some of the strength and stamina we had in our younger days. All it takes is a sensible and regular dose of strength training to prevent sarcopenia.

BENEFITS OF STRENGTH TRAINING

Although there are numerous benefits that arise from strength training, perhaps the most obvious benefit is maintaining existing strength. Doctors Bortz and Nelson, experts in the field of older adult wellness, agree that the best way to stay out of a nursing home and maintain or regain independence is to keep legs strong.

Recent information suggests that strength training once a week is all we need to do to maintain strength. Strength training three times a week provides optimal results. However, performing strength training twice a week yields 80 percent of the benefits that you gain from working out three times a week.

In addition to maintaining existing strength, we can also increase muscle mass and regain lost muscle with regular strength training. Improvements in muscular strength and endurance make everyday tasks, such as opening jars and getting up from the floor, easier. Don't become too concerned with looking like a body builder, though. Most women and people over the age of 50 lack the amount of testosterone needed to develop large muscles.

Strength training also slows aging. One study asked college-age students to identify which older adults, all belonging to the same age group, looked most youthful: those who strength-trained, those who swam, or those who ran. The overwhelming response was that those who lifted weights looked the youngest.

Strength training, when combined with sensible eating habits and moderate aerobic exercise, facilitates weight loss, decreases body fat, and helps keep weight off. Muscles are a furnace that burns calories. Some experts suggest that 1 pound of fat burns only 3 to 5 calories a day whereas a pound of muscle burns 35 to 50 calories a day. Thus, the more muscle mass we have, the more calories we will burn while at work or rest. People who have a higher percentage of muscle mass have a higher resting metabolic rate than sedentary individuals and thus are burning more calories.

Here are some additional benefits derived from strength training.

- **Decreases arthritic and lower back pain.** Muscles provide structure around the joint, creating an internal brace to support and also lessen the load on the joint.

- **Increases bone density.** When strength training, the muscle pulls on the bone, requiring the bone to remodel itself to get stronger and provide a more solid base of support. The integrity of the bone is directly related to the forces applied to it. If a person lives a slothlike existence, their fragile bones will break easily against the slightest force.

- **Improves glucose tolerance and insulin sensitivity.** Diabetes is increasing in the United States at alarming rates. The physical activity that strength training provides improves the way the body utilizes sugar and will lessen the risk of developing diabetes.

- **Improves mobility and functional ability.** Maintaining or regaining strength allows us to do what we want to do, when we want to do it.

- **Improves balance and prevents falls.** Having adequate leg strength allows us to catch ourselves when we trip, preventing a fall and perhaps a broken bone. Strength training also increases bone density so that the bones can withstand the impact of a fall better. In addition, it will be easier to get up if we do fall.

- **Improves posture and self-image.** Strength training correctly can reverse the Dowager's hump and other outward manifestations of poor posture. Proper strength training can assist us in regaining an upright, youthful appearance.

- **Combats depression.** Studies have found that older people who strength-trained for 10 weeks had reductions in depression and improvements in self-esteem. This suggests that strength training gives a sense of empowerment and the idea that it is never too late to improve.

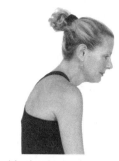

Kyphotic curve

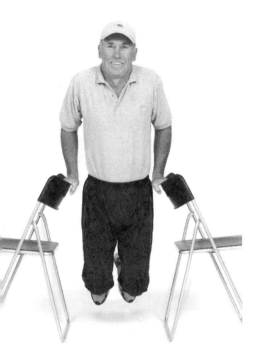

WHAT IS STRENGTH TRAINING?

According to the National Strength and Conditioning Association, strength training is defined as the use of progressive resistance methods to increase one's ability to exert force or resist a force. Basically, strength training is challenging your muscles in a sensible and progressive manner.

It is critical to use muscles in the manner they were designed to be used; unused muscles will no longer work efficiently. "Use it or lose it" has real meaning for older adults. In strength training, it is not where you start that is important but where you end up. I have had numerous students start my class unable to get out of a chair without the use of their hands, but after performing some of the exercises in this book, they can now sit down and get up from a chair with ease, walk around the mall all day, or even get down on the floor and play with the grandkids.

DIFFERENT TYPES

Strength training can take many forms, from lifting your own body against the resistance of gravity to using weights or exercise bands to challenge your muscles. Many people confuse the terms *weight lifting, weight training, strength training*, and *progressive resistance exercise.*

- Weight lifting is a competitive form of strength training using Olympic-style lifts such as the "snatch" and the "clean and jerk."
- Weight training is the process of lifting weights, whether they are dumbbells, barbells, or weight machines.
- Strength training is the application of resistance to movement to increase one's ability to exert force. The muscle does not know nor care what is providing the resistance, so engaging in a method that you enjoy is the key to success. This can include the use of anything from weights to exercise bands to kettlebells to even the resistance of water.

- Progressive resistance exercise is when a person progressively overloads the muscles (by making the load and movement more difficult) by adding more resistance as the move gets easier. The load can be applied several ways: with weights, exercise tubing, or, in water, hand paddles.

The following is a cute example of progressive resistance exercise:

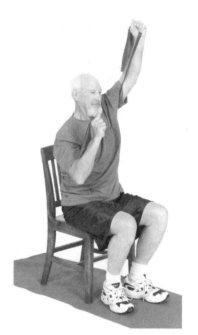

Begin by standing in a comfortable position with plenty of room to move. With a 5-pound potato sack in each hand, lift your arms out to the sides 10 times. When that gets easy, grab a 25-pound potato sack in each hand and lift your arms 10 times. Once that becomes easy, start placing potatoes in the sack. Or another method is to buy a Great Dane puppy and then lift it every day. As the puppy gains weight, your muscles will get progressively stronger to adapt to the new heavier load.

While that was meant to be humorous, it does represent the theory behind progressive resistance exercise: Start at a comfortable load and slowly try to complete more reps each time, adding more load as your muscles get stronger and the movement gets easier.

Several methods are available to develop strength, muscle mass, and muscular endurance. The most common technique is isotonic progressive resistance exercise. The other methods are called isokinetic and isometric progressive resistance exercise.

Isotonic Progressive Resistance Exercise

Isotonic progressive resistance exercise is the most traditional method of strength training, generally using free weights, barbells, or machines that utilize stacked weights or even exercise bands; isotonic progressive resistance is the style this book predominately uses. Isotonic exercise is convenient; the down side, however, is that it does not accommodate to changes in strength at different angles. Muscles can be challenged differently depending on the angle engaged. As the muscle contracts along the range of motion, the angle of the joint affects the strength at that angle.

To test the concept of your muscle's strength being dependent on the angle used, try placing a heavy jug of milk in each hand with your arms alongside your body. Now try to curl your hands toward your shoulders. Did you notice that at certain points/angles the milk jug seemed heavier than at other angles? The weight did not change but the angle made the weight feel heavier at certain points.

Isotonic moves are involved in most of our daily activities, from lifting a bag of groceries to picking up a grandchild.

Isokinetic Exercise

In isokinetic exercise, you contract the muscle through the full range of motion against a resistance lever at a prescribed speed and load. Generally, isokinetic exercise machines are more expensive than isotonic machines and devices.

Isometric Exercise

Isometric exercise involves exerting muscular force against an immovable object, creating a static contraction. This method is often used with extremely weak individuals and with people with ailments such as arthritis, where movement of the joint is not desired. This type of training will not significantly develop muscle size or muscular endurance but will develop strength at the joint angle in which the exercise is performed. The advantage of isometric exercise is that it does not require equipment. The disadvantages are that it can raise blood pressure to dangerous levels; the strength gain is specific to the angle at which the move is performed; and there is little transfer of strength to functional skills or sports.

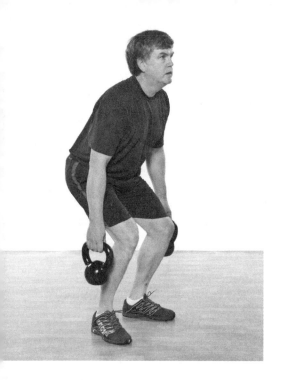

YOUR PROGRAM

Any successful exercise program should be fun, improve function, and assist you in becoming more physically fit and independent. A well-designed strength-training program can address each of these elements, but be aware that strength training can be done incorrectly. When designing a strength-training routine, it is critical that you use the correct dose to get the ideal response.

The first step in designing a safe and sane program is to cater to your health status and personal goals. Pay special attention to your problem areas and do what you feel is best for you. The areas that are at most risk of injury are the neck area, the lower back, the knees, and the shoulders. These areas need to be trained, not strained.

Since so much misinformation abounds about strength training, it is important to use scientifically proven information rather than anecdotal information. Listen to your body and heed what it says. When in doubt, consult your health professional. In fact, it is always wise to inform your health professional before you start any exercise program. However, if you start slow and don't strain, most health professionals will be very supportive of you engaging in a sensible strength-training routine. If you have health issues such as arthritis, heart and blood pressure issues, or bone density concerns, it would be smart to have your health professional review your program before starting.

As you design your program, ask yourself the following questions:

- What is the goal of my strength-training program?
- Do I have joint or other health problems that need special consideration?
- Will my program assist me to function more freely?
- Does my routine address all the major muscle groups of my body?

- Am I addressing only the surface muscles and neglecting the stabilizer muscles and core muscles of the body?
- If I feel worse after working out, am I doing more than I'm ready for or am I doing exercises that don't match my health?

Every exercise program should be customized for your unique characteristics. The questions below are designed for you to do an internal evaluation of how you feel and if you are receiving the benefits that you expect. If not, it is time to reevaluate including the exercise in your program.

- Why am I doing this exercise?
- What are the benefits of this exercise?
- What are the risks of this exercise and can it be modified to make it safer?
- How do I feel while doing this exercise?
- How do I feel after doing this exercise?
- Could I receive the same benefits from doing a different exercise?
- Bonus: Does my doctor and/or therapist support this exercise?

If the exercise fails the above criteria, look for another exercise. There is no perfect exercise.

If exercise is new to you, keep in mind that it'll take 12–16 weeks before you notice any change. It takes at least three months to establish a new habit. Don't quit before you have a chance to see results. If you think getting motivated is hard, staying motivated is just as hard. Make your fitness routine enjoyable and exciting by periodically changing your existing routine with different kettlebell exercises to enhance your desire to exercise. Find movements that match your personality as well as your physical strength and flexibility limits. Research on strength training shows that there's no absolute way to train to improve strength and muscle development. Always listen to your body and heed what it says—no one knows your body better than you.

> **SAMPLE ROUTINE**
>
> A sample routine may look something like this:
>
> | | |
> |---|---|
> | Warm up | 5–10 minutes |
> | Aerobic activity | 20–30 minutes* |
> | Strength training | 20–30 minutes* |
> | Cool down and stretching | 5–10 minutes |
>
> *The order of aerobic activity and strength training can be switched.

THE ROUTINE

A proper exercise program should include a warm-up period to prepare the body for exercise. The older the human machine, the longer and more therapeutic the warm-up should be. A warm-up can take several forms. It can consist of light aerobic activity that limbers up the muscles you plan to engage. It can also be a very light version of the exercise you plan to perform. The best method is to combine the two, doing a few minutes of aerobic exercise to warm up the body and then a light set of each exercise before you do your more formal sets.

The rest of the program should include cardiovascular training, often referred to as "cardio" or aerobics, and then perform muscular strength and endurance training. After the workout, a cool-down period is prudent. This allows your body to taper off from your workout. You do not want to stop abruptly. It is recommended that you walk around slowly then find a place to spend 5–15 minutes stretching the muscles you engaged in your workout. The first section of this book is devoted to stretching as it is the foundation of any strength-training routine.

Cross-training is a good way to avoid injury; an example is strength-training on Monday, Wednesday, and Friday, swimming on Tuesday and Thursday, taking a walk on Saturday, and resting on Sunday. It's okay to break the aerobic exercise into three 10-minute bouts throughout the day. Cross-training does not mean combining aerobic training with strength training by carrying weights while walking or jogging, for instance. While this may sound like a great way to multitask, it is only inviting orthopedic injuries. Wearing ankle weights on the ankles while walking is often linked to hip and knee problems.

An important concept to keep in mind is not to become complacent about your exercise program. Be mindful of your body mechanics at all times. In other words, pay attention to what you are doing. When strength training, it is important that you control the weight and not let the weight control you. About every three to four months, you should change your workout around a bit so that you don't get bored and your body doesn't get accustomed to the work it's performing.

PRE- AND POST-STRENGTH TRAINING

Always start with a 5- to 10-minute warm-up of the body before any strength-training session. Stretch after your workout.

If you find your muscles are very sore after exercising, you are trying to do too much too soon. Muscle soreness results when you cause minor trauma to your muscles and connective tissue by asking them to do more than they are ready to perform. If you start and progress slowly and listen

---

COMMON TERMS

Atrophy: a decrease in muscle size as a result of inactivity

Circuit training: a series of different exercises done with no significant rest in between each set

Contraction: muscles utilizing energy and expending heat to exert a force

Concentric contraction: an isotonic contraction in which muscle length shortens; e.g., bringing a glass of water to your mouth

Eccentric movement: a movement in which the muscle lengthens while resisting the load; e.g., bringing down the glass of water slowly from your mouth

Extension: making the joint angle larger

Flexion: making the joint angle smaller

Rep (or Repetition): the number of times you perform a movement

Set: a grouping of repetitions

to your body, you should be able to avoid what is called "delayed muscle soreness," or next-day soreness. To avoid muscle soreness, always warm up then stretch, and then exercise carefully and again stretch at the end of your workout. Remember the two-hour rule: If you are sore two hours post-exercise, then you overworked and need to back off to an intensity that does not cause discomfort.

SELECTING WEIGHT LOAD

Beginners should choose an amount that enables them to do at least one set of 12 reps; follow this procedure for one to two weeks. After two weeks, add a second set. It is best to do one set then rest for 45 seconds, then do a second set of the same exercise. When you can do two sets of 12 reps without straining, it is time to add just enough resistance so that it is difficult to do 6–8 reps; from here, work yourself back up to 12–15 reps. Add resistance in small increments.

Two ways to improve strength is to add more load or add more reps. The more fit/active the person is when he or she starts, the slower his or her gains will be when compared to a beginner. Remember, you are only competing against yourself.

DECIDING REPS AND SETS

Each workout should not exceed 12 exercises and should engage the major muscles of the body.

Each set should consist of 8–15 reps. The more reps you perform, the more focus you place on muscular endurance. Choosing lower reps emphasizes strength and power. Most experts suggest that older adults should find a load that can be done comfortably six to eight times, gradually increasing the reps until they can do 15 reps with good form before they increase the resistance and then start the sequence all over again. Try to do at least two to three sets of each exercise.

FREQUENCY

The key to a successful strength-training program is to start slow and progress in a sensible manner. Try to strength train a minimum of two days a week; three times a week would be ideal. Overtraining can occur when you are doing too much, working out too often and not allowing your body adequate time to rest and repair itself. This often occurs in newcomers who try to do too many sets with too many reps at a pace that is too fast. To avoid this: Train, don't strain!

TRAINING PROGRESSIONS AND PLATEAUS

Training progression should not exceed 5 to 10 percent a week. In the beginning, your strength increases quickly as you learn how to coordinate the equipment. A beginner can expect to see gains in strength, size, and firmness after six to eight weeks. However, at some point improvement will slow down and then stop. Plateaus in strength often occur after the first few months of training. Don't get discouraged—just realize that improvements will take longer and will not be as noticeable.

As long as you are not feeling bad, good things are still going on inside the muscle. When you reach a plateau, it is time to tweak your routine by changing the exercises or changing the number of reps and/or sets. Athletes who reach a plateau may even take a week off or change their routine completely. But if you stop lifting weights entirely, you can expect to lose 50 percent of your newfound strength in two to three months. Your muscle will atrophy (decrease in size), and if you continue to eat as if you are exercising, the excess calories will be stored as fat. So use your muscle or lose it. You really don't want to start over again, do you? Just keep training at an intensity that feels comfortable.

Change your workout every three to four months if you get bored. Replacing one chest exercise for another chest exercise can do this. Another way is to do more repetitions and lessen the load or decrease rest time between sets.

QUALITY OVER QUANTITY

Never sacrifice quality for quantity. Perform each repetition in a smooth and controlled manner, working through the full range of motion that the joint can comfortably go through.

Training speed should be controlled. It is generally recommended that on the difficult aspect (concentric) of the move, take 2–3 seconds; on the easy part (eccentric), take 4–5 seconds. The bottom line is don't do the move super slowly or too fast. Some new research suggests that well-trained older adults may want to perform the moves a little faster to work on the "power aspect" of strength training. Stay alert to this emerging concept.

Do exercises that use the larger muscles of the body (chest and back, front and back of the legs) before moving on to the smaller muscles (arms and calves). When starting out, do compound exercises that employ multiple muscle groups (bench press) over simple, one-muscle exercises (arm curls).

WELL-ROUNDED PROGRAM

Remember, strength training should be part of a comprehensive fitness routine that includes cardiovascular fitness (which allows you to walk briskly without getting winded), stretching and flexibility (which allows you to reach down and tie your shoes or zip up your dress without pulling a muscle), and balance work (which prevents you from falling down and breaking a bone). You should also incorporate exercises to improve posture (to allow you to stand with a more upright and youthful carriage) and relaxation (to help you reduce stress and lower your blood pressure).

Greatness lies not in being strong, but in the correct use of strength—therefore, every exercise included in your routine should have a specific purpose or a function. To grow strong, not old and feeble, does not require a great deal of time or expensive equipment or even a membership to a gym. Simply follow the simple steps outlined in this book to achieve this.

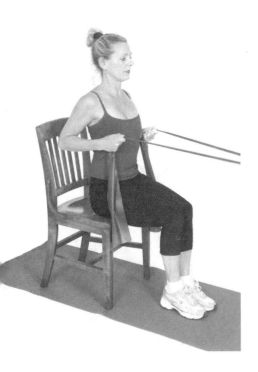

EQUIPMENT

Strength training can be performed with a variety of equipment: barbells, dumbbells, kettle-bells, machines, bands. Which kind you decide to use really has more to do with personal preference and perhaps budget than anything else. Here is a brief list of the pros and cons of each to help you decide on the best equipment for you.

WEIGHTS

The type of weights you choose depends on your needs. Luckily, most options are affordable and readily available from the local sporting goods store.

Dumbbells, which come in predetermined weights, are a safe bet. The main drawback is that you usually need several pairs of differing weights in order to effectively work all parts of your body. If you are careful and follow the guidelines in this book, dumbbells are an inexpensive method to improve strength. They can be used in every manner needed to provide a total-body workout.

Barbells, a bar that is adjusted by switching out weights on each end of the bar, are a hassle to change and come with a higher risk of injury. Unless you already use barbells regularly, I don't recommend using these.

Ankle weights, which can be strapped on to your ankles or wrists, can make certain exercises easier—and safer—to perform. However, don't strap on the weights to "enhance" leisure activities such as walking, jogging, or golfing. Only use them in conjunction with strength exercises.

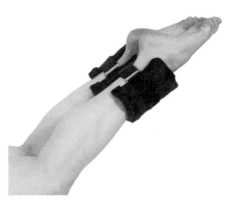

Ankle weights

KETTLEBELLS

The kettlebell is a cast-iron weight that looks like a cannonball with a teapot handle (personally, I think the name should be "kettleball" because of its shape). Kettlebells are part of the plyometric family, which includes exercises such as jumping, bounding, and throwing and catching weighted objects such as medicine balls or kettlebells. These movements involve rapid eccentric (lengthening) and concentric (shortening) actions. Plyometric exercises have their roots in the 1960s, when they were first used in the Eastern Bloc countries to train their weightlifters and track-and-field athletes. A plyometric workout was, and still is, designed to improve explosive muscular power.

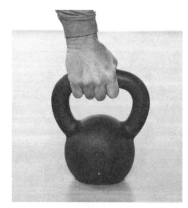
Kettlebell

The reason the kettlebell is gaining favor again is that the motions involved in a kettlebell workout mimic activities of daily living much more than the unidirectional exercise machines seen in most gyms today. The kettlebell is used to perform dynamic exercises that foster power, agility, strength, flexibility, and even aerobic fitness. The shape of the kettlebell places the center of gravity beyond the handle, which allows the bell to be thrown about easily, facilitating swing movements.

EXERCISE BANDS

Every exercise that can be done on a piece of exercise equipment or with weights can be done with an exercise band. They are inexpensive and can be stored anywhere. Some even come with handles to hold on to easily. The bands come in varying resistances. As you get stronger, you may have to purchase more resistant ones in order to accommodate your strength.

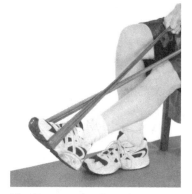
Elastic exercise band

EXERCISE MACHINES

Exercise machines are an excellent way to improve your strength, but often cannot provide a comprehensive workout. If you have the money to purchase a good-quality multi-station machine, or the time and commitment to attend the gym regularly, that's great. If not, this option is not for you.

STABILITY BALL

When choosing a ball, make sure that when you sit on it, your upper legs and lower legs are at 90 degrees, and your shoulders are over your hips. The ball should also be safe for your body weight.

- The firmer the ball, the more challenging the exercise will be.
- Make sure that the floor surface is safe for both you and the ball—avoid sharp objects.
- Don't overestimate your ability—start with the basics.

- Have someone spot you if necessary.
- Only do those movements that are correct for your health status.

FOAM ROLLER

A foam roller is a fun and challenging piece of equipment that can be purchased at most sporting goods stores, gyms, or physical therapy clinics. It has been reported to restore alignment, foster body awareness, and advance proper posture. Foam roller exercises can be done from numerous positions, including supine and kneeling.

The foam roller comes in various shapes, sizes, and densities. The selection of the correct roller depends on your height and body weight. The most common roller used for core-strength training is a full-length roller that's about 3 feet long. It comes in a semicircular or fully circular shape. Beginners do best with the semicircular shape, flat-side down; as they improve, they can flip the roller over. Once that becomes easy, a circular roller is a nice way to ramp up the challenge.

PROPS FOR STRETCHING

A flexibility routine can employ various tools like belts, balls, or a foam roller to enhance the experience. Props offer variety to your stretches. The chair provides support in balance-challenging situations. Often a wall can be used for support and balance as well. Foam blocks are frequently used in yoga to assist in maintaining a position. Blocks can serve as platforms for proper body alignment.

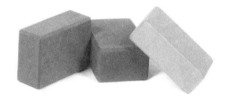

Foam blocks

A pillow can be used in the same fashion as a foam block; it can also be used to support your neck when lying down.

A strap allows you to reach the end stages of a stretch without compromising proper body mechanics. A rope or belt that does not elongate can be used instead of a strap. Other options include TRX suspension straps.

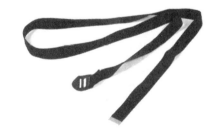

Strap with buckle

A stability ball (also known as the Swiss or Pilates ball) is a popular stretching and relaxation tool. Some balls have knobs to stimulate circulation. Others have bumpy surfaces to promote sensory stimulation, while those with a hard, smooth surface are designed to provide trigger-point tension relief. They range in size from 45 to 75 centimeters.

Smaller, firm therapy balls also facilitate flexibility. The size, shape, and density of the ball you select should be determined by the goal of your session and, if applicable, the area of your

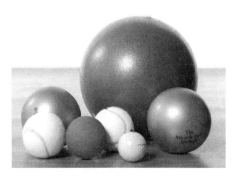

Therapy balls

body you aim to address. In general, tennis balls and other small firm balls (between 1 and 6 inches) with some give are good candidates for self-massage and muscle release.

Finally, it's important that you are comfortable doing stretches. When lying or kneeling on the floor, a mat provides cushioning.

MY RECOMMENDATION

I personally use a combination of dumbbell weights and ankle weights for certain muscle groups and then use exercise bands to complement the rest of the workout. I am also a fan of exercise equipment if you have the space to store it or if you have the money to join a gym. I even use water paddles in the pool to vary my workout on occasion. As discussed earlier, your muscles don't care what is providing the load. You just need to challenge them and change your workout periodically to avoid injury and boredom.

Safety First

No matter which type of equipment you use, always inspect it before using it. Make sure the collars of barbells and dumbbells are on properly, the exercise bands are not worn, and the cables on machines are in good repair. If you are using a machine, also double-check the weight stack: 100 pounds on one machine is not always 100 pounds on another.

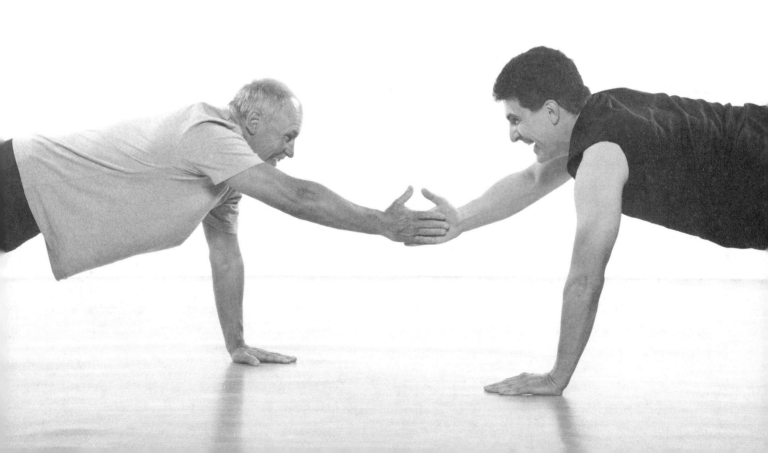

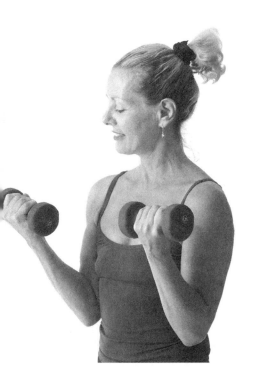

TUNE IN TO YOUR BODY

Strength training involves more than hefting a barbell and curling it to your body a few times. In order to keep your body safe and ensure that you're gaining benefits, not injuries, you must incorporate several things into your training program. The following are important principles that help you train smart.

SAFETY

While strength training has numerous benefits, it is not without risk. Even the best exercise can cause pain and injury if done improperly. In the last two decades, it has been reported that nearly a million people have gone to the emergency room for strength-training injuries. A number of injuries are minor but several deaths have occurred from a barbell choking a person who could not lift the bar off their chest or throat. Most of the injuries are the result of overdoing it and not adhering to safe techniques or using outdated principles and exercises. Paying attention to your body can lower your risks of injuring yourself.

While most strength-training exercises will not kill you or even hurt you if done incorrectly once or twice, the cumulative effects can be damaging. Some exercises have been around so long it seems irreverent to question their efficacy. All too often training methods get adopted and later institutionalized based on anecdotal information rather than sound scientific research—what is scientifically acceptable today may not be acceptable tomorrow after further investigation.

Most people understand that physical activity is good for the human machine. Unfortunately, in their zest to get fit they do more than their body is ready to handle. Remember that it is better to train safer and smarter rather than faster and harder. Think of your 50-plus body as a vintage automobile. A classic car can run just as well as a newer model if well maintained—it just needs a little longer to warm up and more TLC along the way.

Lastly, avoid those well-intended fitness enthusiasts who have all the answers. These people generally base their training methods on popular body-building magazine information rather than scientific information. Stay away from them—these are the people who are going to get you hurt.

PAIN

As you get more familiar with strength training, you may become complacent, and that is when injuries and accidents occur. Learn to listen to your body and trust your ability to distinguish between pain and discomfort.

The old adage "no pain, no gain" is insane. Equally as insane is the adage to work through the pain. Pain is your body telling you that you are doing something wrong. While our bodies are very resilient, misuse, disuse, and abuse can cumulate in an injury. Following proper body mechanics and listening to your body can prevent a problem. Prevention is always cheaper than treatment. Protect your spine and joints at all times and stay mindful of your form.

THE IMPORTANCE OF POSTURE

I work with many 50-plus folks, and they're often concerned about their appearance. They'll spend great amounts of money on hair products, facials, and clothes but spend little or no time on their posture. To better understand posture's role in how we look, check out a local high school play and see how the actor portrays an old person—all hunched over!

If you want to look young, stand tall. If you want to look thinner, stand tall. Core training is all about improving how you look and feel. Every time I do my core-strengthening exercises, I think about how they'll help me stand straight and therefore improve my appearance.

As you can see from the illustration of the human spine on page 23, the neck (called the cervical spine) curves slightly forward. The middle portion of the spine (thoracic spine) is curved outward. The lower portion of the back (lumbar spine) curves inward, presenting a lordotic curve. Although the vertebral column has three natural curves, sometimes as a result of misuse, disuse, or abuse, these curves become overly exaggerated and can contribute to back problems.

A visual that might assist you to better understand the concept is to picture a brand-new tube of toothpaste and stand it on one end. When all the forces are exerting equal pressure, the tube stands up easily. Now squeeze the toothpaste a few times with some spots going in and other parts pushed out. Now try to stand it up. I doubt that it'll stay up.

Learning to sit, stand, and move in the most biomechanical manner is foundational. A properly aligned back has a gentle "S" curve. When it's in the safest position to avoid excessive forces to the spine and discs, it's called *neutral spine*. Everyone has their own neutral spine position. This is how you find it while standing:

- Stand with your weight evenly distributed over both feet and your knees slightly bent.
- Using your abdominal muscles, tilt your hips slowly forward and back. Imagine you have a cup of water resting on your belly and are trying to tip water out of it. Find a position that

feels most comfortable for you (ideally a balanced position from which the water in that cup would not spill). Movement occurs at the hip-hinge joint. Once you locate it, lock in that position.

- Make sure your hips and shoulders are aligned and that the distance from your belly button to your sternum is far apart.
- After this adjustment, you may need to realign the hip-hinge joint again.
- Align your ears over your shoulders, your shoulders over your hips, and your hips over your ankles.

The goal is to put this "feeling" into muscle memory so you can maintain the correct position throughout the day. While this is meant to be natural, it can take some time to get used to.

Another way to find neutral spine is to stand with your spine against a corner or wall and align the base of your skull, your mid-back, and tailbone, allowing for the natural arches. Look in a mirror or ask a friend: Are your ears over your shoulders, shoulders over your hips, and hips over your ankles?

In proper core training, learning proper pelvic positioning is pivotal. Let's review the various positions that the exercises in this book use. The ultimate goal is for you to be able to stand, run, and jump and always have your back in a self-protected position.

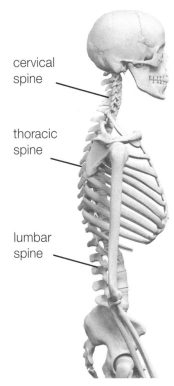

cervical spine

thoracic spine

lumbar spine

Human spine

Lying Position

Whether you're lying on the floor or a roller, flatten and arch your back until you find a comfortable position. Your back shouldn't be completely flat on the ground.

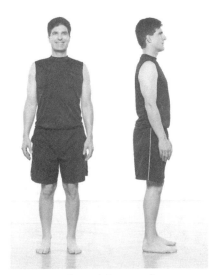

Neutral spine while standing

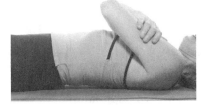

Neutral spine when lying down

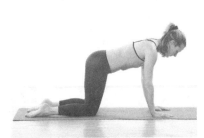

Tabletop position

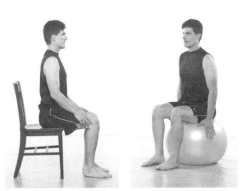

Sitting position on a chair and a ball

Tabletop Position

While on your hands and knees, find neutral position, engage your abdominal muscles, and keep your spine stabilized. Ideally, a broom handle should be able to rest on your back from head to tailbone, with only a small arch in your lower back area.

Sitting Position

Whether you're on a chair or ball, be sure to find neutral spine:

- Sit with both feet on the floor and both bones of your pelvis (not your tailbone) on the chair/ball.
- Your upper legs should be parallel with the floor, and your feet should be shoulder-width apart on the floor. Your weight is evenly distributed over all contact points.
- Your chest, shoulders, and head are up and out, with the maximum distance between your belly button and sternum.
- Avoid sitting with a rounded back and head forward; it could add stress to your discs.

LOWERING AND RAISING YOUR BODY

As basic as the next statement will appear, it's critical that, when performing strengthening and core-stabilization exercises, you understand how to lower and raise yourself to/from the floor in a biomechanically correct manner. Improperly getting up and down from/to the floor contributes to lower back pain. *Remember to maintain control of your torso during every phase of the movement. Think of your shoulders, hips, and spine as one unit.*

1–2. From standing, bend your knees and place both hands on the floor to lower yourself into a tabletop position.

3. Lower one hip to the floor, sitting like a mermaid.

4. Then lower yourself down on that side.

5. Once you're on your side, roll like a log onto your back, keeping your torso in one unit. Use your hands to assist if necessary. Once on the floor, align your spine and neck, and bend your knees and place your feet flat on the floor.

To get up, perform the process in reverse.

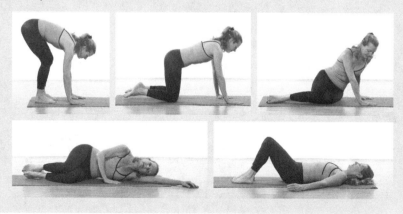

Neck

The old expression "Don't stick your neck out" is excellent fitness advice. The neck is very fragile! Doing anything too fast or too hard can cause serious problems. Never "warm up" your neck by rolling your head around in fast circles—in fact, all quick neck movements are a bad idea. Avoid full neck circles because they strain supporting ligaments and can lead to pinched nerves. Other things to avoid include hyperflexion, when you force your chin to your chest, and hyperextension, when you arch your neck too far back. Neck extensions can also put pressure on the arteries of the neck, which can cause high blood pressure and compromise blood flow to the brain. Some women have had strokes while leaning back to get their hair washed at a salon, hence the term "beauty parlor" syndrome. The exercises in this book will show you safe and sane ways to increase the flexibility of your neck.

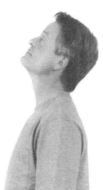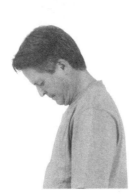

Hyperextension (left) or hyperflexion (right) puts undue pressure on the neck arteries.

Shoulders

Shoulder problems are an increasing concern for the over-50 fitness person. Be careful when you bring your arms above your head, and always control any movement that causes you to raise your arms above shoulder height. Relax your shoulders and don't shrug when you're doing arm exercises. Try your best to keep your shoulder blades pulled together when doing arm moves as well. If your shoulders are tight, don't arch your back to make up for your inflexibility.

Elbow

When exercising, avoid "locking" or hyperextending your elbow joint. You may cause elbow pain and injury if you do. Keep in mind that the elbow is a "pivot," so in most moves the wrist, elbow, and shoulder should be aligned.

Lower Back

Most of us will experience back pain at some time in our lives. It is critical to protect your back when you stretch. Keep your lower back stable at all times. All back exercises should be done in a slow and controlled manner, and if they increase in discomfort, *stop*. Never do stretches in which you bend forward and rotate at the same time: for example, windmill toe touches are a very bad idea. Also avoid bending backward at the waist, such as in yoga stretches that call for you to raise both hands over your head and look up. Quick, uncontrolled trunk twists are not a good idea, either, because torque generated by the twisting action strains the lower back. Be careful when doing fast or forced side bends, too. When sitting on the floor with your legs extended in front of you, be sure to keep your back flat when reaching forward.

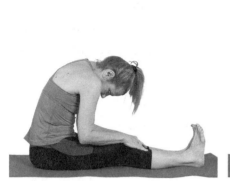 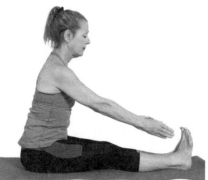 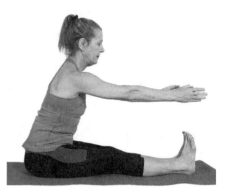

Bad: back is too rounded

Better: back is flat but arms should be parallel to the ground

Best: proper form for reaching

Knees

The knees are designed to straighten and bend; any other movement puts them at some level of risk. The knees and toes should always point in the same direction. Avoid any movements that make your knees rotate or twist, and never twist your body while your feet are planted on the floor. Never straighten your knee so far that it hyperextends, or overly straightens, the leg. Also avoid bending your knees too much. Doing so overstretches the ligaments of the knee and can make the knee joint unstable. Avoid deep knee bends, and make sure you don't squat any lower than the point at which your thighs are parallel to the floor. When lunging, do not allow your knee to extend past your toes. Always remember: Keep your knees "soft" (that is, slightly bent) when strength training.

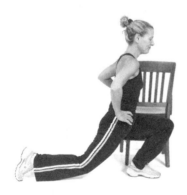 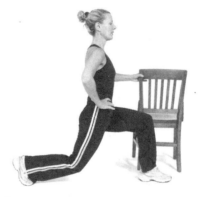

Incorrect: thigh is not parallel to floor and knee is extending beyond the toes

Correct: thigh is parallel to floor and knee is aligned with the ankle

MUSCULAR BALANCE

When performing your workout, think symmetrically. If you do a lot of exercises for your chest, you will notice that your shoulders get rounded. If you work your hamstrings a lot, your quadriceps become weaker in proportion and you will lose flexibility in your legs. Imbalance is the quickest way to injury, so provide balance by exercising both your agonist and antagonist muscle groups. Do unto the front as you do unto the back, and do unto the left as you do unto the right. And remember to stretch what is tight and strengthen what is weak. Keep in mind that you are not just lifting weights to get strong, you are engaging in a body-sculpting activity. When you look at a sculpture of the human body, everything is balanced—no one muscle group is out of proportion. Treat your body like a piece of art.

BREATHING

Never hold your breath—doing so while you perform strength training moves can elevate your blood pressure to dangerous levels. Contrary to popular belief, there is no right or wrong way to breathe. While some trainers suggest that you exhale on effort and inhale on the easy phase, it does not always make sense with certain moves and it does not always feel right with every exercise. The critical aspect is to not hold your breath, whether lifting weights or performing any strenuous maneuver.

Breathe in a manner that feels correct for you, but always include one inhalation and exhalation per repetition. You may want to count out loud or talk while exercising. The key is to breathe freely and effortlessly while strength training.

PART 1

STRETCHING

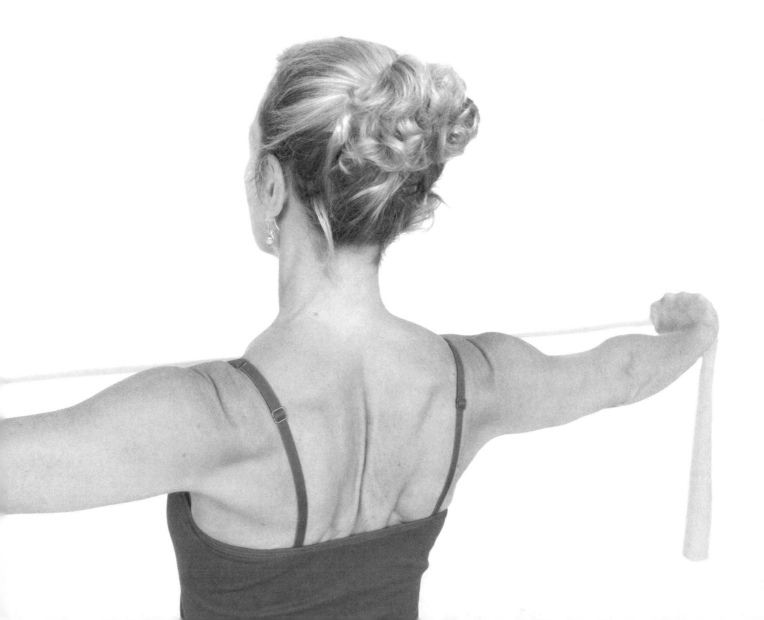

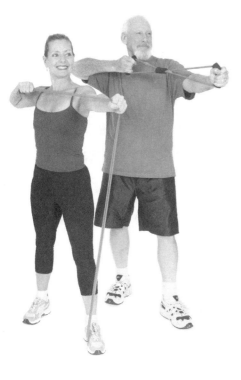

STRETCHING, FLEXIBILITY, AND AGING

The three S's that contribute to creating an atmosphere for positive aging are strength, suppleness, and a sense of humor.

Before we get to the strength-training programs, every routine should begin and end with stretching to warm up and cool down. Have you ever woken up stiff and sore, or found that your shoelaces are a little farther away than they used to be, or that you need help getting your dress zipper pulled up? These are the little signs that your flexibility is decreasing.

Grab the skin on the back of your hand and hold it for a moment. Does it spring right back like it once did? As we age, we lose elasticity in our skin and connective tissue.

The reason for decreased flexibility is the result of many factors, such as muscle imbalances between agonist and antagonist muscles. A properly functioning neuromuscular system relies on the interdependence of muscles, tendons, and bone alignment. An injury, misuse, or abuse of a muscle can disturb this delicate balance, setting up the cycle of inflammation, muscle spasms, and adhesions that cause adaptive shortening of muscles. Chronic malalignments, such as using one set of muscles while not balancing out the opposing muscle group, can lead to poor posture and chronic pain. One example would be a person who lifts weights and does chest exercises but does not balance that out by doing upper back exercises and chest stretches; this behavior would lead to a rounded shoulder appearance.

The key to aging well is to keep the proper balance of strength and flexibility in each joint region. The problem is that, too often, tight muscles get tighter and weak muscles get weaker due to sports or activities of daily living. This is why a daily dose of flexibility work is so critical. A good rule to follow is stretch what is tight and strengthen what is lax.

Aging results in increasing variability in terms of physiologic function. While no two people age in the exact same manner, most people can expect to lose elasticity in their skin and connective tissue with each passing decade. By the age of 60 or 70, we can expect to lose up to 50 percent of normal range of motion if we don't engage in a prudent flexibility routine.

Fit Tip: Most of the things that get worse with age can be positively influenced with proper exercise and stretching.

BENEFITS OF STRETCHING

The most common flexibility limitations seen in the vintage body are osteoarthritis, effects from past injuries, and aftereffects of cancer treatments. If you have any of these, the good news is that poor flexibility can be restored! While it is best to engage in a prudent flexibility program before limited mobility becomes a chronic problem, it's never too late to begin.

A comprehensive stretching program will help you release muscle tension and soreness, as well as reduce the risk of injury. Stretching just a few minutes a day will assist in preventing soft tissue trauma such as muscle strains and ligament injuries.

Enhanced flexibility also fosters greater body awareness and a youthful posture, which leads to an improved connection between the mind and the body. A good relationship between your mind and your muscles allows you a better ability to move your joints within their natural ranges of motion. Keep in mind that the more efficient your movements are, the more easily daily tasks can be performed.

Overly tight muscles can restrict full motion in and around a joint. When muscles are flexible, joints can align themselves in the biomechanical manner in which they were designed. Improved flexibility results in improvements in everything else, from our ability to move, our posture, and even our ability to breathe more completely. Generally, poor flexibility and decreased joint range can be restored more easily if addressed early on, before it becomes a chronic problem. The longer the inflexibility exists, the more difficult it is to restore and the more likely it will become permanent.

It is easy to understand why flexibility training is short-changed. Unlike cardiovascular training, which improves our heart function and assists in weight control, or strength training, which improves our appearance, fosters bone density, and may even improve functional fitness, stretching just seems to be a perfunctory duty. While stretching may not reduce long-term health risks, it does improve posture and our quality of life. In fact, the American Academy of Orthopaedic Surgeons recommends that people of all ages engage in a daily dose of flexibility exercises, which can include yoga, Pilates, and basic stretching.

A sensible flexibility program can benefit the following:

• Osteoarthritis

• Mobility impairments

• Effects of past injuries

- Aftereffects of cancer treatments
- Chronic pain syndrome
- Fibromyalgia

If you have any of these concerns and are looking for a holistic way to decrease pain and improve function, a daily bout of flexibility may be the solution. The longer the inflexibility exists, the more difficult it is to restore and the more likely it will become permanent. However, while it is best to engage in a prudent flexibility program before limited mobility becomes a chronic problem, it is never too late to begin.

WHAT IS FLEXIBILITY?

Flexibility is the range of motion (ROM) around a joint and is specific to each joint—the more you are able to move effortlessly without pain or discomfort, the more flexible you are. Flexibility is influenced by many factors, two of which we have little control over: gender (women are generally more flexible than men are) and anatomy (the shape of our bones and how they form to make a joint). However, we can significantly improve our flexibility by stretching regularly, which this section will help you to do.

The types of physical activity that we participate in can make our muscles tight. Generally, the more muscular a person is, the more inflexible they are. When the same muscles are used over and over again, they become stiffer. We often overuse, misuse, and abuse our bodies in work or even play, which can lead to soft tissue injuries or even osteoarthritis. Joseph Pilates, the creator of Pilates, said, "The stronger the strong muscles get, the weaker the weak muscles become." This imbalance sets us up for injury, which is why stretching is so important. Overworking muscles can make us inflexible if we don't stretch, but being too sedentary may contribute to making us inflexible as well.

WHY IS FLEXIBILITY TRAINING IMPORTANT?

Flexibility is considered an important aspect of a total-body fitness program. Unfortunately, many people neglect this part of their workout in favor of aerobics and strength training. If a person stretches, it is often just a quick series of bouncing toe touches or a few windmills. Unfortunately, as you will see, these types of stretches can cause more harm than good. Instead, stretching should be an integral part of all strength-training and aerobics programs.

As we age, our ability to maintain independence through functional mobility is of utmost importance. Flexibility of our muscles and joints dictates our ability to perform our daily activities and avoid injury. Proper flexibility plays a significant part in how we stand, how we walk, and even how we maintain balance. Balance, in its various guises, is one of the keys to successful aging. This includes keeping your mind balanced with mental stimulation, keeping your center of gravity balanced so you don't fall, and keeping your body balanced by strengthening weak muscles and stretching tight muscles.

The *Guideline for the Promotion of Active Ageing at Primary Level*, published by South Africa's Department of Health, states that lack of flexibility around a joint can cause functional limitations such as a shortened gait and rounded shoulders. Inflexibility can also make daily activities such as tying your shoes or zipping up a dress challenging. These incidents are small warning signs that your flexibility is decreasing and you need a consistent flexibility program.

In most joints, flexibility appears to peak around age 25 for males and somewhere between the ages of 25 and 30 for females. A preventive fitness routine that includes flexibility exercises begun in early adulthood can be the retirement plan for well-being later in life. While flexibility declines with age, studies have found that individuals who follow a consistent stretching program are able to delay and even reverse this degeneration. Most experts agree that loss of flexibility has less to do with aging and more to do with how we live and treat our bodies. You are what you do!

WHAT INFLUENCES MUSCLE FLEXIBILITY?

A muscle is composed of elastic and non-elastic properties. The elastic properties are like springs that lengthen the muscle and return it to its preexisting length. A sustained stretch allows the muscle and tendons to elongate gradually. Over time, biological changes occur in the muscle, allowing greater flexibility in the muscle-tendon unit.

Many factors influence flexibility, including the following:

Joint design. Ball-and-socket joints like the shoulder are more flexible than hinge joints like the knee.

Age. With age, most people undergo a loss of elasticity in the connective tissue and muscles.

Gender. Historically, females tend to be more flexible than men of similar age.

Physical activity. People who engage in a comprehensive exercise program are more flexible than their sedentary counterparts. This may not be true in people who overtrain and neglect a flexibility component of their training.

Temperature. An increase in body temperature or external temperature improves range of motion.

Injury. Injury to an area can compromise the kinetic chain above and below the injury, which can have a negative effect of flexibility.

SPECIFICITY OF FLEXIBILITY

Flexibility is specific to each joint. Unfortunately, this means that doing a stretch for the hamstrings will not keep the shoulder region loose. Another bit of discouraging news is that the benefits of stretching are short lived. This is why a commitment to a long-term stretching program needs to be adopted. A critical consideration is to make sure that the proper balance exists between antagonist and agonist muscles. If one muscle is too lax it can be just as bad as being too tight. The take-home message is that a balanced, slow, and steady stretching program needs to be done regularly.

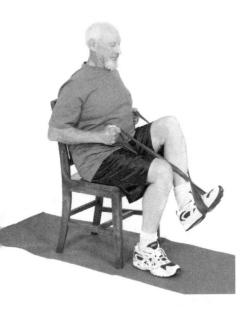

HOW TO STRETCH

Structure follows function—what you do, you become!

We are what we do, so if you do stretches, you can become flexible. As we get older, our bodies recover more slowly from various physical activities. Our 50-plus bodies need more TLC. Too often, active people focus on developing stronger muscles, improving aerobic capacity, or improving sport performance while neglecting the subtle aspects of fitness, such as flexibility. Exercising one particular muscle group without stretching it often causes that area to become less flexible and throws the body out of alignment.

Flexibility training is a planned and deliberate program done consistently with the aim of improving the functional mobility in or around a set of joints. It is an important element of a total-body fitness program. Still, improper stretching techniques can be harmful.

When stretching, always progress slowly and gently. You are unique, so don't compete with anyone else, or even yourself. Some days you will be pliable and some days you will be as stiff as a board—respect that fact, and keep it in mind when stretching. Whenever you are developing a stretching routine, always evaluate the benefits versus risks of each stretch. Not every stretch is right for everyone. Treat the selection of stretches in this book as a menu and pick only those that *feel* good to you. And a reminder: Two hours after stretching, you should not feel worse than when you started. If something hurts, stop immediately; consult your physician for unusual or continuous pain.

Be mindful of your movements. Move slowly between positions of lying down, sitting, or standing—don't overestimate your body's capacity to exercise. However, don't underestimate it either. Remember, your body is designed for movement, but let it adapt slowly and gradually.

WHAT ARE THE BASIC TYPES OF STRETCHES?

There are two basic types of stretches. Ballistic, or bouncing, stretches are generally considered controversial. Research suggests that bouncing does not increase flexibility but can cause the stretched muscle to contract and shorten, which may induce strains or micro-tears of the muscle fibers. Static stretches, which are held for a longer period, are generally believed to be safer and more effective.

---

12 TIPS TO SAFE STRETCHING

When you stretch, keep your movements controlled, maintain good posture, and really listen to your body—especially your neck, back, shoulders, and knees. When you are warming up, use this time to take inventory of your body and heed what it says. If you feel crunches in your joints, please don't ignore them. Listen for snaps, crackles, and pops—if they get louder or cause pain, see a doctor before they turn into real problems. Keeping our vintage car analogy in mind, it is always wiser and cheaper to do preventive maintenance than it is to do major repair work; thus, physical therapy is cheaper than surgery. Also, remember the two-hour rule: Two hours post-exercise, you should not feel worse than you did before you exercised. If you do, reevaluate what you are doing.

1. When stretching, never twist your body quickly while your feet are planted on the floor.
2. Avoid stretches that hyperextend or lock your knee joint.
3. Avoid awkward thigh stretches like the "hurdler's stretch," which places too much torque on the knee area.
4. Avoid movements that force your knee to hyperflex, or bend too far, as seen in full squats. Hyperflexing overstretches the ligaments of the knee and can make the knee joint unstable in the long term.
5. Avoid neck exercises that take the joint to extremes or are done quickly.
6. Always progress slowly and gently.
7. Select stretches that feel good to you. Not every stretch is best for you.
8. Two hours after a stretching session, you should not feel worse than when you started.
9. Make your flexibility session an integrated mind-body experience. Listen to your body and foster body wisdom. Turn your attention inward when you stretch, and try to exclude external distractions. Relax the mind, and many times, the muscles will follow.
10. If something hurts, stop immediately. Consult your physician for unusual or continuous pain.
11. Always warm up the body prior to stretching.
12. You are special, so treat yourself that way. Don't compete with or compare yourself to others.

Remember to stretch opposing muscle groups equally in order to keep your body balanced. Our body is designed with opposing muscles. For example, you have a muscle that brings your hand to your mouth as well as an opposing muscle that takes it in the opposite direction. So if you do a muscle activity that brings your shoulders forward, do a stretch that opens up the chest region to prevent that from occurring. Stretch your tight muscles and strengthen your weak ones.

HOW SHOULD I BREATHE WHILE STRETCHING?

Breathe fully while stretching. We often forget the importance that breathing has on health. Just think about how women use breathing to assist in delivering a baby!

Most of us take shallow breaths rather than deep, full breaths. Teach yourself to inhale slowly and deeply through your nose and exhale slowly through your lips. You will know if you are breathing correctly if your belly expands. Pattern yourself after the way a baby breathes. If you notice your ribs expanding, you are employing the wrong set of breathing muscles.

Breathing fully improves the quality of a stretch. An effective method for stretching a tight muscle is to inhale first and then exhale into the stretch. If you are tight in a certain muscle group, try reaching a comfortable distance, holding that position for a moment, taking in a deep breath, then exhaling and reaching a little farther. This is called the "hold/relax" method of stretching and relaxing.

HOW LONG SHOULD A STRETCH BE HELD?

Most experts from the American College of Sports Medicine (ACSM) suggest that maintaining a stretch for 30 seconds is ideal. After your muscles are warmed up, try to perform each stretch two to five times and gradually try to hold each stretch for 15 to 30 seconds. Start with what you are able to do. If all you can do is hold the stretch for 5 seconds, that is fine! If 30 seconds feels okay, progress to holding the stretch for 1 minute. Once a stretch feels completely comfortable, challenge your body to hold the stretch for longer or to reach farther.

Note that holding a stretch for 15 seconds provides better results than holding it for 5 seconds, and 30 seconds is better than 15 seconds. Some recent studies suggest that holding a stretch for 1 minute or more does not significantly improve the results of a stretching routine, but research has found no ill effects from prolonged stretches. No universal rule exists as to how long to hold a stretch—listen to your body! Aim for the ideal of 30 seconds to 1 minute, but be real. A 5- to 10-second stretch periodically throughout the day is better than no flexibility work. A little bit of any stretching is better than no stretching.

Never hold a stretch to the point of pain. Tweaking the position of the stretch to find the most comfortable position is A-OK. If you have not been stretching regularly for three months, hold the stretch for as long as it is comfortable, working your way from 5 seconds to 30 seconds. Note that you should not hold your breath while holding a stretch. The bottom line is that you should always listen to your body and avoid pain.

WHY WARMING UP IS IMPORTANT

Think of your muscles as taffy. Imagine trying to stretch cold taffy: It would be difficult and snap. The same thing would happen for your muscles. Now imagine stretching hot taffy: It would be pliable and easy to stretch. Again, your muscles respond in a similar manner. If you try to stretch a cold muscle, you are at a greater risk of injury, so you should always increase the temperature of the muscles before stretching. A warm bath or light activity before you stretch is a good idea. Take time to warm up, and then stretch—your body will thank you later. Or, if you can only find time to stretch periodically throughout the day, pick times when your body is most pliable.

As you warm up, use that time to take inventory of your body. Listen to your body and foster body wisdom. Make your flexibility program an integrated mind-body experience. Turn your interests inward when you stretch. Reflect and relax. If your mind is uptight, it will be hard to relax your body. Some people enjoy listening to soft music while performing the stretch-and-relax portion of the program.

SAFE, FUNCTIONAL STRETCHING

First, start with a warm-up. Active warm-up stretches are done slowly to lubricate the joint, increase circulation in the affected area, and make the muscle ready for movement. They should be performed in your pain-free range of motion. The active stretch is usually done as part of the thermal warm-up and as a post-exercise activity. If you have not been stretching regularly for three months, you should start out with 3 to 5 repetitions. If you find that too easy, you may want to shoot for 5 to 10 repetitions; if you are extremely flexible and have no joint disorders, try 10 to 15 repetitions.

Passive, or static, stretches are usually done after your body is warm, such as after a thermal warm-up or after an exercise session. Aim to hold static stretches for 15 to 30 seconds. The ACSM recommends that each stretch be done two to four times to elicit benefits. It is also okay to hold a stretch longer and do fewer reps.

While everyone is unique, the ACSM recommends stretching a minimum of two to three days a week. For best results, stretch five to seven days a week. It would be ideal if you could incorporate stretches in your daily routine, such as when in the shower or while watching TV. The more inflexible you are, the more often you should stretch.

As for which areas of the body need to be stretched, a total-body flexibility routine would be ideal. As you start out, focus on tight areas or problem areas. In most people, the chest, shoulders, backs of the legs, and lower back are often problematic. (In the Flexibility Self-Evaluations section starting on page 40, it is strongly advised to perform a basic flexibility assessment to help you ascertain where you are loose and tight.) As mentioned earlier, the human body is designed with opposing muscles, which are called agonist and antagonist muscles. A general rule of thumb is to stretch opposing muscle groups equally in order to keep your body balanced. The muscle illustration on page 37 will assist you in seeing the opposing muscle groups.

When stretching, think functional! Stretch those joints that you need in everyday life. For example, keep your shoulders flexible so that you can reach the cereal box easily. You don't have to be able to tie yourself into knots, but you want to be able to perform your daily activities without undue discomfort. Stay within your comfort zone, and don't ever force a move!

Remember, stretch what is tight, and strengthen what is lax. If, for example, you do an exercise that tightens your chest muscles, spend time stretching those chest muscles. As noted earlier, flexibility is specific to each joint. Try to stretch all the major joints of your body then focus on your particularly tight areas.

If you stretch correctly, you can avoid injury. It is safer and more effective to go slow; sustained stretches are superior to fast or bouncing stretches. If you ever become lightheaded while stretching, move slowly between positions of lying down, sitting, or standing. Don't overestimate your body's capacity to exercise. Let your body adapt slowly and gradually.

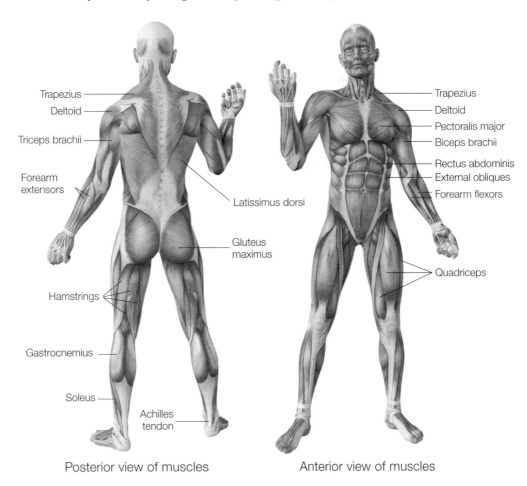

Posterior view of muscles   Anterior view of muscles

BE YOUR OWN MOTIVATION!

The more objections to stretching that you can come up with, the more you need to step up and be a leader in your health. The most common objections for not being involved in a flexibility program are not having enough time and being afraid of failure. However, we all have the same 24 hours to use in a day. The key to being a successful person is how you use those 24 hours. A stretching routine can be done in bed, in front of the TV, or even at work.

Goal Setting: Aim for Ideal, but Be Real

A flexibility plan without goals and objectives is much like a road trip without a map. While a trip without a plan might be enjoyable, it may not take you to your desired destination. If you want to get to where you want to go with regard to flexibility, you need to set goals.

Hopefully, you are currently motivated to start a flexibility habit. But, unfortunately, most people lose the excitement of staying engaged in a stretching program after just a short period. Most experts believe it takes 60 to 90 days to develop a habit, or 10,000 hours to be proficient in a new skill, so be patient with yourself as you develop your healthy stretching habit. Reaping the benefits of a stretching routine requires a long-term commitment. Setting lofty goals sounds impressive, yet it often leads to frustration. It is best to start by setting attainable short-term goals.

What you do today will determine how you feel tomorrow!
Nothing succeeds like success.

Methods to Foster Motivation

Starting a stretching program is easy, but maintaining it on a regular basis is difficult. A daily stretch program is drudgery for most people and agony for those of us who are inflexible. However, with time it should get easier. In this way, stretching is like flossing your teeth: You know it is good for you and easy to do, but it is much easier to neglect. The tips below will help you stay motivated and keep you on track with your stretching goals.

Aim for ideal, but be real. An ideal goal might be, "I will do the basic stretch program from this book every day." A realistic goal would be, "I will do the Wake-Up Routine (page 45) three days a week." Not everyone will become a "Gumby" after reading this book. The purpose of this book is to encourage you to be the best you that *you* can be! Once you see progress, it becomes self-motivating.

Sneak a stretch in as a regular part of your daily routine. Do calf stretches while brushing your teeth, do a cross-leg stretch while sitting in a meeting, or do the zipper stretch while scratching your back.

Set up a support team. Surround yourself with supportive people. Even a million-dollar football player has a support team of coaches and cheerleaders.

Set up a reward system. Everybody enjoys rewards, so reward yourself! It is vital to establish a reward system as you continue to make progress. Set attainable objectives or milestones. Once you stretch daily for a month, treat yourself to a nice dessert. Once you can touch your hands together in the zipper stretch, buy yourself something nice.

Chart your progress. Some people like to keep a log of their progress to aid in staying motivated. Taking before and after photos is a visual way to see how much farther you can stretch than you could two months before.

Variety is the spice of life. Doing the same thing day after day is boring—even when we know it is good for us. If you change your routine periodically, you can keep stretching for a lifetime! Your hamstring muscle does not care if you stretch it while sitting in a chair or while lying on the floor using a strap. The body does not care if you stretch during commercial breaks of your favorite TV show or at some trendy yoga studio—just make sure you stretch! And remember: "No pain, no gain" is insane, so do what's comfortable for you.

DOS AND DON'TS OF STRETCHING

DON'T stretch to the point of pain. Mild discomfort or tension is OK, but pain is not! Remember to breathe. Proper stretching should not cause pain.

DON'T engage in ballistic or sudden movements until fully limbered up.

DON'T rush and perform stretches incorrectly. You will only increase your risk of injury!

DON'T stretch if you have had a recent fracture, sprain, or strain, or suspect you have one.

DON'T overstretch a joint.

DON'T stretch if you suspect that you have osteoporosis or osteopenia. Speak with your doctor about what is best for you.

DON'T stretch if you have pain, discomfort, or an injury in a joint and around a muscle.

DON'T stretch if you have an infected or inflamed joint. (When in doubt, speak to your health professional.)

DON'T take joints to extremes, especially those on your neck or back.

DO warm up before stretching.

DO set realistic goals.

DO engage in static stretching.

DO change it up every now and then—don't get bored!

DO hold the stretch for 10 to 30 seconds.

DO design a flexibility program that focuses on tight muscles and incorporate the use of props to add variety to your program.

DO stretch daily, and enjoy!

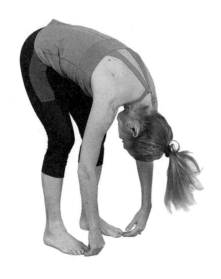

FLEXIBILITY SELF-EVALUATIONS

Determining your current state of activity will provide you a baseline from which to start. Of course, it does not matter where you start but where you end up. The journey of many miles starts with the first step. Take a moment to assess your current level of activity. The following chart is a useful tool.

FITNESS LEVEL	ACTIVITY LEVEL
Athlete	Exercises, plays competitive sports, or has an active job
Currently Active	Exercises at least two times per week
Mildly Active	Weekend warrior; does yard or house work; exercises when time allows
Thinking about Exercise	Knows physical activity is good, but has health or time issues
On the Couch	Too busy to exercise; feels fit enough not to need regular exercise

Using the following pre-stretching assessments will help you better understand how flexible you are currently and provide you with an idea of which areas need to be addressed. With this information in hand, you can design an effective stretching routine. Assess yourself periodically to see how your body is responding to your routine. Being honest with yourself is the first step to achieving your goals. Taking the time to evaluate your current level of flexibility will provide you with a point of reference to design a realistic flexibility plan and achieve your long-term goal. A simple assessment is if you find a stretch uncomfortable or tight, it may be an indication that you are in need of addressing that set of muscles. Most people who find a stretch uncomfortable will forgo working that area only to notice that region get tighter and more uncomfortable.

If you have health issues or concerns, consult your health provider for assistance and support. If you have had an injury, seek professional advice.

SIDE POSTURE EVALUATION

Taking time to review your posture will give you an indication of how your tight muscles are manifesting themselves in a practical way. You can do this evaluation either standing or sitting.

Standing: Stand in front of a mirror and view yourself from the side. Your ears, shoulders, and hips should be aligned.

Seated: Sit normally in a chair and view yourself from the side. Your ears should be aligned over your shoulders, and your shoulders should be aligned over your hips.

WALL POSTURE EVALUATION

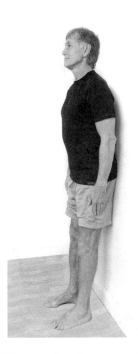 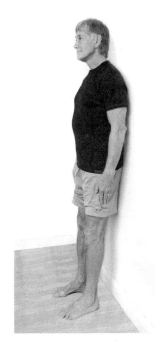 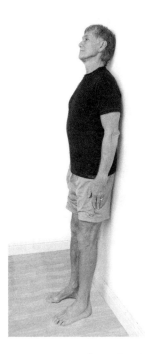

1. Stand with your heels 3 to 5 inches from a wall. Try to place your rear end against the wall.

2. If you are able to complete the first step, try to place your upper back against the wall.

3. If your rear and upper back can touch the wall, try to touch back of your head against the wall.

Posture Analysis

If the back of your head does not comfortably touch the wall, you probably spend a lot of time texting or leaning too far forward, which can lead to neck pain and headaches.

Intervention: Stretch the neck area gently and try the Side-to-Side Neck Stretch (page 57).

If you cannot get your upper back flat against the wall, your shoulder and chest region is too tight. You may notice that when you stand, your shoulders are hunched over. This rounded-shoulder posture can contribute to neck and shoulder pain and is often seen in people who sit at a computer or drive for long periods. This poor posture is common in people such as swimmers and weightlifters who do a lot of chest work.

Intervention: Strengthen upper back muscles, pectorals, and shoulder region.

If you have a significant arch in your lower back (also called a lordotic curve) when standing against the wall, it's possible that your hip flexor muscles at the tops of your thighs are overly tight. People with tight hip flexors often have a greater potential for lower back pain.

Intervention: Stretch out hip flexor muscles with Standing Hip Flexor (page 95) and hamstring stretches like the Sit & Reach (page 99).

HAMSTRING EVALUATION: SIT & REACH

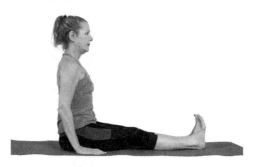

If you want to quantify your results, have someone use a ruler to measure the distance between your fingertips and your toes.

1. Sit on the floor with your feet straight out in front of you.

2. While keeping your back straight, attempt to touch your toes.

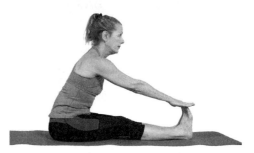

If you can touch your toes, that's good. If you can reach past your toes, that's fantastic! Keep up what you are doing. However, if you are like most people, you are not anywhere near touching your toes. If that's the case, this test is telling you it is time for a hamstring and lower back stretching intervention.

Intervention: Select several hamstring exercises, such as Figure 4 (page 104) or Straight-Leg Stretch (page 102).

SHOULDER GIRDLE EVALUATION: ZIPPER STRETCH

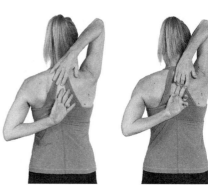

If you want to quantify your results, you can have someone use a ruler to measure the distance between your fingertips.

1–2. Stand facing straight ahead. While standing, place your left hand, palm facing out, up your back as high as possible. Then reach your right hand, with your palm facing your body, over your right shoulder and down your back as far as possible. Repeat on the other side.

Can you touch your hands together? If so, great! If you can't touch your hands, you need to work on shoulder flexibility.

Intervention: Try shoulder stretches like The Zipper (page 71).

STRETCHING PROGRAMS

PROGRAMS OVERVIEW

Generally, as we get older, we lose flexibility. Many common chronic conditions cause us to "guard" or protect the joint, leading to further loss of mobility. Additionally, habitual overuse, either from work or from play, can hasten our loss of flexibility. This section provides you with some sample stretching routines for many common chronic conditions seen in the 50-plus group. It also includes stretching routines to accompany recreational pursuits older adults enjoy, as well as activities done day to day.

Feel free to do some or all of the suggested stretches. Try your best to stretch daily, whether you've been very active or have been sitting for a long time. It is better to do a little bit of anything than to do nothing at all. Just remember to listen to your body!

It was not that long ago that we were instructed to stretch before engaging in sports. Even today, if you attend a high school football game, you will see the players still performing bouncing stretches before a game, which is bad for the body, whether you're 18 or 80 years of age. To prevent injury, the stretches in this book are all of a sustained nature.

It is ideal to warm up the muscles you plan to use with active stretches and a light jog or quick walk prior to doing any activity. Another good time to stretch is after a warm shower or bath, especially if you have osteoarthritis. Treat yourself like an expensive racehorse—no horse owner would ever allow her horse to go out on the track without being completely warmed up. So don't do anything, from shoveling snow to golfing, without warming up your body first. Note that warming up is *not* the same as stretching! Do a few minutes of light activity before ever attending to your daily chores or doing your favorite sport.

GENERAL FLEXIBILITY

The warm-up stretches I recommend in this program are good to do before any activity. However, the best results are achieved if the body is warm, thus a few minutes of light activity or a warm shower or bath will make the stretching session easier and more enjoyable. Start slowly and mindfully. The cool-down stretches, done after activity, will help your body release any tension or tightness you accumulated. In fact, some research suggests that post-activity is actually the best time to stretch to gain lasting results. If you're looking for variety, I've included a general flexibility program that incorporates props.

GENERAL FLEXIBILITY WARM-UP

GENERAL FLEXIBILITY COOL-DOWN

GENERAL FLEXIBILITY WITH PROPS

NOVICE

To get you started on the right foot, the next two programs are like the bunny slope in skiing, designed to see how your body responds to stretching. If you are flexible, you will find these programs very easy and sail through them. But for safety's sake, spend a week testing them out. If you find these stretches challenging, it is perfectly OK to stay at this level forever. It is also OK to modify the program to your skill set. Keep in mind there are no "musts" in this book. It is for your body, so personalizing the program for *you* is perfectly fine! Always prepare the body with a warm-up before any activity. Start slowly and mindfully. Once the body is warm, engage in gentle, active stretches.

STRETCHES, NOVICE LEVEL 1

Side-to-Side Neck Stretch	page 57	Gas Pedals	page 118
Seated Knee to Chest	page 88	Shoulder Rolls	page 68
Rear Calf Stretch	page 116		

STRETCHES, NOVICE LEVEL 2

Sit & Reach	page 99	Elbow Touches	page 73
Seated Knee to Chest	page 88	Picture Frame	page 70
Apple Pickers	page 63		

WAKE-UP ROUTINE

Many of us with chronic pain or stiffness wake up tight in the morning. Many times, it is a good idea to take a few moments while warm and snuggly in bed to make note of which joints and muscles are clicking and clunking, and limber out those creaks. Slowly move your body through a comfortable range of motion. Use your cat or dog as a model. Animals often stretch before they jump up and play. If dogs and cats do it, why don't humans do it? Sometimes getting up and taking a warm shower and then doing this easy routine back in bed is a good way to start the day, or even to end the day when you're ready to go to sleep.

BED STRETCHES

Knee Roll	page 86	Double Knee to Chest	page 90
Single Knee to Chest	page 89	Gas Pedals	page 118
Rock 'n' Roll	page 92	Pec Stretch	page 75

CHRONIC CONDITIONS

Most physical therapists and exercise physiologists agree that most of the common chronic physical conditions can be positively influenced with sensible, regular exercise. Research has shown that everything from arthritis to multiple sclerosis can benefit from a gentle stretching program.

Many of the common conditions seen in older adults make the person stiffer, which can increase pain. Flexibility training can reduce muscle injury, decrease lower back pain, improve biomechanics, and reduce the stiffness of arthritis and other muscular-skeletal issues.

Although all the stretching exercises in this book can be done by anyone, this section offers routines for many common chronic conditions seen in mature adults.

Nothing you do should make you feel worse; if it does, cut back a bit and reevaluate what you are doing. Don't be afraid to consult your health professional for a selection of stretches specific to your ailments.

Arthritis/Fibromyalgia

Stiffness is a common characteristic of osteoarthritis and fibromyalgia. Sensible stretching is of paramount importance in managing arthritis. Unfortunately, many people with arthritis complain of decreased flexibility, which results in a loss of range of motion. "Use it or lose it" really pertains to arthritis: If you don't move the joint, it will become stiffer and more painful, which can impair function. This is why a water exercise program designed specifically for people with arthritis would be an excellent complement to a safe and sane stretching program approved by your health professional.

When stretching with arthritis, follow these recommendations:

- always follow medical advice
- never over-exercise
- don't mask pain with medication
- never stretch a swollen or "hot" joint
- keep movement within the pain-free range of motion

Gentle stretching can be useful, as long as you stretch the parts you're using (stretching your legs will provide little or no benefit to the shoulder region). Lastly, remember the two-hour rule: If something hurts more than two hours after exercise, back off and do less next time.

STRETCHES FOR ARTHRITIS

Side-to-Side Neck Stretch	page 57	Finger Tap	page 80
Seated Knee to Chest	page 88	Rotator Cuff	page 66
Sit & Reach	page 99	Shoulder Rolls	page 68
Rear Calf Stretch	page 116	Windmills on Roller	page 62
Ankle Circles	page 120	Hamstring Massage	page 106
Gas Pedals	page 118	Foot Massage	page 121
Seated Wrist Stretch	page 76		

Frozen Shoulder

A frozen shoulder usually results from non-use of the shoulder because of a painful shoulder condition such as tendinitis or bursitis. If your arm is not used for a while, adhesions (tightness) may form on the sleeve-like structure that holds the ball-and-socket portion of your shoulder joint together. If the shoulder is not moved for two to three weeks, these adhesions will become very dense and strong and will result in a shoulder that cannot move freely—thus the term "frozen shoulder." If you have not been able to use your shoulder for a few months, consult a health care professional and follow a program under his or her supervision. Let pain be your guide: If stretching increases your pain, back off and follow the two-hour rule. It might be wise to warm up the joint with a heating pad prior to stretching and using ice after stretching.

STRETCHES FOR FROZEN SHOULDER

Shoulder Rolls	page 68	I, Y & T	page 72
Double Wood Chops	page 64	Prone Reverse Flyes	page 69
Hands Behind Back	page 74	Neck Massage	page 60

Hip Problems

Designed to support the load of our body, the hips are often called the workhorse of the body. Unfortunately, some people overuse them at their jobs, or in the weight room with heavy lifts. Sometimes, years of being overweight can put too much load on the joint and cause good hips to go bad. Consult your health professional for specific exercises for the hip joint. Avoid flexion past

90 degrees (allowing your knee to get too close to your chest) or crossing the midline of your body (when you swing your leg in front of or behind the other leg).

STRETCHES FOR HIP PROBLEMS

Sit & Reach	page 99	Hamstring/Hip Release	page 105
Inner Thigh Stretch	page 97	Quad Massage	page 113
Standing Hip Flexor	page 95	Hamstring Massage	page 106
Rear Calf Stretch	page 116	Side Bend with Band	page 85
Gas Pedals	page 118		

Knee Problems

Chronic knee problems can be the result of poor anatomical design. If you are bowlegged or knock-kneed, you are at a mechanical disadvantage that can set you up for injury. Foot misalignments can also contribute to knee problems. In addition, injuries from sports such as football or soccer, or even too many step aerobics classes or badly executed stretches, can harm your knees. Your knee is an engineering marvel but can still break down if used incorrectly. Be careful to keep the knee in biomechanical alignment: Your knees and toes should always point in the same direction, and you should never over-bend your knees or over-straighten your legs.

STRETCHES FOR KNEE PROBLEMS

Sit & Reach	page 99	Hamstring Massage	page 106
Straight-Leg Stretch	page 102	Quad Massage	page 113
Standing Hip Flexor	page 95	Inner Thigh Massage	page 98
Rear Calf Stretch	page 116	Side Bend with Band	page 85
Rear Calf Stretch with Strap	page 117		

Lower Back Pain

Lower back pain is caused by a variety of sources, including weak abdominals, tight hamstrings and quadriceps, improper body mechanics, poor posture, overuse, facet and joint problems, and herniated discs. Many arm movements affect the lower back, and activities such as overhead reaching affect the lumbar lordosis. Back problems should be diagnosed by a health care professional. A healthy back program includes exercises that strengthen the abdominals and stretch the hamstrings and lower back muscles. For people with back problems, learning about and performing the good neutral spine technique is very important (see The Importance of Posture on page 22). All exercises should be done from this stance unless otherwise instructed by your health professional.

STRETCHES FOR LOWER BACK PAIN

Single Knee to Chest	page 89	Piriformis Stretch	page 92
Double Knee to Chest	page 90	Windmills on Roller	page 62
Sit & Reach	page 99	Hamstring Massage	page 106
Mad Cat Stretch	page 122	Double-Leg Stretch	page 107
Standing Hip Flexor	page 95		

Repetitive Wrist Strain

Repetitive injuries are caused from—just as they sound—doing any detailed task repeatedly without taking a break. The pathology that causes the problem is complex and needs to be explained by your doctor. It is interesting to note that carpal tunnel wrist syndrome really increased when computers became popular.

STRETCHES FOR REPETITIVE WRIST STRAIN

Inward/Outward Wrist Stretch	page 76	Standing Wrist Stretch	page 77
Seated Wrist Stretch	page 76	V-W Stretch	page 81
Forearm Massage	page 78	Band Roll-Up	page 78

RECREATIONAL PURSUITS

This series is designed to prevent possible injuries, rehabilitate existing injuries, and balance out the negative results of one-sided activities, such as golf and tennis.

Biking/Cycling

Most people would assume that biking is a lower body activity, but think of your posture as you're on the bike. Your body is rounded over the handlebars, with much of your weight resting on your wrists and hands. Start out with an easy warm-up ride. If you're very inflexible, get off the bike and stretch. Otherwise, stretch after your ride and ice sore joints if necessary. If you can, have your bike professionally adjusted to fit you.

STRETCHES FOR BIKING/CYCLING

Single Knee to Chest	page 89	Gas Pedals	page 118
Standing Quad Stretch	page 109	Ankle Circles	page 120
Double Knee to Chest	page 90	I, Y & T	page 72
Kneeling Hip Flexor	page 94	Torso Relax	page 86
Piriformis Stretch	page 92	Hamstring/Hip Release	page 105
Figure 4	page 104	Quad Massage	page 113
Rear Calf Stretch	page 116	Foot Massage	page 121

Bowling

Many people don't think bowling is a sport, yet it can be very hard on the hips, knees, shoulders, and back. One problem that bowling presents is that it is one-sided, and you are asked to throw a heavy ball with full force. All this can lead to injuries. Practice with a few easy rolls before going full strength.

STRETCHES FOR BOWLING

Sit & Reach	page 99	Shoulder Rolls	page 68
Standing Hip Flexor	page 95	Side-to-Side Neck Stretch	page 57
Gas Pedals	page 118	Side Bend	page 84
Heel Raise/Heel Drop	page 119	Seated Knee to Chest	page 88
Inward/Outward Wrist Stretch	page 76	Twister	page 83
Seated Wrist Stretch	page 76	Windmills on Roller	page 62
Finger Tap	page 80	Drop-Off Stretch	page 117
Finger Spreader	page 80	Forearm Massage	page 78

Canoeing, Kayaking, or Stand-Up Paddle Boarding

Stand-up paddle boarding (SUP) and paddling sports like canoeing and kayaking are primarily upper body tasks, so pay attention to not getting overly tight through the chest region. Perform a light walk or jog beforehand. If you tend to use only one side to stroke, try to switch sides in order to balance out your muscle use.

STRETCHES FOR CANOEING, KAYAKING, OR SUP

Twister	page 83	Windmills on Roller	page 62
Side-to-Side Neck Stretch	page 57	Neck Massage	page 60
Pec Stretch	page 75	I, Y & T	page 72
The Zipper	page 71	Standing Quad Stretch	page 109
Picture Frame	page 70		

Golf

Many people say they play golf, yet I am still waiting to speak to someone who "plays" golf. Most people actually *compete* at golf, and often make an enjoyable pastime a stress-laden event. Golf is tough on the body and hard on the knees, hips, and especially the lower back. One problem with golf is that it is asymmetrical, meaning only one side of the body gets used repeatedly. The other issue is that the worse at golf you are, the harder it is on your body due to more repetition and bad form.

Walk for a few minutes before the match starts; walk the course, if possible. Don't always pull your clubs with the same arm. Similarly, try taking an equal number of swings to the left and right to even out all the one-sided swings you'll be executing in the game. Try to stay as balanced to the left as you are to the right. And, finally, avoid the food and drink at the 19th hole!

STRETCHES FOR GOLF

Side-to-Side Neck Stretch	page 57	Finger Spreader	page 80
Turtle	page 58	Shoulder Rolls	page 68
Side Bend	page 84	Hands Behind Back	page 74
Palm Tree	page 82	The Zipper	page 71
Double Knee to Chest	page 90	Elbow Touches	page 73
Rear Calf Stretch	page 116	Windmills on Roller	page 62
Standing Wrist Stretch	page 77	Prone Reverse Flyes	page 69
Inward/Outward Wrist Stretch	page 76	Neck Massage	page 60

Skiing/Snowboarding

Skiing can be an explosive sport that asks you to perform hard for short spurts, stand around for a while in line, and then exert at full force again. With skiing, you have to contend with the cold at high altitudes, and our 50-plus tendons and ligaments often gel up when left alone in the cold. Skiing is a total-body sport and can be hard on shoulders, knees, and tendons. Always warm up, and stop when you are fatigued. Listen to your body. Don't over-ski your ability or fitness level. Ski a couple of bunny slopes before you start the day, and finish with a stretch after a warm shower.

STRETCHES FOR SKIING

Skyscraper	page 58	Finger Spreader	page 80
Palm Tree	page 82	Double Wood Chops	page 64
Side Bend	page 84	Choker	page 70
Sit & Reach	page 99	Picture Frame	page 70
Standing Quad Stretch	page 109	Over the Top	page 69
Standing Hip Flexor	page 95	Kneeling Hip Flexor	page 94
Rear Calf Stretch	page 116	Inner Thigh Massage	page 98
Ankle Circles	page 120	Hamstring Massage	page 106
Seated Wrist Stretch	page 76	Foot Massage	page 121

Swimming

Water exercise is gentle on the body and everybody should do it. But swimming is not as kind. Over time, swimming laps can contribute to shoulder problems, and breathing to one side repeatedly can aggravate lower back problems. A few gentle laps to warm up is always a good idea. Stretch after your laps. It would be wise to have your swim skills analyzed if you swim a lot.

STRETCHES FOR SWIMMING

Gas Pedals	page 118	Windmills on Roller	page 62
Shoulder Rolls	page 68	Neck Massage	page 60
Double Wood Chops	page 64	Prone Reverse Flyes	page 69
Choker	page 70	I, Y & T	page 72
Over the Top	page 69	Torso Relax	page 86
Pec Stretch	page 75		

Tennis/Pickleball

Tennis and pickeball are fun sports, but they often take a significant toll on the body. The knees take a pounding and the shoulders are asked to perform some difficult moves. The load placed on the spine, not to mention the cardiovascular system, is tremendous. The fact that these are mostly asymmetrical games (meaning both sports are done mostly on one side of the body) sets you up for misalignments.

Stretching is very important if you are a tennis or pickleball player. Take a few minutes to walk around the court then gently hit the ball back and forth to lubricate the affected joints. Once you're warmed up, take a few moments to stretch before the game starts. Stretch between sets and after the game as well. It's important to always cool down after your pickle ball or tennis match.

STRETCHES FOR TENNIS/PICKLEBALL

Walking/Jogging

Jogging, running, and walking are primarily lower body activities. To incorporate a stretching routine into your regular activities, start out at a slower pace than you usually do. Once you feel warmed up, stop and stretch your hips, legs, knees, and ankles. Don't forget to stretch your chest and shoulders, because often your upper body becomes hunched over. After you exercise, take time to stretch some more.

STRETCHES FOR WALKING/JOGGING

Double Knee to Chest	page 90	Side Bend with Band	page 85
Standing Hip Flexor	page 95	Kneeling Hip Flexor	page 94
Rear Calf Stretch	page 116	Quad Massage	page 113
Gas Pedals	page 118	Hamstring Massage	page 106
Ankle Circles	page 120	Inner Thigh Massage	page 98
Windmills on Roller	page 62	Foot Massage	page 121

DAILY ACTIVITIES

The following are some simple stretching routines for daily activities that seem innocuous enough but can cause problems when performed abruptly or for too long.

Gardening

Gardening sounds like fun to some and work to others. If you are not fit to bend, squat, or lift, perhaps window box gardening may be a better option. Warm up the body before you start gardening. If it is spring planting season and you have been sedentary all winter, use caution and don't overdo it.

STRETCHES FOR GARDENING

Side-to-Side Neck Stretch	page 57	Finger Tap	page 80
Side Bend	page 84	Apple Pickers	page 63
Twister	page 83	Double Wood Chops	page 64
Standing Hip Flexor	page 95	Mad Cat Stretch	page 122
Rear Calf Stretch	page 116		

Housecleaning/Lifting

Doing housework can be strenuous physical activity and should be performed with caution because it is very easy to strain muscles. Areas of special concern should be the lower back and knees. Walk around for a few minutes before doing chores and then stretch afterward. Protect your back and ask for help when needed. Use stepladders rather than a chair to reach high places. Be careful when vacuuming or making the bed, as those tasks can be hard on your lower back.

STRETCHES FOR HOUSECLEANING/LIFTING

Seated Knee to Chest	page 88	Heel Raise/Heel Drop	page 119
Sit & Reach	page 99	Finger Tap	page 80
Inner Thigh Stretch	page 97	Shoulder Rolls	page 68
Rear Calf Stretch	page 116	Double Wood Chops	page 64
Ankle Circles	page 120	Picture Frame	page 70

Long Drive or Plane Flight

A long drive or plane flight can cause muscles to get tight. Often the upper and lower back start to ache, and the shoulders and lower legs will get cramped. Sitting for a long time will not only make you inflexible but can be hazardous to your health. There is a condition called "economy class" syndrome, when people sit for a prolonged period; the worst-case scenario is death. Get up as often as possible, drink water, avoid alcohol, and stretch regularly.

STRETCHES FOR LONG DRIVES OR PLANE FLIGHTS

Side-to-Side Neck Stretch	page 57	Heel Raise/Heel Drop	page 119
Turtle	page 58	Seated Wrist Stretch	page 76
Standing Hip Flexor	page 95	Finger Tap	page 80
Rear Calf Stretch	page 116	Finger Spreader	page 80
Gas Pedals	page 118	Shoulder Rolls	page 68

Shoveling Snow

Anyone who has ever shoveled snow knows how tough this task can be. How often do you pick up the paper to read about someone dying because of shoveling snow? Shoveling is hard on the whole body, but especially your lower back. Always warm up first. Don't hurry or strain—doing so could kill you! This may be an activity that you should hire a kid to do, rather than doing it yourself and then paying a doctor to fix your back or after an heart attack. If you feel that your heart and breathing rate are elevated as you're shoveling, stop and check them. If they are high, slow down or stop.

STRETCHES FOR SHOVELING SNOW

Side Bend	page 84	Apple Pickers	page 63
Sit & Reach	page 99	Double Wood Chops	page 64
Roll into a Ball	page 91	Windmills	page 61
Standing Hip Flexor	page 95	Mad Cat Stretch	page 122
Heel Raise/Heel Drop	page 119		

Working at a Desk or Computer

Sitting still and doing anything for a long time is not good for the body. Sitting over a computer causes you to have rounded shoulders, a protruding head, and wrist problems. Get up and move around as often as possible. Stand while on the phone. Walk to deliver a message whenever possible. Set your computer alarm to remind you to get up once every hour. Drink plenty of water or juice to make you get up often. At lunch, don't work at your desk—take a walk. Park as far away from your office as you can and take the stairs when possible.

If you, like many older adults, find yourself spending hours in one position (at a desk or in an airplane seat, for example), you may feel tired and stiff. The following is a simple way to stay limber:

- get up and walk around
- slowly look left and right
- squeeze your shoulder blades together
- sit in your chair, place your legs straight out in front of you, and reach forward toward your toes
- reach for the sky several times

STRETCHES FOR WORKING AT A DESK OR COMPUTER

Side-to-Side Neck Stretch	page 57	Double Wood Chops	page 64
Side Bend	page 84	Mad Cat Stretch	page 122
Standing Hip Flexor	page 95	Foot Massage	page 121
Rear Calf Stretch	page 116	Hamstring Massage	page 106
Finger Tap	page 80	Forearm Massage	page 78
Apple Pickers	page 63		

STRETCHING EXERCISES

Side-to-Side Neck Stretch

Target: neck

CAUTION: If you have a history of neck problems (e.g., herniated discs, arthritis of the neck), consult a health professional before performing this move.

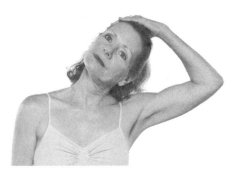

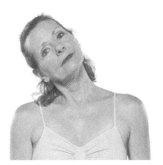

1. Stand with proper posture. While inhaling deeply through your nose, slowly tilt your head to the left. Once in this position, place the fingertips of your left hand on the right side of your head. While exhaling through your lips, gently pull your head to your left shoulder. Keep your shoulders relaxed and down. Hold this position and continue to breathe deeply in through your nose and out through your lips.

2. Release and return to starting position before switching sides.

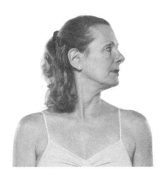

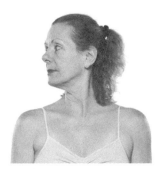

3. Inhale slowly through your nose and look to your left as far as you can without feeling discomfort. Exhale slowly through your lips and hold this position for a moment, feeling the stretch.

4. Inhale slowly through your nose and look slowly to the right. Exhale slowly through your lips and hold this position for a moment, feeling the stretch.

Skyscraper

CAUTION: Avoid hyperextending and hyperflexing the neck. If you have a history of neck problems, do not do this move. You can also try this stretch sitting with proper posture.

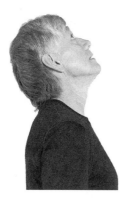 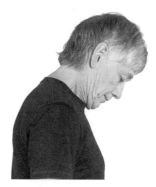

1. Stand with proper posture. Position your chin so that it's parallel with the floor. While inhaling slowly through your nose, tilt your head just slightly to look up at the ceiling. Don't arch your neck. Hold this position for a moment, feeling the stretch.

2. Exhale through your lips and lower your chin to your chest just slightly.

Repeat as many times as feels comfortable.

Turtle

This exercise is designed to reverse the effects of "forward" head, a common result of sitting in front of a computer for hours. You can also try this stretch sitting with proper posture.

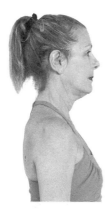 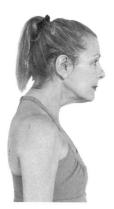

1. Stand with proper posture. Pretend you're holding an apple under your chin, or keep your chin parallel with the floor. Inhale deeply.

2. While exhaling through your lips, push your chin forward.

Now inhale through your nose and slowly pull your head back to the neutral position. The focus of this exercise is to pull the head back.

Repeat this move as many times as feels comfortable.

Hold/Relax Turtle

Target: neck

This exercise is designed to reverse the effects of "forward" head, a common result of sitting in front of a computer for hours. You can also try this stretch standing with proper posture.

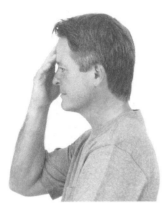

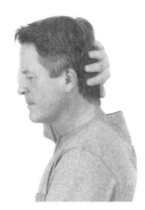

1. Sit with proper posture. Pretend you're holding an apple under your chin, or position your chin so that it's parallel with the floor. Position the fingertips of your right hand on the center of your forehead. Focus on your deep breathing techniques. Gently press your forehead into your fingertips. Stay mindful of your breathing and hold this position for a comfortable moment.

2. Return to starting position, then place your right hand on the back of your head.

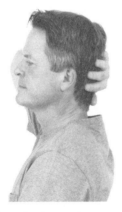

3. Now inhale deeply through your nose and push your skull into your hand. Place more emphasis on this phase of the exercise. Stay mindful of your breathing and hold this position for a comfortable moment.

Release and return to starting position.

VARIATION: Instead of using your fingertips, you can press your head into a pillow held in your hand. If your right shoulder is tight, use your left hand, and vice versa.

Neck Massage

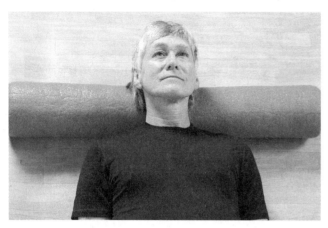

1. Lie on your back with your knees bent, feet on the floor, and arms along your sides. Position a foam roller under the base of your head. Slowly breathe in through your nose and out through your mouth as you allow your back to settle and relax.

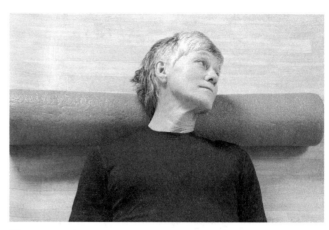

2. Inhale as you gently and slowly look to the left.

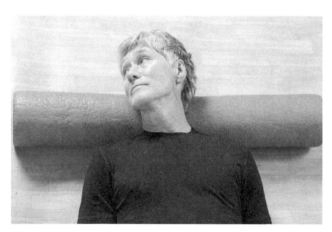

3. Exhale as you return to starting position. Inhale as you look to the right.

Exhale as you return to starting position.

Windmills

Target: shoulder region

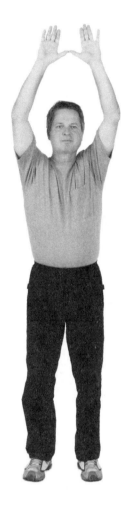

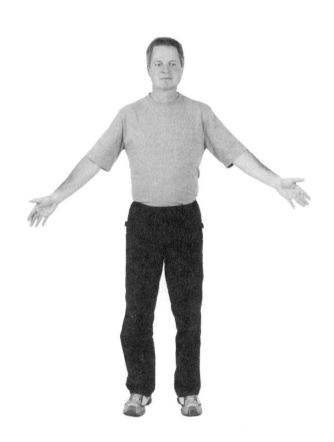

1. Stand with proper posture with your arms at your sides, palms facing forward. Inhale deeply through your nose and slowly raise your arms out to the sides as high as is comfortable. Try to touch your thumbs.

2. Exhale and slowly lower your arms.

Repeat as desired.

VARIATION: This exercise can also be done one arm at a time.

Windmills on Roller

Target: shoulder girdle

This exercise increases the range of motion in your shoulders and helps stabilize your muscles. Note that this is a more advanced move and makes use of a foam roller.

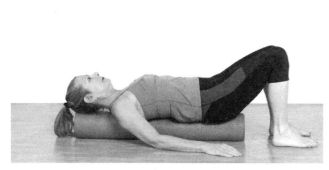

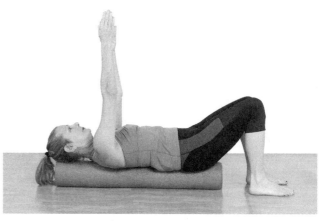

1. Lie on a foam roller, resting your head and the entire length of your back on it. Bend your knees and place your feet on the floor; place your arms on the floor alongside your body for balance. Breathe naturally and allow adequate time for your chest and shoulder region to relax and open up. For many people, this is an adequate stretch and it's OK to stop here without progressing to the following steps.

2. Once comfortable and stable, extend both arms up to the ceiling while maintaining balance on the roller; your palms should face each other. Be sure to stabilize your core the entire time by contracting your abs.

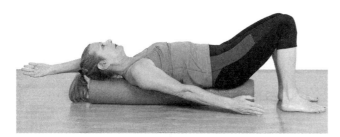

3. Allow one arm to move forward and the other backward. Stay within your comfortable range of motion.

Reverse directions.

Release and relax.

Apple Pickers

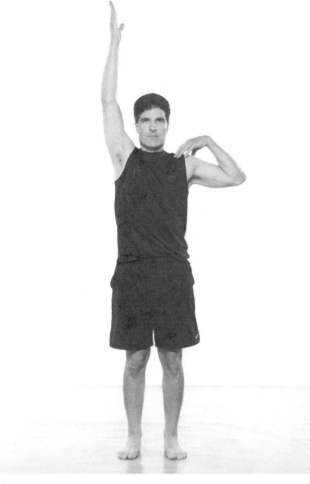

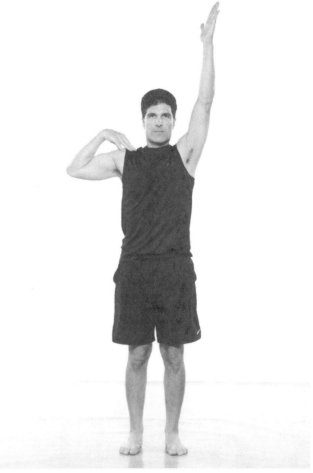

1. Stand with proper posture and place your hands on your shoulders. Reach your right hand as high as is comfortable.

2. Place your right hand back on your shoulder. Now reach up with your left hand.

Repeat as desired.

Double Wood Chops

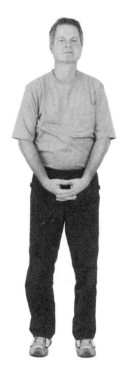

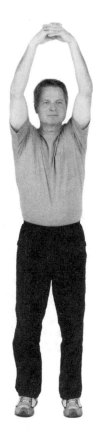

1. Stand with proper posture. Position your hands in front of your body and interlace your fingers.

2. Inhale deeply through your nose and slowly raise both arms in front of you to a comfortable height. Hold 1 to 2 seconds.

Slowly lower your arms to starting position.

Repeat as desired.

Soup Can Pours

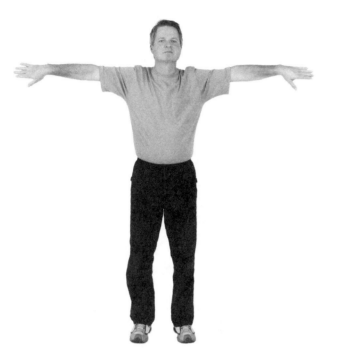
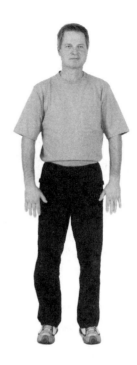

1. Stand with proper posture, your arms at your sides and your palms facing back. Inhale deeply through your nose and bring both arms slightly forward as your raise them out to the sides, keeping your palms facing back. Raise your arms no higher than shoulder level.

2. Exhale as you lower your arms.

Repeat as desired.

Rotator Cuff

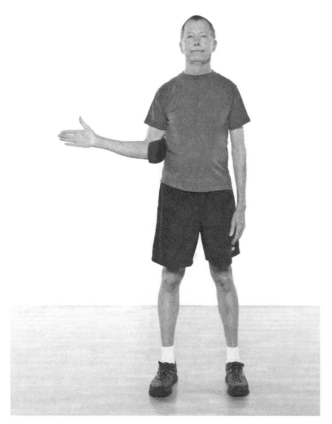 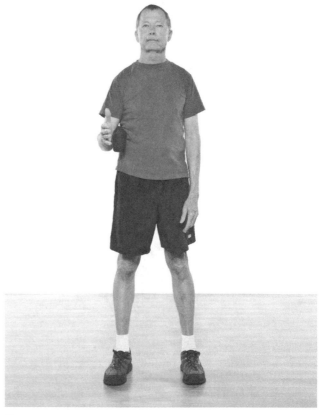

1. Stand with proper posture with your arms at your sides. Squeeze a rolled-up towel or block between your right arm and your torso and bend your right elbow 90 degrees. Point your thumb up.

Keeping the towel against your body and your forearm parallel to the floor, rotate your forearm out to the side.

2. Rotate your forearm back in toward your body. Repeat, then switch sides.

VARIATION: Try this with your palm facing down or up.

Arm Circles

Target: upper body

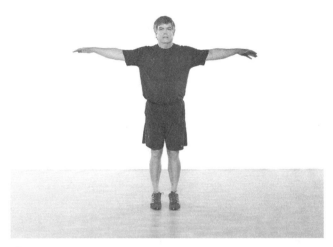 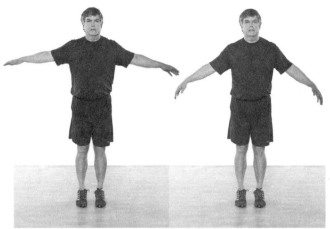

1. Assume a regular stance and raise both arms out to the sides at shoulder height.

2–3. Keeping your arms straight, slowly circle your arms forward, starting with small circles and progressing to larger ones.

Reverse direction.

Arm Swings with Neck Turn

Target: shoulders, neck

Caution: Perform this move slowly and with control. If you have neck issues, get clearance from your doctor before doing this.

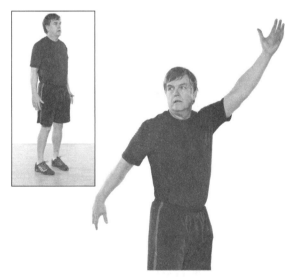 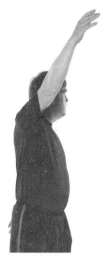

1. Stand tall with your arms along your sides. Gently swing your left arm forward as you swing your right arm backward, moving your arms as high as they can easily go. Gently look to the right.

Return to the starting position.

2. Gently swing your right arm forward and look to the left while your left arm moves backward. Gently look to the left.

Shoulder Rolls

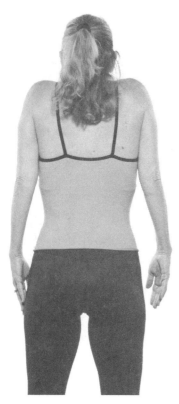 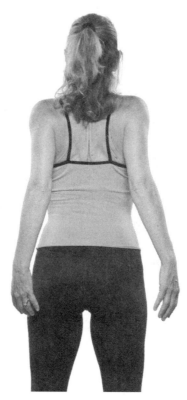 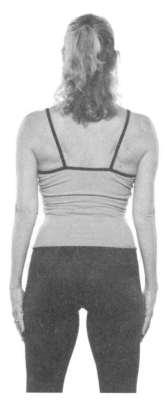

1. Stand with proper posture. Inhaling deeply through your nose, slowly shrug your shoulders.

2. Now pull your shoulders back and squeeze the shoulder blades together and down.

3. Exhaling through your lips, drop your shoulders and return to starting position.

Repeat as desired.

Prone Reverse Flyes

Target: shoulders, upper back

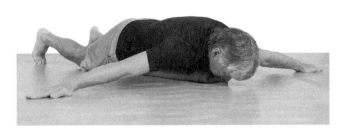 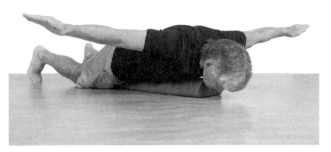

1. Carefully lie face-down on a half foam roller with its flat side down; your toes should rest on the ground. Extend your arms out to your sides in a "T."

2. Keeping your abs tight, slowly lift your arms a comfortable distance off the floor. Hold.

Return to starting position.

Over the Top

Target: shoulders, rotator cuffs

You can also try this stretch standing with proper posture.

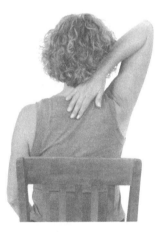 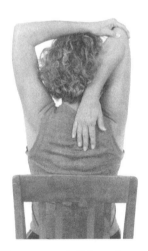

1. Sit with proper posture in a stable chair. Raise your right arm and place your hand on your back, over your right shoulder.

2. Place your left hand on your right elbow and gently press your right arm down your back as far as feels comfortable. Hold the position for a comfortable moment.

Switch sides and repeat.

VARIATION: In Step 2, press your right arm down as you push your right elbow up into your hand. Hold this position for a comfortable moment, remembering to breathe. Then release and allow your hand to slide a little further down your back.

Choker

You can also try this stretch standing with proper posture.

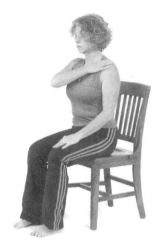
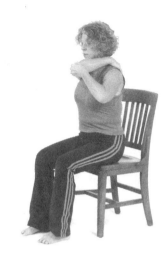

1. Sit with proper posture in a stable chair. Place your right hand on your left shoulder.

2. Place your left hand on your right elbow and gently press your right elbow toward your throat. Hold for a comfortable moment.

Switch sides and repeat.

VARIATION: In Step 2, press your right elbow into your left hand. Hold for a comfortable moment, remembering to breathe. Then release to reach the right hand a little farther back.

Picture Frame

Target: shoulders

Remember not to let your lower back arch. You can also try this stretch sitting with proper posture.

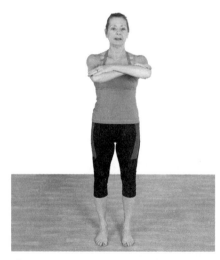
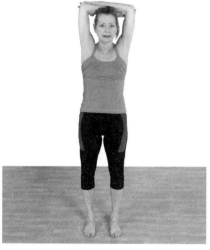

1. Stand with proper posture. Place your right hand on your left elbow and your left hand on your right elbow.

2. Slowly lift your arms overhead, raising your arms as high as feels comfortable. Hold the position for a moment. You are now framing your face in a picture frame created by your arms — smile! Repeat as desired.

The Zipper

You can also try this stretch sitting with proper posture.

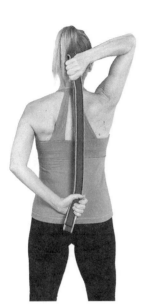

1. Stand with proper posture. Hold a strap in your right hand and raise your arm above your head. Bring your right hand down behind your head and grab the dangling end of the strap with your left hand.

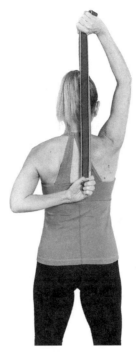

2. Raise your right hand up as high as possible to lift the lower hand, staying in your pain-free zone. Hold the position for a comfortable moment.

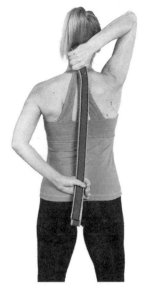

3. Pull down with your left hand to bring down the right hand. Hold the position for a comfortable moment.

Switch sides and repeat.

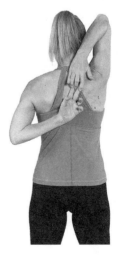

ADVANCED VARIATION: As you become more flexible, eliminate the use of the strap and try to grab your fingertips.

I, Y & T

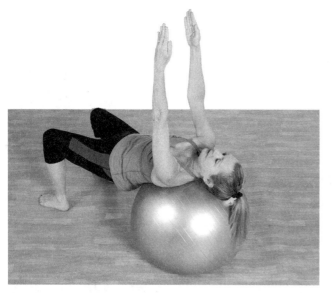

1. Sit on a stability ball and then slowly move your feet forward until the ball is comfortably supporting your upper back, neck, and head. Your feet should be shoulder-width apart and bent 90 degrees. Extend your arms toward the ceiling with palms facing each other.

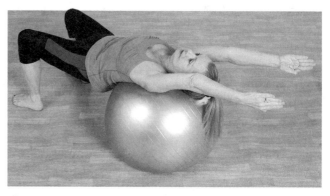

2. While engaging your core muscles, slowly and deliberately take both arms back by your ears, making your body look like an "I" from a bird's-eye view.

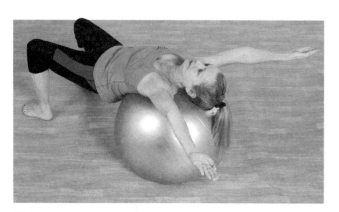

3. Return to starting position and then slightly take your arms back and to the sides, as if making a "Y."

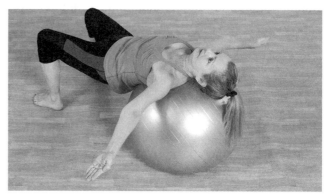

4. Return to starting position and then open your arms out to the sides to make a "T."

Elbow Touches

You can also try this stretch standing with proper posture.

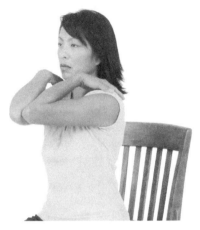
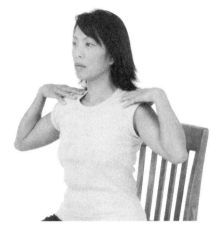

1. Sit with proper posture in a stable chair. Place your hands on your shoulders. Slowly bring your elbows together in front of your body.

2. Bring your elbows back and squeeze your shoulder blades together. Hold for a moment, focusing on opening up your chest.

Bring your elbows back to the starting position and repeat as desired.

VARIATION: Once you've done Step 2, draw circles with your elbows.

Elbow Touches Against Wall

Target: chest

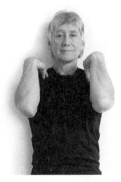
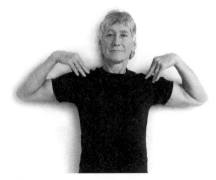
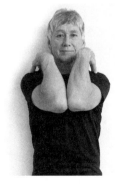

1. Stand with your back and head against the wall. Place your hands on your shoulders and point your elbows forward.

2. Carefully move your elbows toward the wall. Don't arch your back to increase your range. Touching the wall is not critical; the goal is to feel a gentle stretch in your chest and shoulders.

3. Slowly move your elbows back to center until you can touch them together.

Return to starting position.

Hands Behind Back

Target: shoulders, chest

You can also use a bar instead of a strap. CAUTION: Be careful not to exceed safe range of motion; don't force an uncomfortable position.

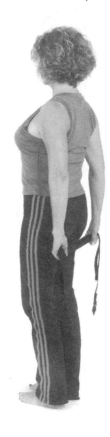
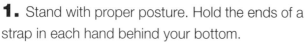
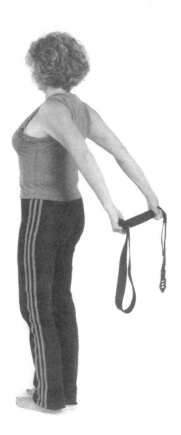

1. Stand with proper posture. Hold the ends of a strap in each hand behind your bottom.

2. Attempt to straighten your arms behind you. Focus on squeezing your shoulder blades together. Hold this position for as long as is comfortable.

ADVANCED VARIATION: Instead of using a strap, interlock your hands behind your back.

Pec Stretch

You can also try this stretch standing with proper posture.

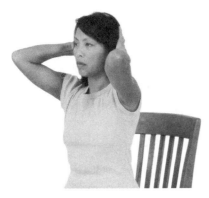 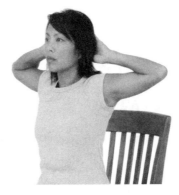 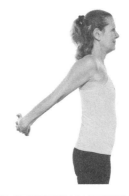

1. Sit with proper posture in a stable chair. Place your hands behind your head.

2. Gently move your elbows back and try to bring your shoulder blades together. Focus on opening up the chest and tightening the upper back muscles. Go as far back as is comfortable and hold for a moment. Repeat as desired.

PEC STRETCH VARIATION: Stand with proper posture and clasp your hands behind your back. Raise both hands up behind you, feeling the stretch in your chest and the fronts of your shoulders. Only go up as high as is comfortable and hold for a moment.

Chest Stretch

Target: chest

CAUTION: Be careful not to extend back too far; stay in your comfort zone.

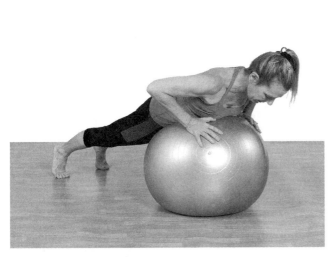 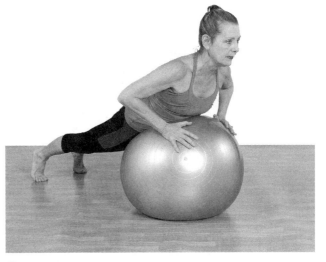

1. Kneel in front of a stability ball and place your belly and chest on the ball. Rest your hands and forearms on the ball. Extend your legs behind you, making a straight line from head to heels.

2. Keeping your head and neck neutral, gently raise your chest off the ball. Don't come up too high.

Return to starting position.

Inward/Outward Wrist Stretch

Target: forearms, wrists

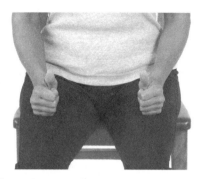 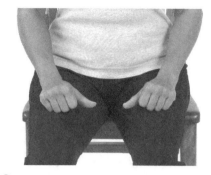 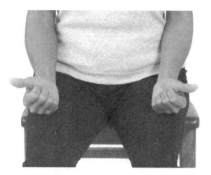

1. Sit with proper posture in a stable chair. Rest your fists on your thighs with your thumbs pointing up toward the ceiling.

2. Slowly turn your fists so that your thumbs point inward.

3. Slowly turn your fists so that your thumbs point outward.

Repeat as desired.

Seated Wrist Stretch

Target: forearms, wrists

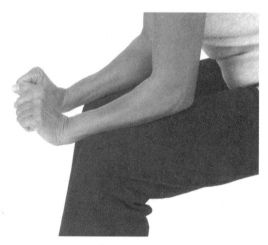 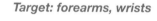 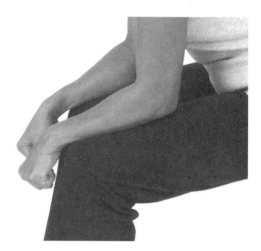

1. Sit in a stable chair. Rest your forearms on your thighs so that your wrists hang off. Your hands should be in loose fists. Slowly lift your knuckles toward the ceiling and hold 1 to 2 seconds.

2. Slowly lower your knuckles toward the floor and hold 1 to 2 seconds.

Repeat as feels comfortable.

ADVANCED VARIATION: After you lift your knuckles upward in Step 1, extend your fingertips, then make a fist, lower your knuckles, and extend your fingers downward.

Standing Wrist Stretch

Target: forearms, wrists

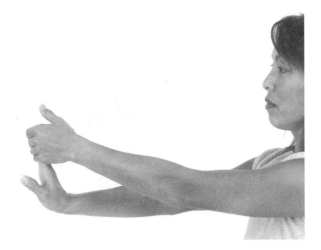

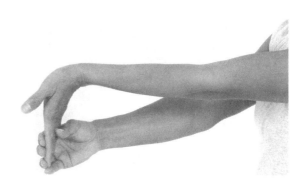

THE POSITION: Stand with proper posture. Extend your right arm in front of you to shoulder height, with your palm facing forward and fingers pointing toward the ceiling.

Gently pull your fingers back with your left hand until a desired stretch is felt under your wrist. Hold the stretch for several seconds. Repeat as desired then switch sides.

ADVANCED VARIATION: Try doing the exercise with the fingertips pointing down.

Kneeling Wrist Stretch

Target: forearms, wrists

This is a very advanced exercise.

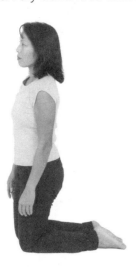

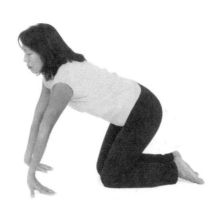

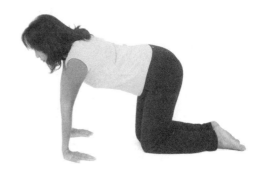

1. Kneel on the floor, using a mat as necessary.

2. Slowly place your fingers on the floor so that your fingers are pointing toward you.

3. Slowly lower your palms to the floor without discomfort in your wrists. Be sure to keep your elbows soft. Hold the stretch for a comfortable moment.

Forearm Massage

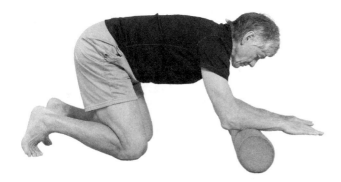 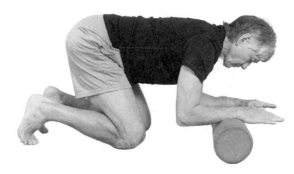

THE POSITION: Kneel in front of a foam roller and place your forearms on the roller with your palms down.

Slowly move your arms forward and back across the roller. Along the way, stop and apply pressure wherever additional attention is needed.

Band Roll-Up

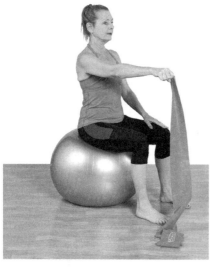 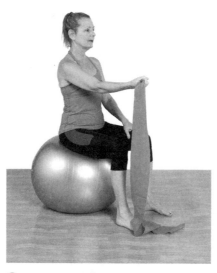 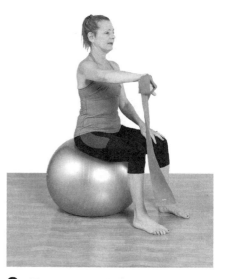

1. Sit with proper posture on a stability ball. Hold the end of a resistance band in your right hand and extend the right arm straight out in front of you, palm down.

2. Turn your palm up and grab more band in your hand.

3. Turn your palm down and grab more band, balling up the band in your hand as you go. Continue until you've grabbed as much band as you can, then squeeze tightly several times.

Switch hands and repeat.

Squeezer

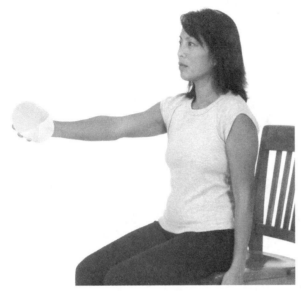 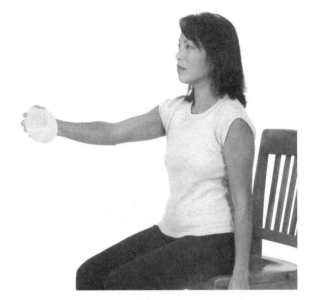

1. Sit with proper posture in a chair. Hold a small, soft, squeezable object in your right hand and extend that arm straight out in front of you. Keep your left arm by your side.

2. Slowly squeeze the object and hold for 1 to 2 seconds.

Repeat until the hand has done a comfortable number.

Switch hands and repeat.

MODIFICATION: You can also try doing this with an object in both hands.

VARIATION: Try this on something more difficult to squeeze, like a tennis ball.

Finger Tap

Target: hands, forearms, fingers

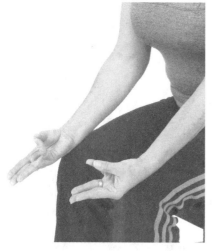 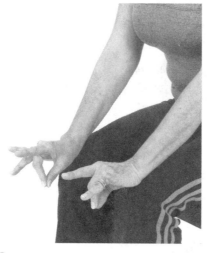 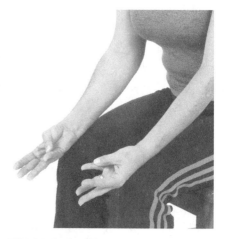

1. Sit at the edge of a stable chair. Rest your hands on your thighs with your palms turned up. Touch the tip of your little finger to your thumb then progress through each finger until you reach your index finger.

2. Now turn your palms down and repeat the exercise.

FINGER BASE TAP VARIATION: Touch the thumb to the base of your little finger, then progress through each finger until you reach the index finger. Now turn your palms down and repeat the exercise.

Finger Spreader

Target: hands, forearms, fingers

This exercise can also be done standing.

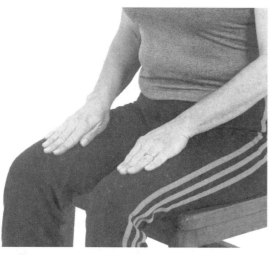 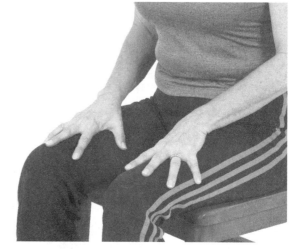

1. Sit with proper posture in a stable chair. Rest your hands on your thighs with your palms down and fingers gently spread. Squeeze your fingers and thumb together.

2. Now separate all fingers and thumb as far apart as possible.

Turn your palms up and repeat Steps 1 and 2.

V-W Stretch

This exercise can also be done standing.

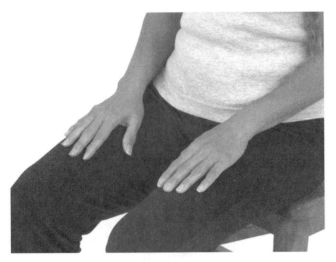

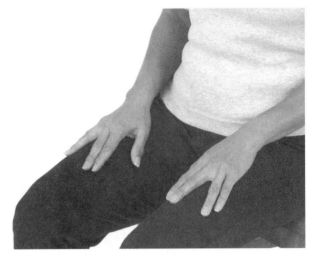

1. Sit with proper posture in a stable chair. Rest your hands on your thighs with your palms down. Squeeze all your fingers together.

2. Separate one finger at a time, starting with the little finger, then the ring finger, until you've separated all your fingers. Squeeze your fingers together and repeat the exercise.

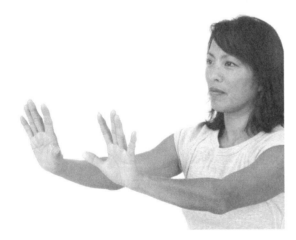

ADVANCED VARIATION: Increase the challenge by holding your arms straight out in front of you. Instead of just separating your fingers, try to make a "V" and "W." To make a "V": Spread your little finger and ring finger away from your index finger and middle finger. To make a "W": Put your ring finger and middle finger together and separate the little finger and index finger from the group.

Palm Tree

Target: torso

CAUTION: If you have poor balance or lower back problems, avoid this move. You can also try this stretch standing with proper posture.

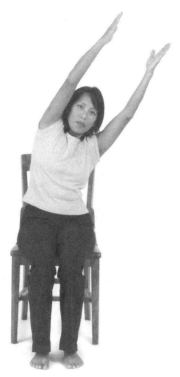

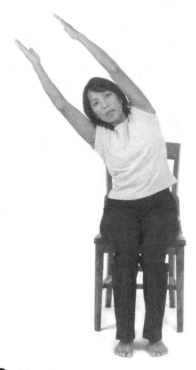

1. Sit with proper posture in a stable chair. Raise your hands overhead with your arms as straight as feels comfortable. Inhale deeply through your nose. While exhaling through your lips, slowly lean to your left. Hold the position for a comfortable moment, feeling the stretch along the right side of your body.

2. Now inhale fully and deeply through your nose and lean to your right. Hold this position for a comfortable moment.

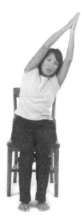

ADVANCED VARIATION: Try pressing your hands together as you do the side bends.

Twister

CAUTION: Be careful if you have lower back problems. You can also try this stretch standing with proper posture.

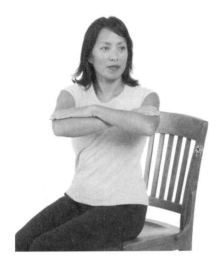 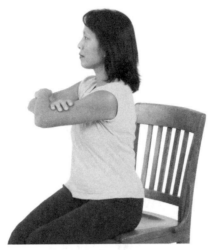 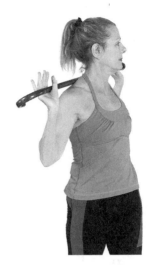

1. Sit with proper posture in a stable chair. Cross your arms in front of your chest and inhale slowly and deeply through your nose. While exhaling through your lips, slowly twist to your left. Hold the position for a comfortable moment and feel the stretch in your torso.

2. Inhale and return to the starting position before exhaling and twisting to your right. Hold the position for a comfortable moment and feel the stretch in your torso.

VARIATION: Rest a broom handle across the back of your shoulders and perform Steps 1 and 2 smoothly and gently.

Side Bend

CAUTION: Be careful if you have lower back pain. You can also try this stretch sitting with proper posture.

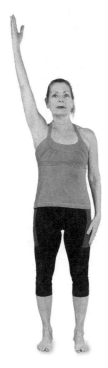 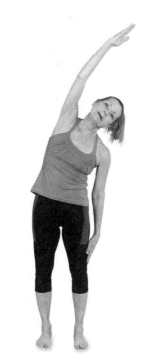

1. Stand with proper posture. Raise your right arm over your head to a comfortable height. Inhale deeply through your nose.

2. Now exhale through your lips and slowly and carefully lean to the left. Once you have leaned over enough to feel a gentle stretch along the right side of your body, hold this position for a comfortable moment.

Switch sides and repeat.

VARIATION: If your shoulder is stiff, place your hand on top of your head.

Side Bend with Band

CAUTION: Be careful if you have arthritis of the spine.

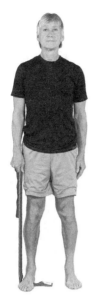

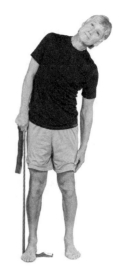

1. Stand with your feet shoulder-width apart and place a band under your right foot. Grasp the band near your right hip with your right hand.

2. Lean your body to the left.

Return to starting position and repeat.

Switch sides.

Torso Rotation

Target: torso

This exercise makes use of a resistance band to increase the stretch and strengthen the torso.

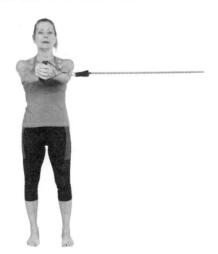

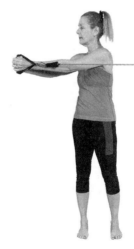

1. Secure the band to a door with the proper strap so that the band is at chest height. While standing with your left side to the door, grab the band with both hands and step away from the door with your arms fully extended until the band is taut. Stand with your feet shoulder-width apart.

2. Slowly twist to the right and hold for 1 to 2 seconds.

Return to starting position and repeat as desired.

Switch sides.

Torso Relax

Target: torso, spine, neck

This releases back tension and lengthens the spine and neck. Use a large stability ball. CAUTION: If you're pregnant or have stomach issues, speak to your health professional before doing this movement.

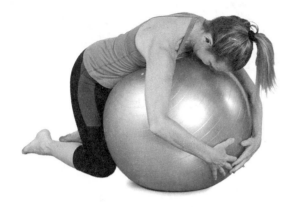

THE POSITION: Kneel in front of a stability ball. Drape your upper body over the ball, hugging the ball or placing your hands on the floor in front of you as necessary. Breathe slowly and fully.

To get off the ball, shift your weight back toward your hips so that you return to kneeling.

Knee Roll

Target: torso, hips

CAUTION: If you have lower back problems, avoid this move.

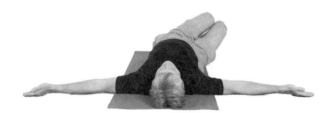 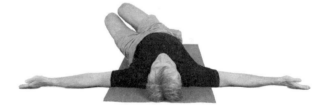

1. Lie on a mat with your knees bent and your feet flat on the floor. Place your arms straight out to your sides in a "T" position. While inhaling through your nose, allow your knees to drop gently to the right without discomfort. Exhale and hold this position for a comfortable moment.

2. Inhale and bring your knees back to center, then gently drop them to your left. Exhale and hold this position for a comfortable moment.

Cross-Leg Drop

Target: torso, piriformis

CAUTION: Be careful if you have lower back problems.

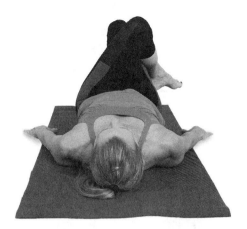 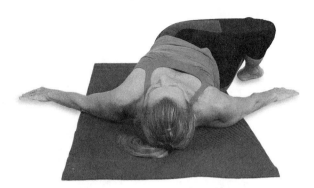

1. Lie on a mat with your knees bent and your feet flat on the floor. While focusing on your breathing, place your left knee on top of your right knee.

2. Slowly allow your left knee to gently fall toward the right side. Stop when you feel tightness. Hold this position for a comfortable moment. The stretch should be felt near the rear pocket area of the left leg. Focus on the stretch, not on how close you can bring your knees to the floor.

Switch sides and repeat.

Diagonal Knee to Chest

Target: torso, gluteus maximus

CAUTION: Avoid this stretch if you have hip problems.

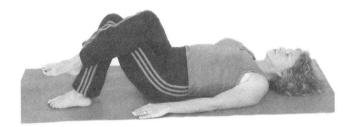 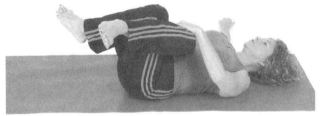

1. Lie on a mat with your knees bent and your feet flat on the floor. Place your right knee on top of your left knee.

2. Draw your knees in toward your chest and pull your right knee toward your left shoulder using your left hand. Hold for a comfortable moment, focusing on the sensation of the stretch, not on how close your knee comes to your shoulder.

Switch sides and repeat.

VARIATION: You can also use a strap to draw in your knees.

Seated Knee to Chest

Target: lower back, gluteus maximus

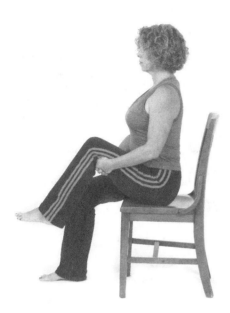
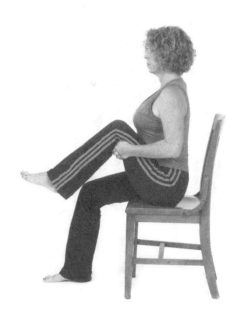

1. Sit with proper posture in a stable chair and place your feet on the floor. Clasp both hands beneath your left leg.

2. Bring your left knee toward your chest. Hold this position for a comfortable moment, feeling the stretch in the gluteal region.

Release the knee, switch sides, and repeat.

Single Knee to Chest

Target: lower back, gluteus maximus

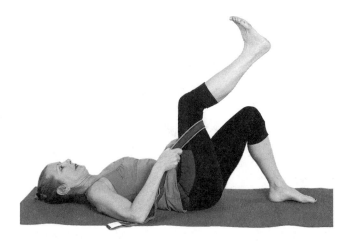

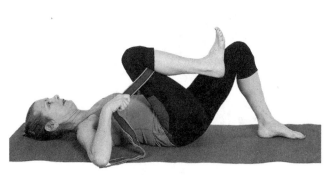

1. Lie on a mat and, if needed, place a pillow under your head. Bend your knees and place both feet flat on the floor. Loop a strap behind the back of your right leg and hold an end of the strap in each hand.

2. Gently pull the straps to bring the knee toward your chest. Hold this stretch for a comfortable moment.

Release the knee, switch sides, and repeat.

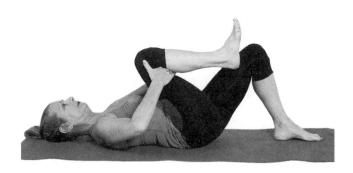

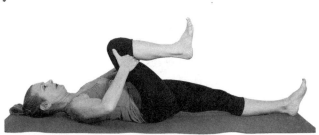

INTERMEDIATE VARIATION: This can also be done using just the hands to bring in the knee.

ADVANCED VARIATION: Extend one leg straight on the floor and bring one knee to your chest.

Double Knee to Chest

Target: lower back, gluteus maximus

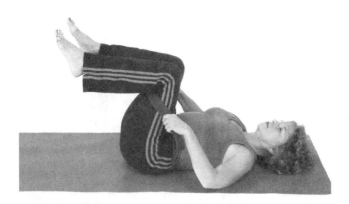

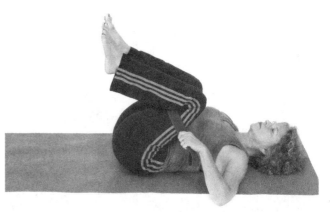

1. Lie on a mat and, if needed, place a pillow under your head. Bend your knees and place both feet flat on the floor.

Loop a strap behind the backs of both legs and hold an end of the strap in each hand.

2. Gently pull the straps to bring your knees to your chest. Hold this position for a comfortable moment, feeling the stretch in your bottom and lower back.

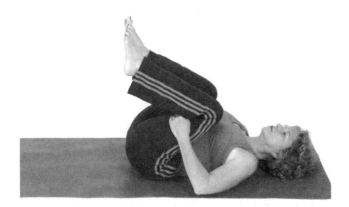

ADVANCED VARIATION: Use just your hands to draw in your knees.

Roll into a Ball

Target: lower back, gluteus maximus, torso

CAUTION: Do not do this stretch if you have knee problems.

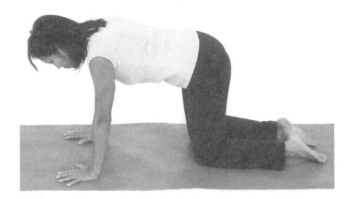

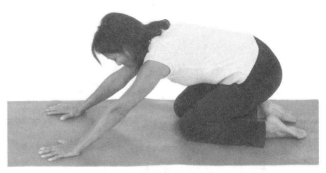

1. Place your hands and knees on the floor. Inhale through your nose.

2. While exhaling deeply through your mouth, slowly allow your bottom to drop toward your heels. If you feel discomfort, you may place a pillow between your heels and bottom.

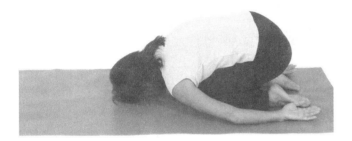

3. Place your forehead on the floor or a pillow, and position your arms alongside your body. Hold this position for a comfortable moment, enjoying the sensation of the stretch up and down your back.

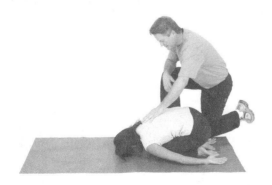

VARIATION: If you can find a friend to rub up and down your back while doing this stretch, it will enhance the stretch.

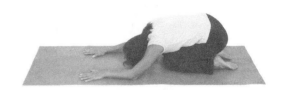

ADVANCED VARIATION: Stretch your arms out straight in front of you.

Piriformis Stretch

The piriformis muscle is a deep-lying muscle in the gluteal region, through which the sciatic nerve passes. When the piriformis is too tight, it can cramp the sciatic nerve, causing the symptoms of sciatica.

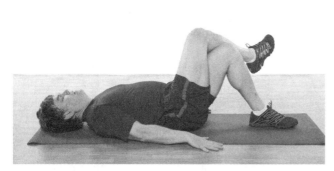

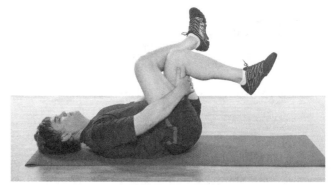

1. Lie on a mat with your knees bent and your feet flat on the floor. Cross your right knee on top of your left knee.

2. Place your hands under your left thigh and pull your knees in toward your chest. Stop when tension occurs. Hold this position for a comfortable moment, focusing on the sensation of the stretch.

Switch sides.

MODIFICATION: Loop a strap around both legs to assist in pulling in your knees.

Rock 'n' Roll

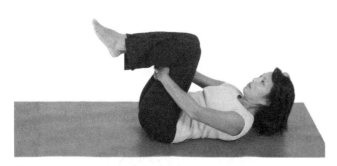

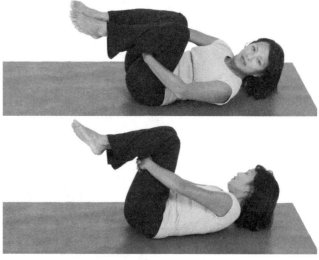

1. Lie on a mat and slowly bring both knees toward your chest. Gently reach around both legs and allow your shoulders to lift off the mat.

2–3. While inhaling deeply through your nose and exhaling through your lips, slowly rock left and right, enjoying the relaxing feeling.

Rock 'n' Roll on Roller

Target: lower back, torso

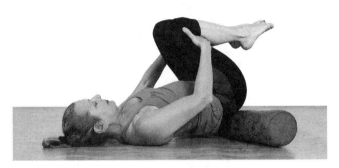
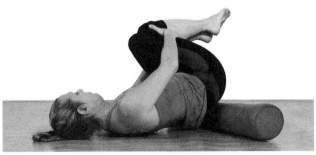
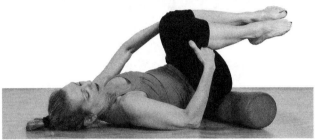

1. Lie on your back and place a foam roller under your tailbone. Slowly bring both knees toward your chest with your hands.

2–3. While inhaling deeply through your nose and exhaling through your lips, slowly rock left and right, enjoying the relaxing feeling.

Ab Stretch

Target: abdominals, lower back, torso

This stretch requires a large stability ball and a medium-sized therapy ball. If you don't have a medium ball, you can use two small therapy balls, firm or hard. Placing both your fists (instead of balls) under your back also works.

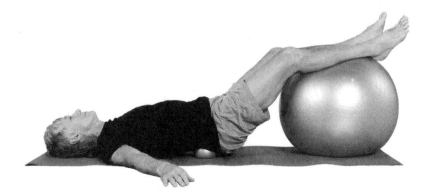

THE POSITION: Lie on your back and place your legs on top of a stability ball. If you can tolerate it, place a medium-sized therapy ball under your lower back. Place your hands anywhere they're comfortable (along your sides, under your head). Breathe and relax, allowing your abdominal area to elongate.

Kneeling Hip Flexor

Target: hip flexors

CAUTION: Avoid this stretch if you have poor balance or bad knees.

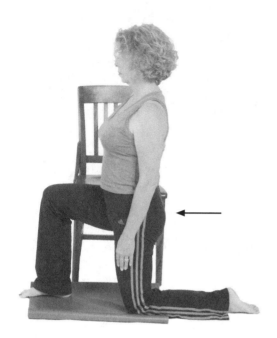

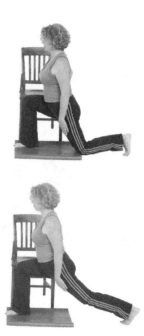

THE POSITION: Kneel on a mat with a chair on your right side. Move your right knee forward so that you can place your right foot flat on the floor. Maintain an erect position by pulling in your chin, squeezing your shoulder blades together, pulling in your belly button, and contracting your gluteals.

Slowly press your hips forward until you feel a comfortable stretch in front of your kneeling leg. Hold this stretch for a comfortable moment.

Switch sides and repeat.

INTERMEDIATE VARIATION (top): Slide your left knee back and press up onto the ball of your foot.

ADVANCED VARIATION (bottom): You can rise onto the ball of your rear foot to lift your knee off the floor and intensify the stretch.

Standing Hip Flexor

Target: hip flexors

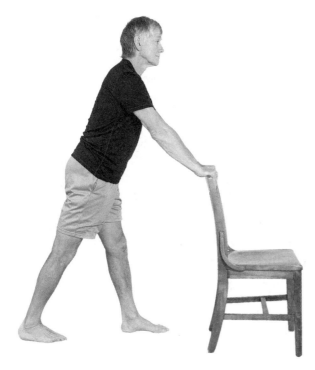

THE POSITION: Stand behind a chair and place your hands on the back of the chair. Slide your right leg back a comfortable distance. Keeping your rear heel down, gently tuck your tailbone under and press your hips forward. Hold this stretch for a comfortable moment, focusing on feeling the stretch in the upper leg/ hip region rather than in the calf area.

Switch sides and repeat.

Supine Hip Flexor

Target: hip flexors

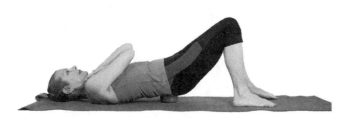
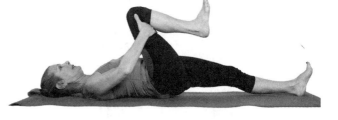

1. Lie on your back with your knees bent and feet flat on the floor. Place a medium-sized therapy ball under your tailbone. Adjust the ball so that you balance comfortably on it.

2. Once you've settled your weight into the ball, inhale and bring your right knee to your chest and clasp your hands beneath your knee. Exhale and straighten your left leg as far as is comfortable along the floor. Hold, breathing slowly and fully, feeling the stretch in your extended leg.

Slowly switch sides.

The Butterfly

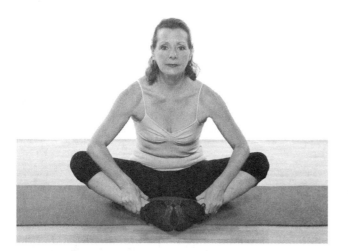 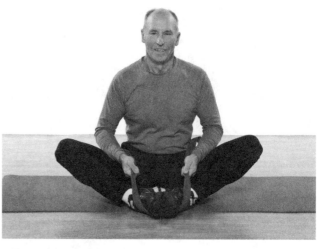

THE STRETCH: Sit on a mat with your knees bent and your feet flat on the floor. Place the soles of your feet together and gently allow your knees to drop to the floor. Place your hands on your ankles and gently pull yourself forward, not down. Hold this stretch for a comfortable moment.

MODIFICATION: Loop a strap around your feet and gently pull yourself forward.

Seated Inner Thigh Stretch

Target: inner thighs

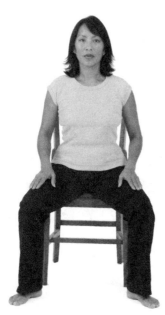 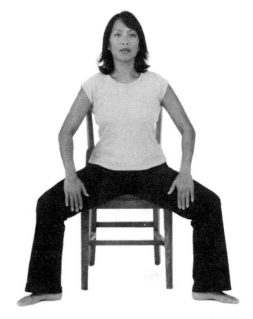

1. Sit at the edge of a stable chair and place both feet flat on the floor. Spread your legs apart and point your knees and toes 45 degrees out to the sides.

2. Place your hands on the insides of your thighs and gently push your legs a little wider. Hold this stretch for a comfortable moment.

Repeat as desired.

Inner Thigh Stretch

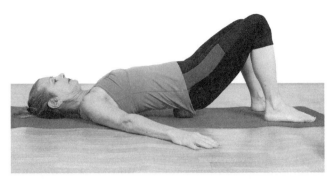

1. Lie on your back with your knees bent and feet flat on the floor. Place a medium-sized therapy ball under your tailbone. Adjust the ball so that you balance comfortably on it.

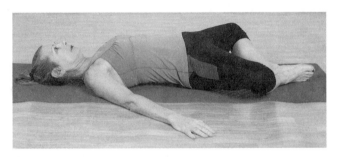

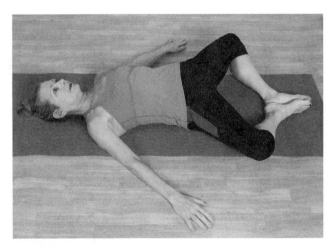

2. Once you've settled your weight into the ball, exhale, and slowly let your knees drop open to the sides. Hold, breathing slowly and fully, feeling the stretch in your inner thighs.

Inner Thigh Massage

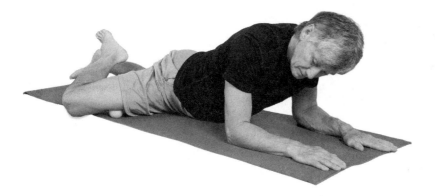

1. Resting on your forearms, lie face-down with both legs extended. Bend your right leg and take your knee to the right side, opening up your hip. Place one or two firm small balls (in a sock) under the inside of your right thigh.

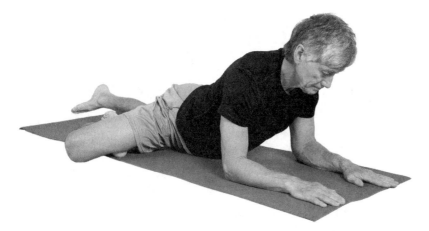

2. Gently roll the ball(s) around under your thigh, controlling the pressure by shifting your weight. Breathe slowly and fully.

Switch sides.

Sit & Reach

Be careful not to tip the chair over.

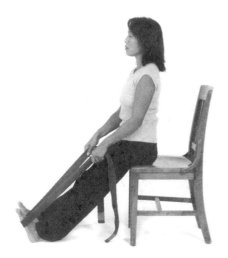

1. Sit at the edge of a stable chair. Loop a strap around the ball of your left foot and hold an end of the strap in each hand. Extend your legs straight out in front of you and place your heels on the floor with your toes pointing up 90 degrees.

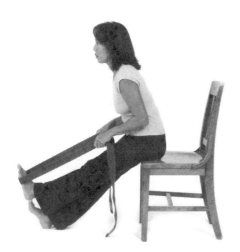

3. Now exhale through your lips and gently pull yourself forward by leading with your chest rather than rounding your back.

Switch sides and repeat.

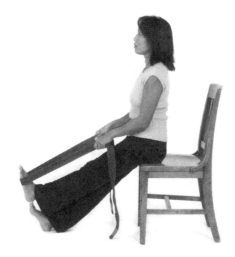

2. Stack your left heel on top of your right foot, keeping your legs as straight as possible. Inhale deeply through your nose.

INTERMEDIATE VARIATION: Instead of using the strap, you can extend your arms forward and gently reach forward with your fingertips.

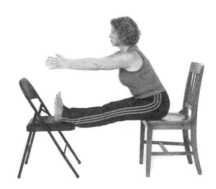

ADVANCED VARIATION: Place both heels on a chair in front of you.

Bent-Over Toe Touch

CAUTION: Stop if you notice undue compression in your knee or experience any lower back discomfort. If you feel a cramp coming on, do a hamstring stretch.

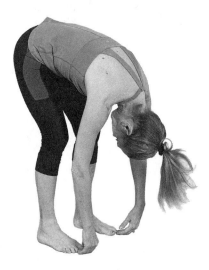 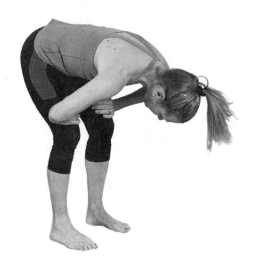

1. Stand upright in proper posture with a slight bend in the knees. Slowly bend over from the waist with knees slightly bent and attempt to touch your toes.

2. Stop when you feel tension in the hamstring muscles; place both hands on your thighs to take the load off your lower back. Hold 30 seconds to 1 minute.

Return to upright posture by slowly rounding your back.

MODIFICATION: If you have balance issues, place hands on a chair for support.

ADVANCED VARIATION: Cross your right leg over your left leg and perform the stretch, then try with your left leg over your right.

V Stretch

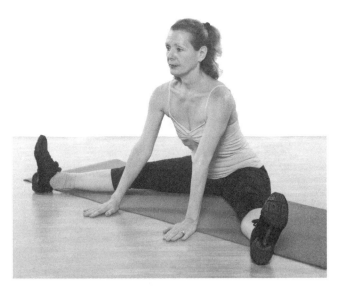

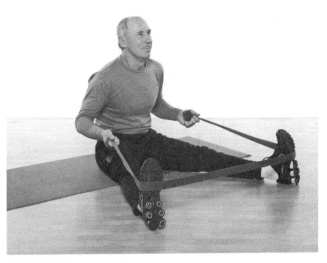

THE STRETCH: Sit on a mat with both legs extended into a "V" position and place both hands on the floor in front of you. Keep your head and torso tall, taking care not to round your back. Inhale and then exhale, allowing your weight to fall forward until you feel a comfortable stretch in the hamstrings and inner thighs. Hold this stretch for a comfortable moment, focusing on the sensation of the stretch, not on going as far as possible.

MODIFICATION: If you have trouble sitting up tall, try looping a strap around both feet.

Straight-Leg Stretch

Target: hamstrings, lower back

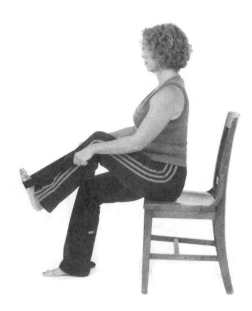

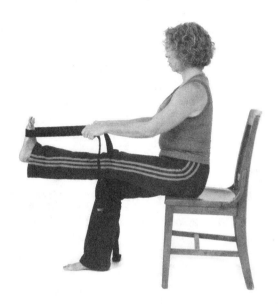

1. Sit at the edge of a stable chair and place both feet flat on the floor. Position a strap around the sole of the left foot and hold an end of the strap in each hand.

2. Inhale deeply through your nose and straighten your left leg. Now exhale through your lips and attempt to straighten your left leg as far as is comfortable. Hold this position for a comfortable moment.

Switch sides and repeat.

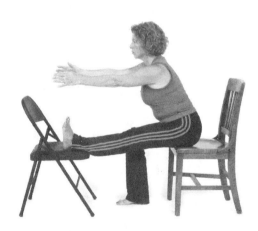

ADVANCED VARIATION: Place one heel on a chair in front of you.

Inverted Figure 4

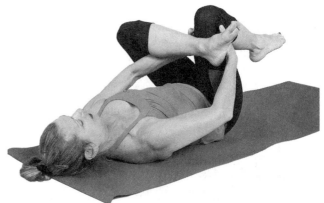

Target: hamstrings

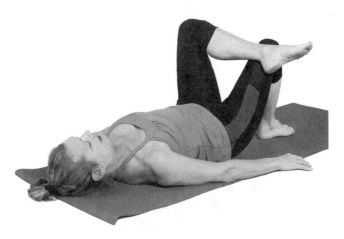

1. Lie on a mat with your knees bent and your feet flat on the floor. Place your left ankle on top of your right knee. Inhale deeply through your nose.

2. Wrap both hands around your right leg and bring your knee and ankle to your chest while exhaling.

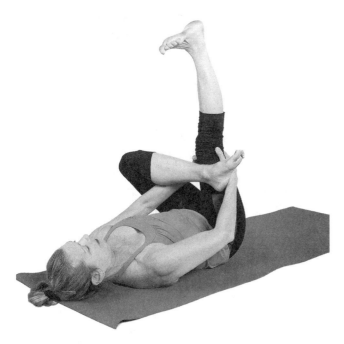

3. Now straighten your right leg toward the ceiling as much as is comfortable. Focus on inhaling and exhaling fully and hold this stretch for a comfortable moment.

Switch sides and repeat.

Figure 4

CAUTION: Avoid this move if you have knee problems.

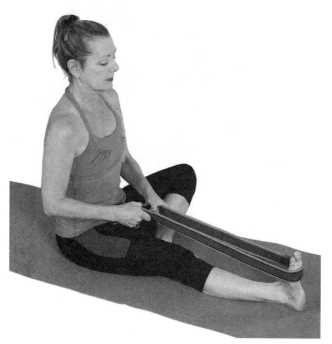 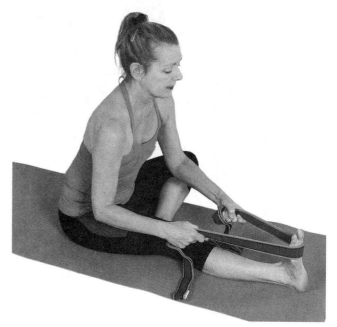

1. Sit on a mat with both legs extended straight out in front of you. Keep your torso as tall as possible. Place your left foot against your right knee. Loop a strap around the sole of your right foot and hold on to the ends of the strap. Inhale deeply through your nose.

2. While keeping your head and torso tall, exhale and pull yourself forward until you feel a comfortable stretch in the backs of your legs. Hold this stretch for a comfortable moment, focusing on the sensation of the stretch, not on going as far as possible. The goal is to hold the stretch for 60 seconds. Exhale through your lips and return to the starting position.

Switch sides and repeat.

Hamstring/Hip Release

Target: hamstrings, lower back, hips

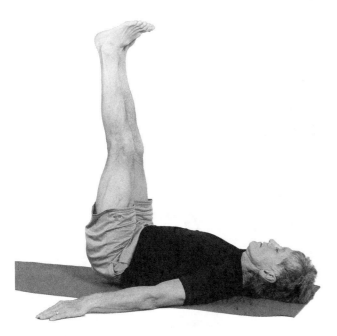

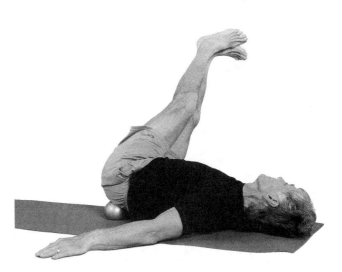

1. Lie on your back with your knees bent and feet flat on the floor. Place a medium-sized therapy ball under your tailbone. Adjust the ball so that you balance comfortably on it. Inhale and bring your knees to your chest and then exhale and extend your legs up to the ceiling, as if sliding your legs up an imaginary wall.

2. Keeping your legs together, gently shift your weight to your right hip. Hold, feeling the stretch in your hip.

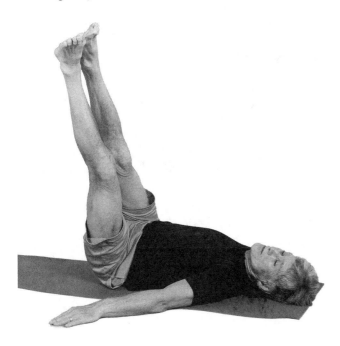

3. Gently shift your weight to your left hip and hold. Repeat as necessary.

Hamstring Massage

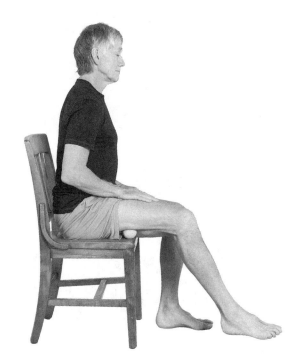

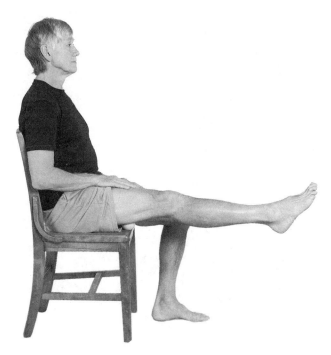

THE POSITION: Sit upright in a chair and place one or two firm balls (in a sock) under the back of one leg. Roll the ball(s) around under your thigh, from above your knee to under your buttock, controlling the pressure by shifting your weight. Use your intuition to guide you on how hard to press and where and how long to roll. Breathe slowly and fully.

Switch sides.

VARIATION: If rolling the ball is too painful, try slowly extending the leg, staying mindful of the pressure.

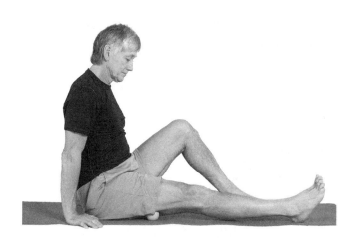

FLOOR VARIATION: Sit on the floor with one or both legs extended. To make rolling easier, support yourself with your hands or with a bent leg to lift your bottom off the floor.

Double-Leg Stretch

Target: hamstrings, lower back

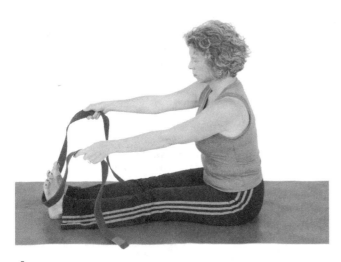

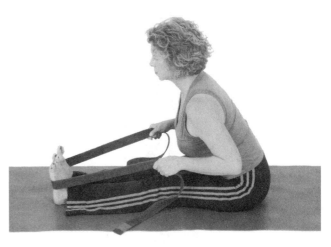

1. Sit on a mat with both legs straight out in front of you and your toes pointing up. Loop a strap around your feet and hold an end of the strap in each hand.

2. Gently pull yourself forward, keeping your back straight while you reach as far forward as is comfortable. Hold for as long as is comfortable, feeling the stretch in your lower back and the backs of your legs. Focus on keeping the legs straight.

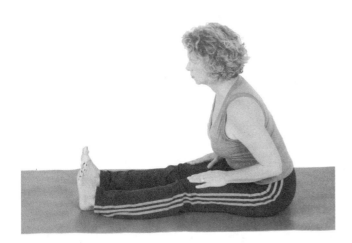

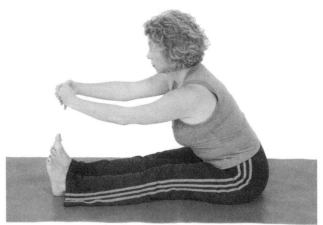

VARIATION: If you don't have a strap, you can gently press your thighs to the floor, your palms down on your thighs. If you have a partner, have him/her gently push you forward.

ADVANCED VARIATION: Interlace your fingers and reach forward, keeping your arms parallel to the floor.

Quad Stretch

CAUTION: Avoid this exercise if you have poor balance. STOP if you notice undue compression in your knee or experience any lower back discomfort. If you feel a cramp coming on, do a hamstring stretch.

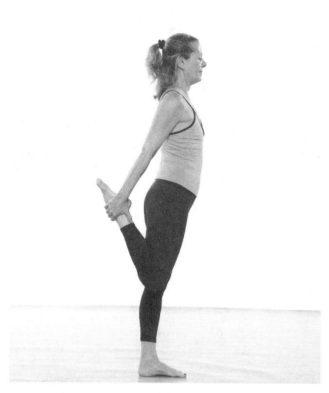 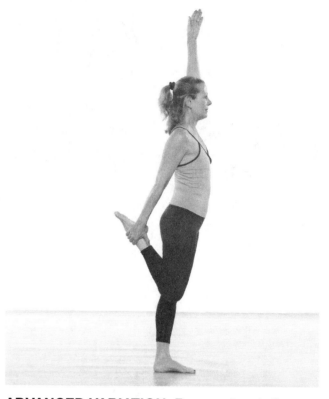

THE STRETCH: Stand with proper posture. Bring your right heel toward your bottom and hold your ankle with your right hand. Keep both knees as close together as possible. Gently pull your heel closer to your bottom. Hold this stretch for a comfortable moment.

Switch sides.

ADVANCED VARIATION: For an extra challenge, raise your free arm toward the ceiling.

Standing Quad Stretch

Target: quadriceps

CAUTION: Avoid this exercise if you have poor balance. Stop if you notice undue compression in your knee or experience any lower back discomfort. If you feel a cramp coming on, stretch your hamstrings.

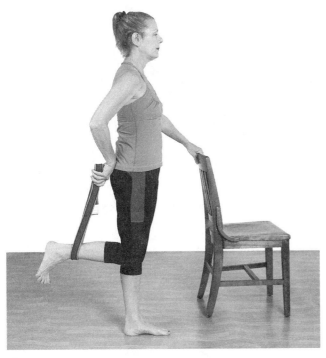 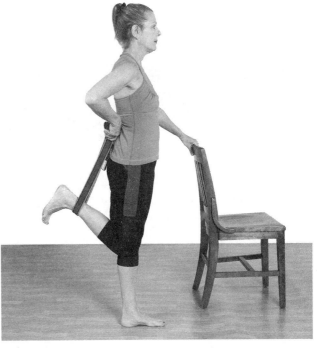

1. Stand with proper posture facing a chair. Loop a strap around your right ankle and bring your right heel toward your bottom. Keep both knees as close together as possible.

2. Gently pull your heel closer to your bottom, using the back of a chair for balance if necessary. Hold this stretch for a comfortable moment.

Switch sides and repeat.

INTERMEDIATE VARIATION: Try this without the strap by grabbing your foot with your hand.

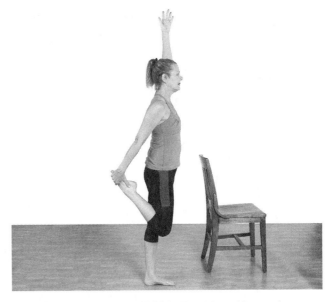

ADVANCED VARIATION: Try this without the strap and the chair, raising your free arm toward the ceiling.

Side Quad Stretch

CAUTION: Stop if you notice undue compression in your knee or experience any lower back discomfort. If you feel a cramp coming on, stretch your hamstrings.

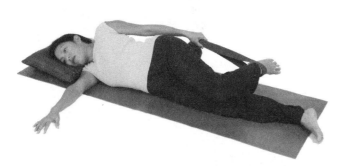

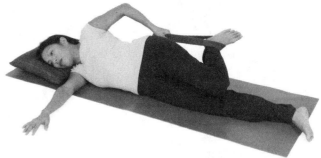

1. Lie on the right side of your body on a mat. Keep your body in proper alignment: your left hip should be stacked on top of your right hip, your left knee on top of your right, your left shoulder on top of your right. Extend your bottom arm for balance. Loop a strap around your left ankle.

2. Gently bring the foot back, pulling your heel toward your bottom. Hold this stretch for a comfortable moment.

Switch sides and repeat.

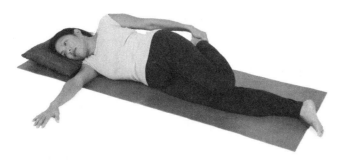

ADVANCED VARIATION: You can try this without the strap by grasping the top of your foot.

Prone Quad Stretch

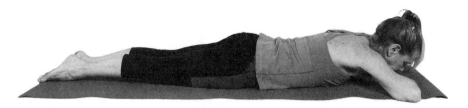

1. Lie face-down on the mat with your legs straight.

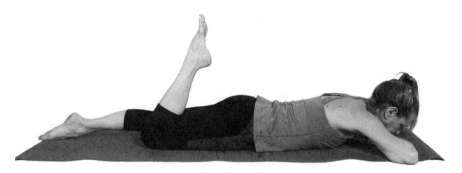

2. Bend your right leg toward your bottom and hold. If you feel a cramp coming on, stretch your hamstrings.

Switch sides and repeat.

Kneeling Quad Stretch

Target: quadriceps

CAUTION: Avoid this move if you have knee problems. You may want to kneel on a pad or mat to protect your knees.

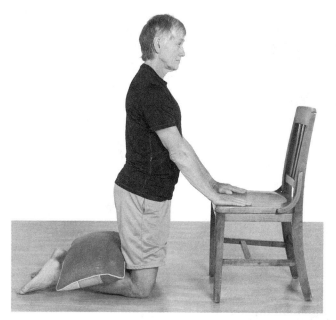 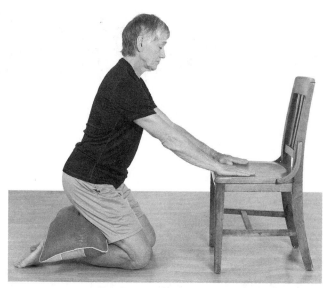

1. Kneel in front of a chair. Place a pillow between your heels and your bottom, and place your hands on the chair.

2. Keeping both hands on the chair, slowly allow your bottom to drop toward your heels. Stop when you feel tension. Hold this stretch for a comfortable moment.

VARIATION: To increase the intensity of the stretch, use a flatter pillow, or eliminate the pillow altogether.

Quad Massage

CAUTION: Avoid arching your lower back too much.

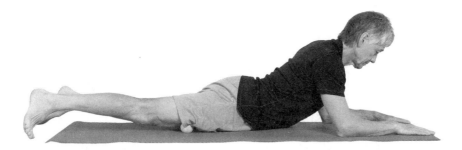

1. Lie face-down with your arms placed in a comfortable position to provide support. Place one or two small, firm balls (in a sock) under your thigh and just above your kneecap.

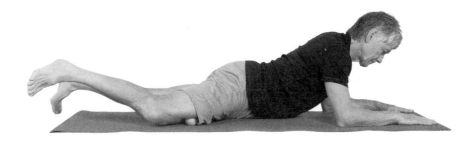

2. Roll the ball(s) around under your thigh, controlling the pressure by shifting your weight. Use your intuition to guide you on how hard to press and where/how long to roll. Breathe slowly and fully.

Switch sides and repeat.

Pretzel

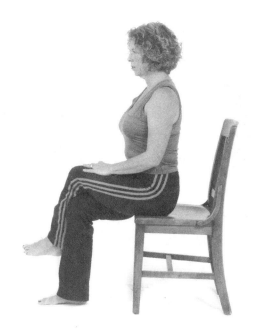

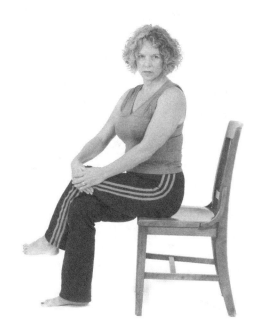

1. Sit at the edge of a stable chair. Cross your left knee over your right.

2. Reach both hands around the top of your left knee. Gently twist to the left while pulling the knee toward the midline of your body. Hold this stretch for a comfortable moment.

Switch sides and repeat.

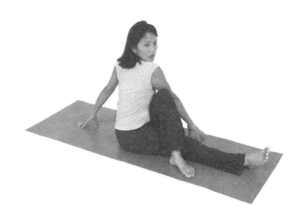

ADVANCED VARIATION: This exercise can also be done sitting on the floor with your legs straight out in front of you. Bend your left knee and place your left foot on the outside of your right leg, as close to the right knee as possible. Then gently twist to the left as you look right.

Outer Thigh Stretch

CAUTION: If you've been advised by your doctor or therapist not to cross your legs, do not do this exercise.

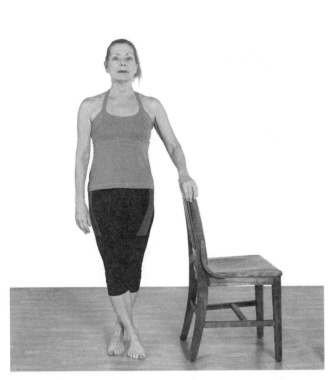

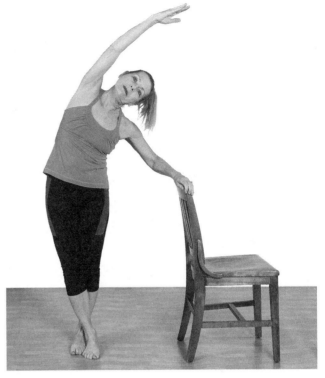

1. Stand with proper posture next to a chair on your left side. Cross your right leg in front of your left leg.

2. Raise your right arm up overhead and lean to the left, gently pressing your right hip outward to the right. Use the chair for balance. Hold this stretch for a comfortable moment.

Switch sides and repeat.

VARIATION: If your shoulders are tight, just place your hand on your hips.

ADVANCED VARIATION: If balance is not an issue, try this without the chair.

Thigh Twist

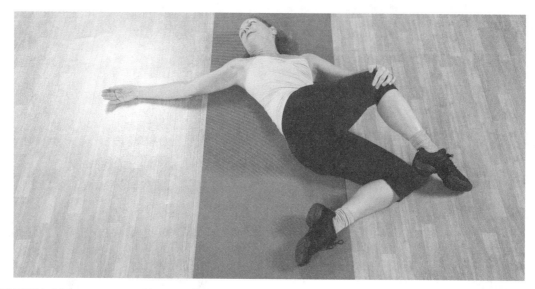

THE STRETCH: Lie on a mat with both legs straight. Using your left hand, gently bring your right knee across your center and toward your left side. Hold for a comfortable moment, focusing on the sensation of the stretch, not on how close your knee comes to the ground.

Switch sides.

Rear Calf Stretch

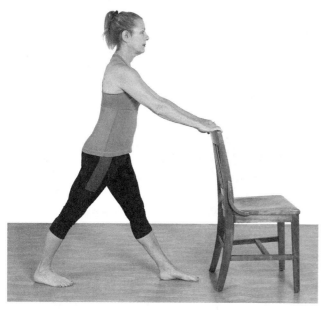 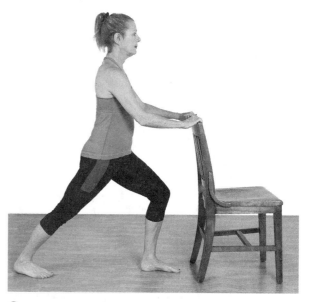

1. Stand behind a chair, placing both hands on the back of the chair. Keeping the heel down, slide your right leg as far back as you can.

2. Bend your left knee until the desired stretch is felt in the calf area. Hold this stretch for a comfortable moment.

Switch sides and repeat.

Rear Calf Stretch with Strap

Target: calves

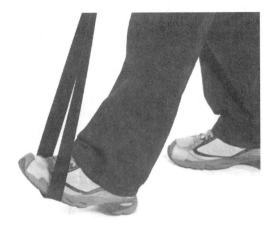 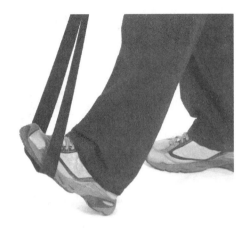

1. Stand with proper posture, holding a strap in your left hand. Step your left foot forward and loop the strap around the ball of the foot.

2. Keeping your heel on the floor, gently pull your toes up until you feel the desired stretch in your calf. Hold for a comfortable moment.

Switch sides and repeat.

Drop-Off Stretch

Target: calves

CAUTION: Only do this exercise if you're fairly flexible. Do not force anything, do not do this move if you have a history of Achilles' heel injury, and do not do this stretch if you're unsure of your balance.

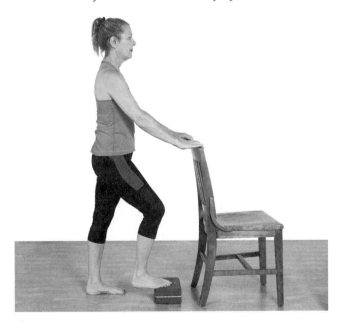 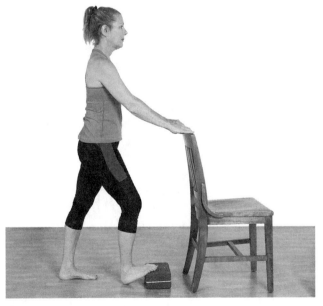

1. Stand behind a chair, using the back for support. Place your right foot on a block.

2. Gently and slowly lower your right heel toward the floor until you feel the desired stretch in your calf area. Hold this stretch for a comfortable moment, using the chair for balance if necessary.

Switch sides and repeat.

Gas Pedals

Target: ankles, calves

CAUTION: Do not force your toes in either direction. Be aware that your calf may cramp when extending your toes. Be careful not to tip the chair over.

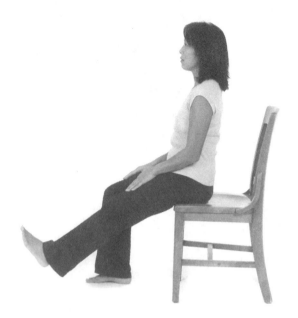

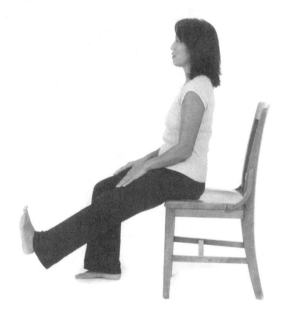

1. Sit at the edge of a stable chair. Extend your left leg straight out in front of you and lift it off the ground.

2. Point your toes up and hold for several seconds.

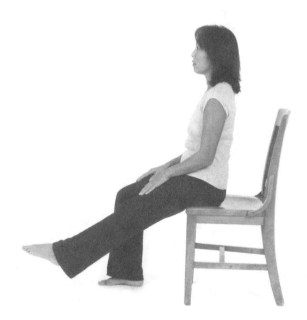

3. Extend your toes away from you and hold for several seconds.

Repeat a comfortable number of times then switch sides.

RESISTANCE BAND VARIATION: Wrap a resistance band around the ball of your foot once to keep it in place. Then perform the exercise.

Heel Raise/Heel Drop

Target: ankles

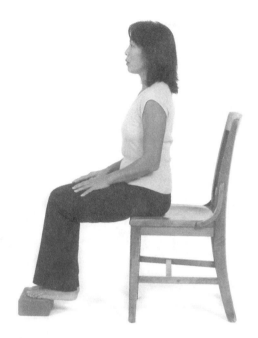

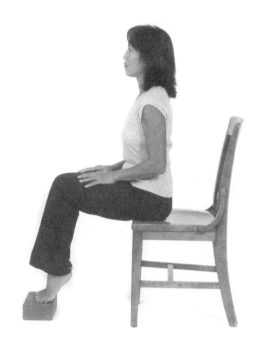

1. Sit at the edge of a stable chair and place a block under the balls of your feet.

2. Keeping the balls of your feet on the block, raise your heels and hold the stretch for several seconds.

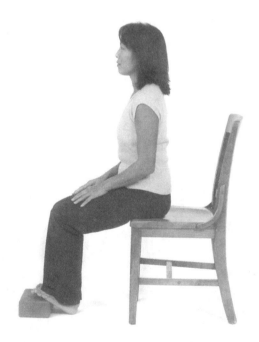

3. Drop your heels toward the floor and hold the stretch for several seconds.

Repeat a comfortable number of times.

Ankle Circles

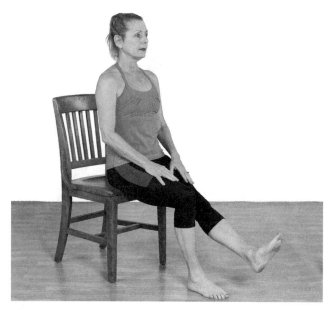 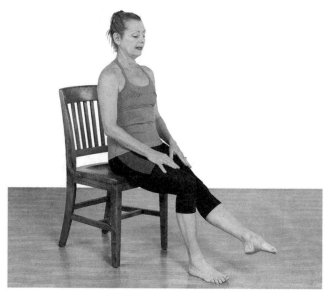

1. Sit at the edge of a stable chair. Extend your left leg straight out in front of you and lift it off the ground.

2. Keeping your leg stationary (using your hands for support, if necessary), point your toes and draw several circles with your foot in both directions.

Switch sides and repeat.

ANKLE WRITING VARIATION: Point your toes and write your address and phone number with your foot. Switch sides and repeat.

Self ROM

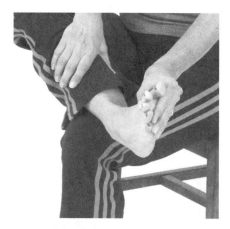 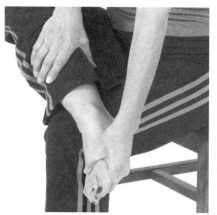 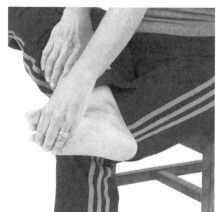

THE POSITION: Sit at the edge of a stable chair. Cross your right ankle on top of your left knee and gently grasp your right foot with your left hand. Slowly use your hand to move your foot gently in comfortable circles as well as forward and backward.

Switch sides and repeat.

Ankle Roller

If you do not have a rolling pin, you can also use a frozen orange juice container (good for icing sore feet) or a can of soup.

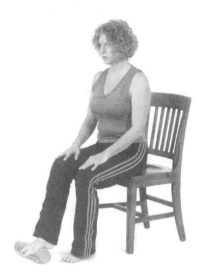 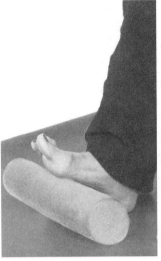 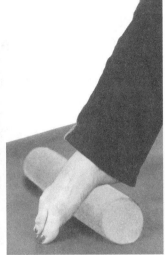

1. Sit at the edge of a stable chair and place both feet on the floor, directly below your knees. Place a rolling pin under the arch of your right foot.

2. Slowly move your foot back and forth over the roller.

Switch sides and repeat.

Foot Massage

This can be done while standing or sitting. If you have balance issues, standing by a wall or sitting are recommended.

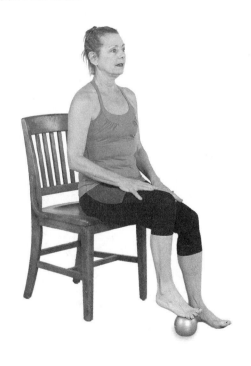

THE POSITION: Sit at the edge of a stable chair. Place a small, firm ball under the ball of your foot. Roll the ball around under your entire foot and along the sides. Use your intuition to guide you on how hard to press and where/how long to roll. Breathe slowly and fully.

Switch sides.

Mad Cat Stretch

Target: lower back flexibility

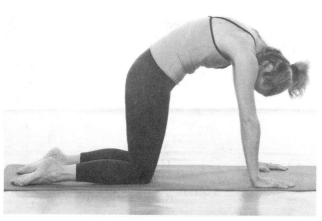 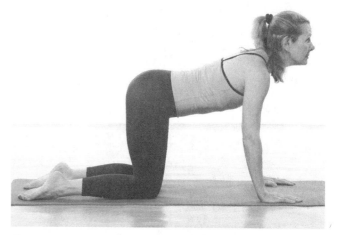

1. Assume the tabletop position. Draw your belly button in, causing your back to round. Inhale deeply.

2. Now exhale and slowly relax your body to the starting position.

Repeat as desired.

Long Body Stretch

Target: total body

For this stretch, try listening to some relaxing music.

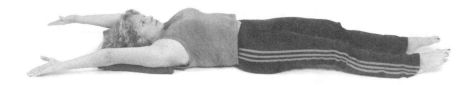

THE POSITION: Lie on a mat, with your head on a pillow if needed. Focus on breathing slowly in and out through your nose. Reach your arms as far back as is comfortable. Lengthen your legs as far as is possible. Try to make your body as long as possible while breathing in a comfortable fashion. Remember to focus on your breath.

PART 2

CORE STRENGTH

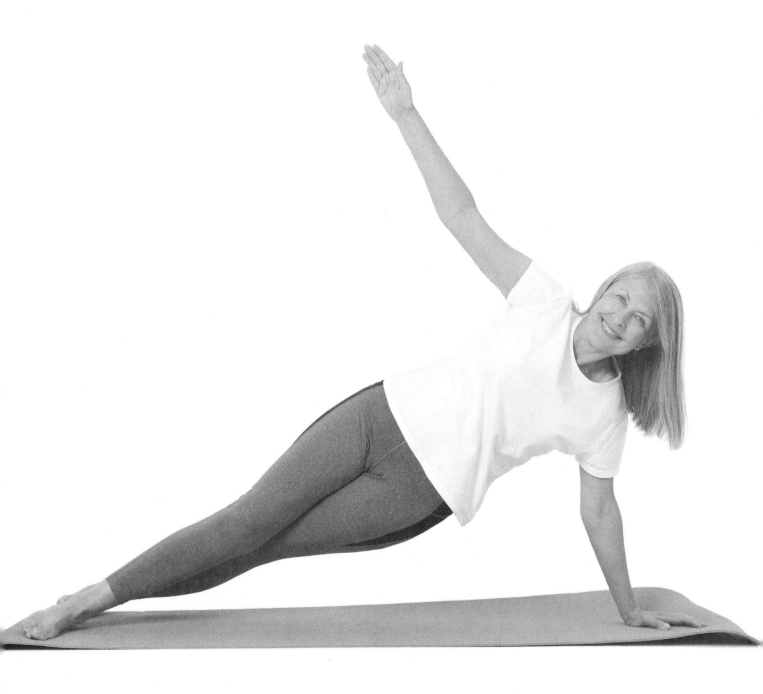

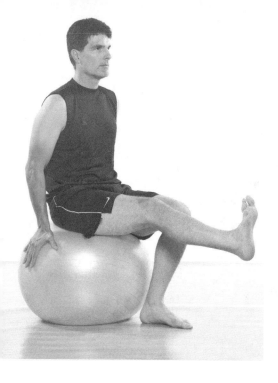

THE IMPORTANCE OF CORE STRENGTH

The "core" is the powerhouse of the body. When the concept of "core strength" training was first introduced, the core was considered to be only the abdominal region and the lower back area. Nowadays, some experts consider the core to be the region from the tops of the legs to the shoulder area. With its roots in back rehabilitation, core training was later thought to be useful in sports performance. Today, core training needs to be a part of everyday exercise programs.

Having an aligned and strong yet flexible core can take the load off the vertebral column and discs, which results in improved function and less discomfort and pain. It'll also assist you in activities of daily living, help improve posture, and maybe even boost appearance and foster athletic performance.

Consider a tower of blocks: If the blocks aren't lined up properly and a load is placed on top of it, the middle portion often buckles and collapses. This is also what happens when we don't have a solid core. Some experts maintain that true core strength is the interaction of the total body. It's about improving functional fitness and reducing the strain on the spinal region. Core strengthening goes far beyond just having a flat stomach and six-pack abs.

This program is very different from other core-training programs because it focuses on providing comprehensive, total-body core-strengthening options. The exercises described in this book are based on the most recent scientific knowledge of how the spine responds to corrective exercise. Any exercise that doesn't have both superior benefits and minimal risks was not included. Additionally, some traditional core exercises were transformed a bit to accommodate balance and joint issues often seen in the 50-plus person. By incorporating the core-strengthening program in this book, you're well on your way to enhancing your spine's stability and reeducating correct muscle-activation patterns.

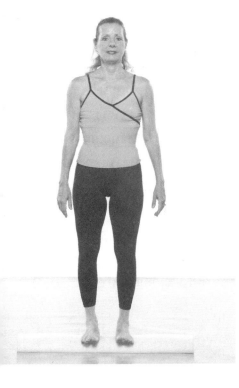

WHAT IS CORE STRENGTH?

Fitness fads come and go, but core-strength training is not a passing trend. "Core strength" is *not* achieved by just doing a bunch of sit-ups; in addition, using heavy resistance is counterproductive. Rather, core strength is an integrated approach of systematic conditioning and correcting of muscular imbalances.

Too often people exercise their abdominals (or "abs") for aesthetic reasons, but correct core strength is gained through proper activation of specific muscles in a coordinated fashion. Proper core training teaches you to engage and protect your back even when you're not thinking about your core. You'll know you've mastered core training if you automatically engage your core muscles when you open a door, swing a golf club, get up from sitting, or lift something.

The roots of core training stem from sound back rehabilitation. The average fitness follower or anyone who has ever had a bad back is familiar with the terms "core stability" and "core training." Core training is also known as "dynamic lumbar stabilization."

Core training became very common in the early 1980s and received acclaim when used by San Francisco 49er quarterback Joe Montana. It remains a pillar of exercise programs to this day. The belief was that stabilization of the lumbar region would guard your lower back by using your own body to build your own lumbar support. Patients were taught how to find the most balanced, pain-free position while in a static position and then progress to being able to locate that position in a variety of dynamic movements. This approach was so successful with clients who had intervertebral disc problems as well as facet joint involvement and other muscular imbalance issues that it was incorporated into fitness and sports conditioning routines for the young and old.

CORE STRENGTH VS. CORE STABILIZATION

Core training goes by many names, such as core stabilization and core strengthening, to name the most common ones. They all generally agree that the abdominal and lower back muscles must have the right amount of strength, endurance, and flexibility, as well as the muscle memory of knowing automatically when and how to engage and relax the core set of muscles. However, people often overlook the muscular balance that's required for a strong core, and only do sit-ups and back extensions without addressing all the subtle changes of posture and deep-lying muscles. This may lead to physical problems down the line. When strengthening your core, be sure to train both the superficial and deep-lying muscles in the front, back, and sides of the body. Your body needs a combination of muscular endurance to handle prolonged sitting and standing, and enough strength in that region to keep your posture long and tall.

EQUIPMENT

The beauty of core training is that it requires no equipment. If you don't have the space for a ball, don't buy one. If you don't feel safe on a roller, don't use it. Balance balls, foam rollers, and other tools can all be used to challenge the system, but they're not necessary to strengthen the core. In fact, if they're not used properly, they'll only contribute to muscle imbalances. Too often people rush to use a piece of equipment before they're ready. In core-strength training, perfect technique is vital.

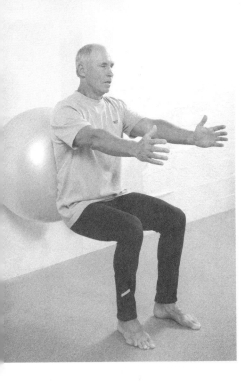

WHERE IS THE CORE?

The "core" of anything is the central foundation of the structure, whether it's the core of an apple or the core of a nuclear reactor. Although no one universal definition of "core" exists, most people refer to the abdominal wall muscles in the front of the body and the muscles of the back that run up and down the spine as the core of the human body. Sometimes the gluteal region gets included.

The core is a complicated arrangement of bones, nerves, ligaments, tendons, and supporting muscle configurations. Understanding the locations and roles of the muscles that comprise the core will motivate you to keep participating in a core-strengthening routine day in and day out.

The core team is made up of a pole (the vertebral column) and guide wires (the muscles), and each member of your core team has a specific role. The core muscle group includes the transverse abdominis, internal and external obliques, rectus abdominis, and erector spinae.

The *transverse abdominis* is the deepest-lying layer of fibers of the abdominal wall. The transverse abdominis provides compression to the internal organs and serves as nature's back brace. Some physical therapists believe that the transverse abdominis is the most important element of core training.

The *internal and external obliques* are the muscles on the sides of the body. They're engaged when you twist to reach and grab something.

The *rectus abdominis* is the muscle that flexes the vertebral column. We're most familiar with this muscle because it gives us the six pack. It also helps stabilize the pelvis when walking.

The *erector spinae* group is responsible for extending the back. It's made up of three distinct muscles: the iliocostalis, the longissimus, and the spinalis. The erectors add stability to the trunk area and are also the primary muscles that help us stand erect.

When the core muscles are properly trained, they lead to improved posture and back protection.

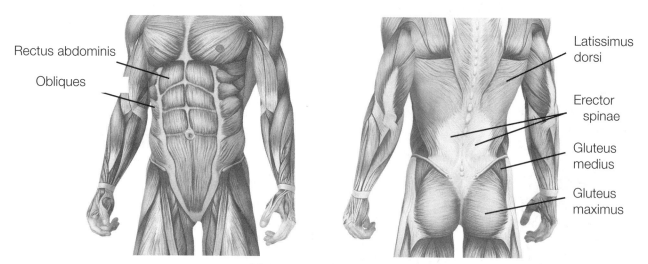

Rectus abdominis

Obliques

Latissimus dorsi

Erector spinae

Gluteus medius

Gluteus maximus

Major Muscles of the Core

Current research also suggests that the diaphragm assists spinal stability via a hydraulic consequence on the abdominal hollow space by increasing intra-abdominal pressure, often seen in weightlifters who bear down when doing a heavy lift. For years the transverse abdominis was considered the key component for spinal stabilization training. However, today it's understood that the "deep core" muscles and the diaphragm need to work in a coordinated manner to provide an ideal platform from which the more superficial muscles can operate.

Author Karl Knopf makes some adjustments

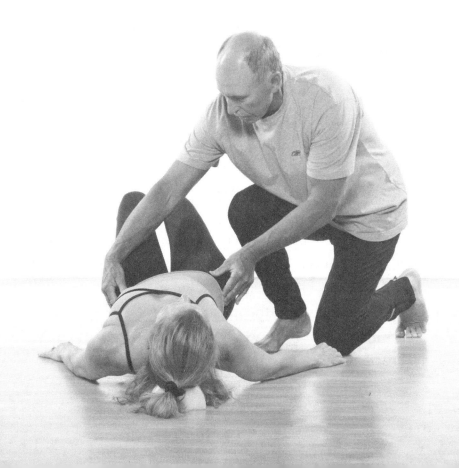

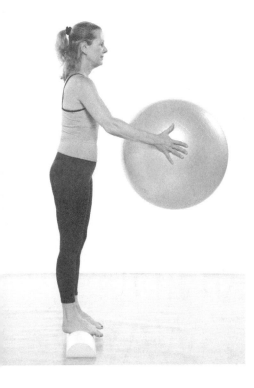

BENEFITS OF A STRONG CORE

Much like replacing the plumbing under your house, core strengthening is often not visible. No one will ever see what you've done but if it's not working, things can really become a mess. Being fit doesn't necessarily translate into being highly aware of your core muscles. Oftentimes, a fit, athletic person can more easily substitute other muscles to perform the functions associated with the core.

The benefits of having a strong core include improved posture, which allows you to present a more youthful appearance, and balance. It also means less load on the lumbar region of your lower back, reducing the risk of injury to any arthritic joints and discs in addition to pain. Performance in sports and recreational pursuits is also boosted.

CORE STRENGTH AND BACK PAIN PREVENTION

Having a solid core is like keeping a radio tower upright. A radio tower is installed with guide wires to keep the tower straight and tall. If one set of wires is lax and another set is too tight, the tower becomes misaligned. The same applies to the back, with the spine being the radio tower and the muscles of the body being the guide wires. If one set of muscles is too tight from overuse and the others too lax from lack of use, the spine becomes unstable and is at high risk for injury. Muscle imbalances, along with poor body mechanics and age, are believed to be a factor in lower back issues.

Keep in mind that "back pain" is a very generic term and can range in severity from simple over-exertion to a herniated disc to something very serious (e.g., pain referred from a major organ). That's why a medical doctor should evaluate persistent, unrelenting lower back pain. That said, certain kinds of back pain can be prevented or reversed by proper core strengthening. A comprehensive core-strength program can be thought of as building your own back brace to protect your spine, along with learning proper biomechanics and maintaining flexibility to avoid muscle spasms.

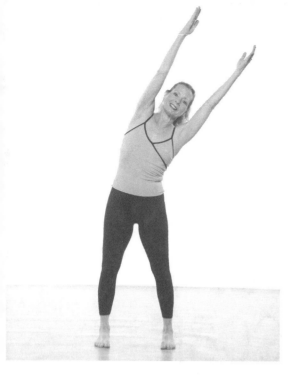

CORE TRAINING THE RIGHT WAY

Core strengthening is all about improving functional fitness and reducing the strain on the spinal region. A well-designed core-strength program requires a delicate balance of core strength, core muscle endurance, proper body mechanics, and flexibility of the surrounding muscles (such as the hamstrings, quadriceps, iliopsoas, and the iliotibial band) that often contribute to lower back imbalances.

Complete core-strength training requires a balanced multiplanar approach that includes a combination of isometric and dynamic exercises. While many of the exercises in this book look simple, it's critical that you master the subtleties of the movements through concentration and practice them until they become automatic before moving on to the next level.

Proper core stabilization has four basic stages:

Stage 1   Learn to contract deep-lying muscles.

Stage 2   Focus on endurance of the deep-lying muscles.

Stage 3   Challenge the core with arm movements once stabilization can be maintained.

Stage 4   Continue challenging the core.

The beauty of a core-strength program is that it can be used as both a preventative and rehabilitative back-care wellness tool. The desired outcomes of a good core-strength program are:

• A solid core that will protect the lower back, reduce back injuries, and foster better lower back health

• Improved sports performance

• A better interdependence between the muscles on the front of the body and the back of the body, which will reduce fatigue and improve posture

To achieve these aspects, you can progress to performing the exercises in a supported position, such as supine, prone, kneeling, and standing, before finally incorporating dynamic movement. To truly improve core strength, meticulous body awareness is needed. Talking or listening to music while doing these exercises can detract from learning core stabilization, so no distractions are recommended. Core training requires total mind-body interaction. Just pounding out sit-ups to the latest tunes is not what core-strength training is all about.

10 CORE-TRAINING TIPS

Here are 10 tips that will help you make the most of your core-training workout.

1. Core training can and should be done daily. If you're pressed for time, exercise the front side of your body one day and then exercise the posterior side of your body the next day.

2. Concentration and practice and then more concentration and more practice are the axiom of core training.

3. Train, don't make pain. Follow the two-hour rule: If you hurt more than two hours post-exercise, reevaluate your exercise program and back off.

4. Better results occur when you cross-train—in addition to core training, include a regular walking program with comfortable shoes or participate in a water-exercise program.

5. Avoid doing core exercises first thing in the morning. It's believed that intervertebral fluid pressure in the spinal region is higher in the morning and can cause problems.

6. Focus on core muscle endurance rather than aiming to make the muscles overly strong.

7. Sad but true, there's no ideal set of exercises for everyone. Your exercises need to evolve and adapt according to your functional goals and pain issues. Some people will do core exercises for rehabilitative purposes and others for general fitness and prevention, while others do them to enhance athletic performance. Therefore, use your inner wisdom when selecting and designing a core-strength program.

8. Don't expect quick results. It'll take a long time to learn to perform the exercises correctly and mindfully. The goal of core training is instinctually knowing how to properly engage your core muscles while performing activities of daily living.

9. Practice braced breathing and learn diaphragmatic breathing (see page 142).

10. When performing static exercises, don't hold your breath. If you have any cardiovascular issues, avoid static exercises.

TRAIN SMART!

The keys to correct core-strength training are as follows:

- Concentration and perseverance
- Quality over quantity of movement
- Slow, purposeful progression to more challenging movements
- The ability to perform every action from a neutral spine

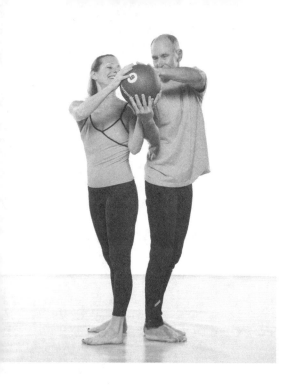

BEFORE YOU BEGIN

Before embarking on a core-training program, first make sure that you're healthy enough to participate. If you have any existing health concerns, always consult with your health professional. Given that you're indeed healthy, make sure you're fit enough to get up and down from the floor. If not, please check out weights and kettlebell sections of this book to help you get stronger.

Core training is usually best done when the body is properly warmed up. Many people participate in this routine at the end of their exercise session or after a warm shower. Pay attention to your body and figure out the best times for it. The key is not to force your body to do things it's not ready for—train, don't strain.

To train safely, please keep these additional simple tips in mind for a core workout:

- Listen to your body: If it hurts more two hours post-exercise than it did before you started, you did too much. Be smart and do less next time. Only YOU know your body best.

- If an exercise hurts, stop and reassess if that exercise is right for you. In addition, please note that not every exercise is right for everyone. What might be a perfect exercise for one person can contribute to further issues for another.

- If you experience numbness, please see a health care professional.

- Research has shown that unstable-surface training results in increased core muscle recruitment. However, do not progress to an unstable surface until you have the requisite balance skills. You can obtain adequate core conditioning without ever doing unstable-surface exercises. Always consider your safety first.

CORE-STRENGTHENING PROGRAMS

CORE-STRENGTHENING BASICS

The key to a well-aligned core is to strengthen that which is weak and lengthen that which is inflexible. This section of *The Strength Training Bible for Seniors* has eight different core-strengthening programs to help you improve your posture, prevent chronic lower back issues, improve performance in recreational pursuits, and have a more youthful stature. Choose from equipment-free programs or those that use a variety of stability-building tools or pick and choose from the exercises in this section and create your own routine.

The programs have more exercises than you're expected to do. Focus on the particular aspects that are relevant to you, then select 5–6 exercises and do them for several weeks. Most people will be fine just doing a daily dose of levels 1 or 2. After that period, select another 5–6 exercises from the same level or the next. It's okay to select exercises from different levels as long as you're able to safely and properly perform them. This method keeps your routine more vibrant and prevents burnout. By inserting new exercises on a regular basis, you also continue to challenge your core. When I teach classes, we never do the same core exercises every single time. Again, core training isn't like weight training, where each exercise works a specific muscle. Core training essentially works the entire core.

Keep in mind that you're encouraged to select those exercises that you enjoy or feel your body requires—this is *your* program. Some readers will need more back stabilization/strengthening exercises while others may need more mobility of the lower back and pelvic area. If you're having a particular concern, you may want to take this book to your health provider and ask them to select the exercises that meet your current health issue.

Every reader should start at the baseline of "beginner." Whether and how quickly you progress to the next level is determined by your particular competence at each level. The progression from one level to the next is very subjective and not at all like progression levels seen in weight training.

Unlike traditional strength training (which is all about numbers of reps), core-strength training blends the concepts of both strength training and endurance training (which focuses on how long you can perform a move before the muscular system fatigues). Perfect form and mindfulness are extremely important. If you can't perform a movement without maintaining stability, you're not performing the exercise correctly and are wasting your time. That said, when it comes to training the core, you can utilize a combination of both reps and/or duration:

Beginner: 10 reps or 30 sec

Intermediate: 15 reps or 45 sec

Advanced: 20 reps or 1 min

Super-Advanced: 30 sec or as many/as long as tolerated

These parameters are just suggestions. Determining whether you use duration or reps is a personal choice. It's always prudent to start with just a few and progress only as you feel confident to do so. As always, listen to your body and enjoy the process of strengthening your core.

The beauty of core-strength training is that it can be done anytime and anywhere with or without equipment. Some people perform core strengthening at the end of their exercise session. This can serve as a cool-down portion of their routine and is an ideal time to also stretch the muscles that influence core alignment. Regardless of when you do your core training, make sure to properly warm up your body for movement.

Everyone should start with the *supine floor exercises*, which focus on the muscles of the anterior side of the body. Master these moves before moving on to the *prone* (face-down), *tabletop* (hands-and-knees), and *plank* exercises. Once the tabletop and plank exercises become easier, you can challenge yourself some more by placing an unstable surface such as a pillow under your hands and/or knees or feet.

Safe positioning is paramount in performing the *foam roller exercises*. It'll take time to get used to maintaining proper alignment and stability on the roller. For this series, you may want to start with a half roller and place the flat side down. As you become more comfortable, flip the roller over and perform the movement with the rounded side down. Once you're proficient at that stage, try a full circular roller, and then progress to resting your feet on a pillow while doing the exercises to challenge yourself even more.

The major focus of the standing roller exercises is to encourage greater static and dynamic core stability. Since these moves require a good level of balance, you may want to place a chair alongside you or work next to a wall. Don't perform these moves if you're not 100 percent confident in your skill level. These are very advanced exercises and are not needed to obtain good core stability.

The *ball exercises* are a fun way to challenge yourself, but make sure you have adequate balance as well as space to perform the exercises. Doing exercises on an unstable surface is an excellent way to engage greater core muscular activation.

The *partner exercises* are for the extremely advanced person. Partner exercises require cooperation and communication between partners. It's not about competition. Partner training when done cooperatively can target specific muscle groups and functional movements. If you choose to do partner exercises, make sure you both understand the movement patterns of the drill and are willing to adjust to each other's level.

Remember, you don't need to do all of the exercises listed in each program during each session if you don't have time. However, if you do an exercise that addresses the muscles on the front of the body, try to follow it with an exercise that addresses the muscles on the back of the body. Additionally, if the program calls for ball or roller moves but you don't own either, it's fine to perform the equipment-free versions.

EQUIPMENT-FREE PROGRAM LEVEL 1

This level focuses on mastering the movements and toning your deeper-lying muscles. It'll meet the basic needs of anyone wishing to add a core-strengthening element to their existing fitness routine.

EQUIPMENT-FREE LEVEL 1

Warm up with some light aerobic exercise or a warm shower for at least 10 minutes before performing core training. Then select 5–6 exercises and do them for 10 reps or 30 seconds.

Supine Foundational Position	page 141	Tabletop Arm Raises	page 170
Supine Leg Extensions	page 143	Tabletop Leg Raises	page 171
Supine Arm Swings	page 144	Clam Shell	page 169
Curl-Ups	page 150	Mad Cat Stretch	page 122
Pelvic Lift	page 156		

Remember to stretch after your workout. Select 3–5 exercises and hold for 30 seconds to 1 minute. See stretching exercises starting on page 57 for suggestions.

EQUIPMENT-FREE PROGRAM LEVEL 2

Level 2 introduces dynamic compound exercises that progressively challenge the core.

EQUIPMENT-FREE LEVEL 2

Warm up with some light aerobic exercise or a warm shower for at least 10 minutes before performing core training. Then select 5–6 exercises and do them for 10 reps or 30 seconds.

Remember to stretch after your workout. Select 3–5 exercises and hold for 30 seconds to 1 minute. See stretching exercises starting on page 57 for suggestions.

EQUIPMENT-FREE PROGRAM LEVEL 3

This advanced program places a more rigorous demand on the core by introducing more complex elements. Most readers won't engage in all the exercises in this section. As with all the exercises in this book, form is critical and duration of how long you perform the movement is the goal.

EQUIPMENT-FREE LEVEL 3

Warm up with some light aerobic exercise or a warm shower for at least 10 minutes before performing core training. Then select 5–6 exercises and do them for 10 reps or 30 seconds.

Remember to stretch after your workout. Select 3–5 exercises and hold for 30 seconds to 1 minute. See stretching exercises starting on page 57 for suggestions.

EQUIPMENT-FREE PROGRAM LEVEL 4

This super-advanced program is designed for the highly motivated. It's extremely challenging and also includes a fun partner move.

EQUIPMENT-FREE LEVEL 4

Warm up with some light aerobic exercise or a warm shower for at least 10 minutes before performing core training. Then select 5–6 exercises and do them for 10 reps or 30 seconds.

Prone Double-Double	page 166	Plank to Side Salutation	page 185
Side Plank	page 168	Plank Clap	page 209

Remember to stretch after your workout. Select 3–5 exercises and hold for 30 seconds to 1 minute. See stretching exercises starting on page 57 for suggestions.

Level 1

This level focuses on mastering the movements and toning your deeper-lying muscles. It'll meet the basic needs of anyone wishing to add a core-strengthening element to their existing fitness routine.

LEVEL 1

Warm up with some light aerobic exercise or a warm shower for at least 10 minutes before performing core training. Then select 5–6 exercises and do them for 10 reps or 30 seconds.

Supine Foundational Position	page 141	Tabletop Arm Raises	page 170
Supine Leg Extensions	page 143	Tabletop Leg Raises	page 171
Supine Arm Swings	page 144	Clam Shell	page 169
Curl-Ups	page 150	Pointer Series	page 183
Pelvic Lift	page 156	Ball Sit	page 190

Remember to stretch after your workout. Select 3–5 exercises and hold for 30 seconds to 1 minute. See stretching exercises starting on page 57 for suggestions.

Level 2

This program introduces dynamic compound exercises that progressively challenge the core. It also uses the foam roller, which you may choose to not use.

LEVEL 2

Warm up with some light aerobic exercise or a warm shower for at least 10 minutes before performing core training. Then select 5–6 exercises and do them for 10 reps or 30 seconds.

Supine Leg Extension/Arm Swing Combo	page 145	Prone Single-Leg Lifts	page 162
Supine Foot Presses	page 148	Tabletop Advanced Combo	page 173
Curl-Ups with a Twist	page 152	Roller Seated Orientation	page 174
Figure-4 Half Sit-Ups	page 154	Roller Stabilization—Arms	page 176
Pelvic Lift with Arm Lifts	page 157	Roller Stabilization—Legs	page 177
Pelvic Lift with Leg Extensions	page 158	Mad Cat Stretch	page 122
Pelvic Lift with Arm Lift/Leg Extensions	page 159	Roller Stabilization Arm/Leg Combo	page 178
Prone Single-Arm Lifts	page 161	Pelvic Lift on Roller	page 180
		Leg Press-Out on Roller	page 181

Remember to stretch after your workout. Select 3–5 exercises and hold for 30 seconds to 1 minute. See stretching exercises starting on page 57 for suggestions.

Level 3

This advanced program places a more rigorous demand on the core by introducing more complex elements, and many of the exercises use a stability ball. Most readers won't engage in all the exercises in this section. As with all the exercises in this book, form is critical and duration of how long you perform the movement is the goal.

LEVEL 3

Warm up with some light aerobic exercise or a warm shower for at least 10 minutes before performing core training. Then select 5–6 exercises and do them for 10 reps or 30 seconds.

Supine Heel Slides	page 146	Ball Sit with Foot Lift	page 192
Supine Heel Taps	page 147	Ball Sit with Leg Extension	page 193
Supine 90-Degree Abdominal Isolation	page 149	Ball Sit with Leg Extension & Arm Lift	page 194
Raised-Leg Curl-Ups	page 151	Supine Base Position on Ball	page 195
Opposite Hand-to-Knee Contraction	page 153	Prone Arm Raise on Ball	page 201
Unilateral Contraction	page 153	Prone Leg Raise on Ball	page 202
Supine Double Knee to Chest	page 155	Prone Arm & Leg Raise on Ball	page 203
Pelvic Lift with Heel Taps	page 160	Ball Crunch	page 196
Prone Cross-Body Lifts	page 163	Twisting Ball Crunch	page 197
Prone Double-Arm Lifts	page 164	Reverse Trunk Curl on Ball	page 198
Foam Roller Push-Up	page 184	Ball Roll-In	page 199
Prone Double-Leg Lifts	page 165	Ball Pelvic Lift	page 200
Plank	page 167	Prone Torso Extension on Ball	page 204
Supine Marching	page 142	Ball Wall Slide	page 207
Ball Sit with Hip Movement	page 191		

Remember to stretch after your workout. Select 3–5 exercises and hold for 30 seconds to 1 minute. See stretching exercises starting on page 57 for suggestions.

Level 4

This super-advanced program is designed for the highly motivated. It's extremely challenging and also includes some fun partner moves.

LEVEL 4

Warm up with some light aerobic exercise or a warm shower for at least 10 minutes before performing core training. Then select 5–6 exercises and do them for 10 reps or 30 seconds.

Prone Double-Double	page 166	Ball Plank	page 205
Side Plank	page 168	Ball Push-Up	page 206
Plank to Pike	page 185	Twisting Ball Crunch	page 197
Plank to Side Salutation	page 185	Reverse Trunk Curl on Ball	page 198
Foam Roller Push-Up	page 184	Ball Roll-In	page 199
Foam Roller Stand	page 186	Ball Pelvic Lift	page 200
Standing Slide	page 187	Prone Torso Extension on Ball	page 204
Standing Foam Roller Mini-Squat	page 188	Medicine Ball Twist	page 208
Standing Foam Roller Ball Pick-Up	page 189	Plank Clap	page 209

Remember to stretch after your workout. Select 3–5 exercises and hold for 30 seconds to 1 minute. See stretching exercises starting on page 57 for suggestions.

EXERCISES FOR CORE STRENGTH

Supine Foundational Position

The purpose of this exercise is to gain awareness of core muscles, braced breathing, and proper posture, with the long-term goal of teaching you to be able to locate a neutral spine position with the least amount of effort in any position.

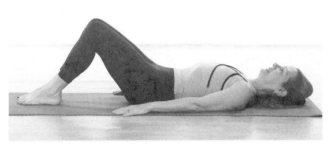

1. Lie on your back with your knees bent and feet flat on the floor.

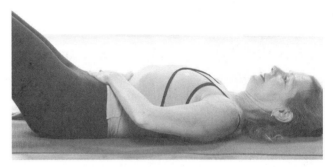

2. Placing one hand on your abs, draw your belly button in as you push the small of your back into the floor. Pretend that you have a sponge in the small of your back and are trying to compress the sponge. Hold for 1–2 seconds.

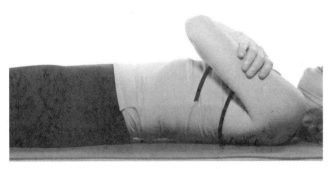

3. Release and allow the small of your back to return to a comfortable position (arms crossed to show space beneath the lower back).

VARIATIONS: You may place your fingers under the small of your back to better feel the move. If it's uncomfortable to place your head on the floor, place a small pillow under your head at first.

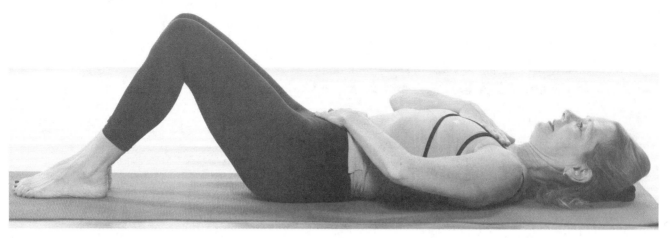

BREATHING OPTION 1 (Diaphragmatic Breathing): Place one hand on your belly and the other hand on your chest. Slowly breathe in through your nose for a count of 1-2-3-4, hold for 4 counts, and then slowly exhale via pursed lips for a count of 4. Repeat several times.

BREATHING OPTION 2 (Braced Breathing): Pretend you're about to be punched in the belly and hold that position for 1–5 seconds and perform slow diaphragmatic breathing. This concept is useful to learn for when doing moderately heavy lifts. It will increase intra-abdominal pressure and may provide some level of stabilization.

Supine Marching

This exercise improves trunk stabilization and abdominal strength.

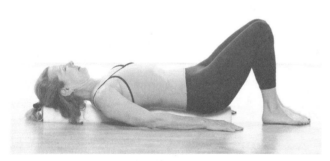

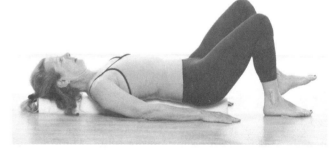

1. Place a full-length roller on the floor and lie on it from head to tailbone. Bend your knees and place your feet on the floor. Extend your arms alongside your body for extra support.

2. Once stable, slowly lift your left foot 1–2 inches off the floor (the less you lift your foot off the floor, the more challenging this exercise is). Hold for 15 seconds. Do not allow your torso or hips to rock.

3. Return to starting position and switch legs.

Continue alternating.

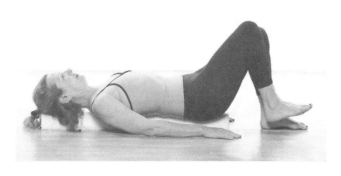

Supine Leg Extensions

While this may appear to be a leg exercise, it emphasizes the engagement of the abdominal muscles.

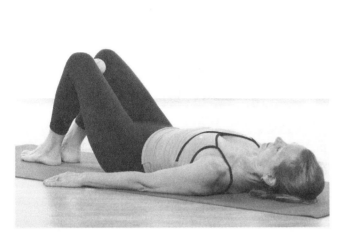 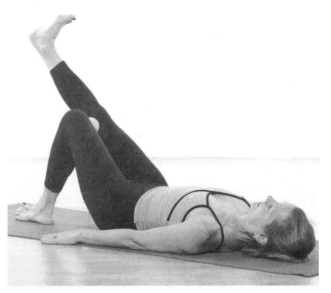

1. Lie on your back with your knees bent and feet flat on the floor. Find and maintain neutral spine position and place a tennis ball between your knees. Extend your arms along your sides.

2. Keeping the tennis ball in place, slowly and purposefully extend your right leg from the knee joint and flex your foot. Mindfully engage your abs while performing the leg movement. Avoid rapid leg motions and keep the arch in your back to a minimum.

Slowly return to the starting position.

Reposition into proper neutral spine position and switch legs.

Supine Arm Swings

This exercise will help you maintain neutral position while moving your extremities.

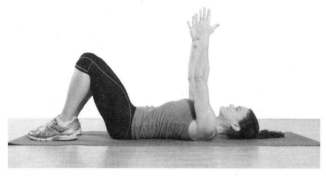

1. Lie on your back with your knees bent and feet flat on the floor; find and maintain neutral spine position. Extend both arms directly above your shoulders with your palms facing each other.

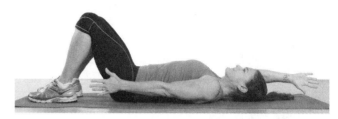

2. Keeping your arms somewhat straight, slowly move one arm forward (lead with the pinky) toward your hip and the other back toward your ear (lead with the thumb).

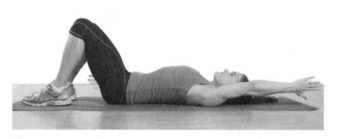

3. Slowly return to starting position and then move the arms the other direction.

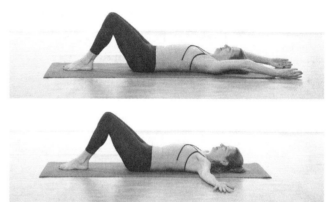

VARIATIONS: Swing both arms back, both arms to the front, and both arms to the sides.

Supine Leg Extension/Arm Swing Combination

This exercise teaches neutral spine position and conditions the abdominal region. Pelvic control is critical in this exercise. Speed is not important, nor is the number of repetitions. Do not perform this move until you can perform the Supine Leg Extensions (page 143) and Supine Arm Swings (page 144) correctly. In addition, if your lower back arch increases, you're not ready for this exercise; continue working on the previous exercises.

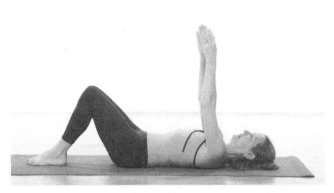

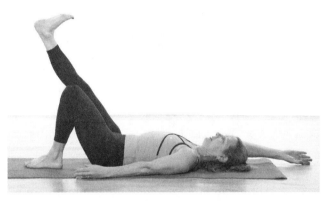

1. Lie on your back with your knees bent and feet flat on the floor; find and maintain neutral spine position. Keeping your knees together, extend both arms directly above your shoulders with your palms facing each other.

2. Slowly move your right arm back toward your ear and your left arm toward your hip, and simultaneously extend your right leg.

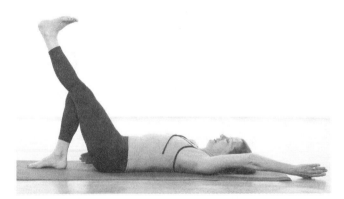

3. Slowly return to starting position and then repeat with the opposite side.

VARIATION: You can also extend the opposite arm and leg (e.g., right leg extends while left arm moves to the ear and right arm moves to the hip).

Supine Heel Slides

This exercise teaches core stabilization. Do not allow your lower back to arch. It's easier to perform on a smooth floor with stocking feet.

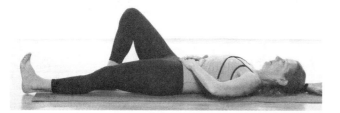 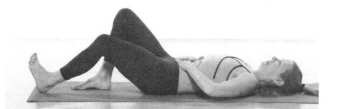

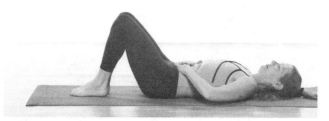

1. Lie on your back with your knees bent and feet flat on the floor; find and maintain neutral spine position. You may place your hands on your abs to remind yourself to engage them throughout the movement.

2–3. Keeping your core engaged, slowly and mindfully slide your left heel forward along the floor. Only move your heel out as far as you can while still keeping your lower back neutral.

Return to starting position and then slide the right heel out.

Supine Heel Taps

This exercise teaches core stabilization and conditions the abdominal region. Do not allow your lower back to arch.

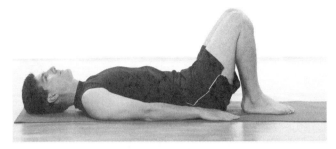

1. Lie on your back with your knees bent and feet flat on the floor; find and maintain neutral spine position. Extend your arms along your sides.

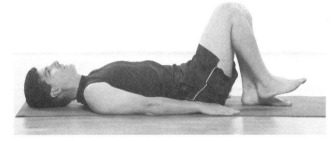

2. Slowly lift your right heel 1–3 inches off the floor. Only lift your heel as high as you can while still keeping neutral spine position. Periodically touch your abdominal muscles to make sure that you're engaging them.

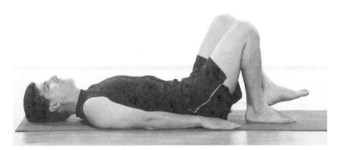

3. Slowly return your heel to the floor, reposition your spine, and repeat with your left heel.

Supine Foot Presses

This exercise conditions the abdominal region and teaches core stabilization. Do not allow your lower back to arch.

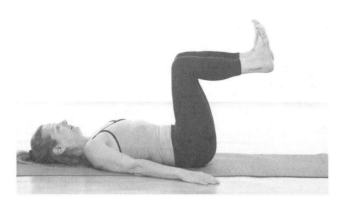

1. Lie on your back with your knees bent and feet flat on the floor; find and maintain neutral spine position. Raise both legs to a 90-degree angle, as if resting your lower legs on a chair. Extend your arms along your sides. Make sure to maintain proper neutral spine position throughout the exercise.

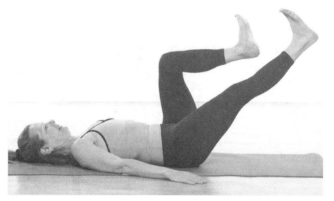

2. Keeping both legs elevated, press your right foot forward and away from you. Only extend your leg as far as you can while still maintaining neutral position.

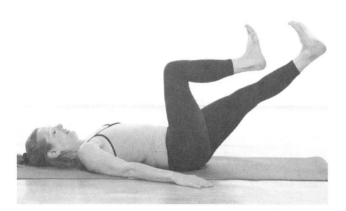

3. Return to starting position and repeat on the other side.

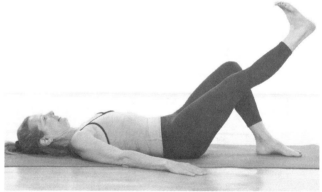

MODIFICATION: You may find it easier to do only one side at a time while keeping the other foot on the floor for better stabilization.

Supine 90-Degree Abdominal Isolation

This exercise strengthens and conditions the abdominal muscles while maintaining core stability.

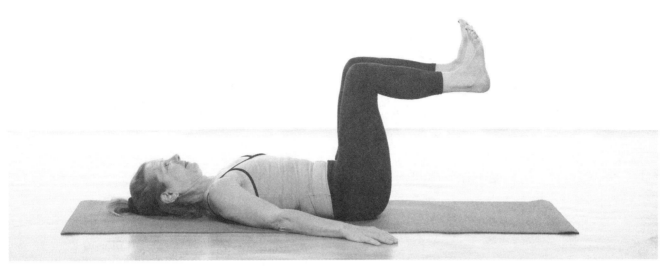

THE POSITION: Lie on your back and lift both legs to 90 degrees. Keep your shoulders on the floor and extend your arms alongside your body. Draw your belly button in and contract your abs hard, as if bearing down. Hold, but don't hold your breath—remember to breathe! Relax and repeat when ready.

Curl-Ups

This half sit-up conditions the abdominal region.

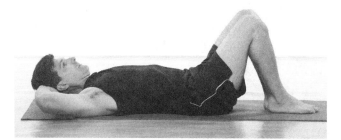 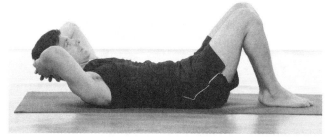

1. Lie on your back with your knees bent and feet flat on the floor; find and maintain neutral spine position. Place your hands behind your head to cradle and support your neck. Tuck your chin to your chest and inhale to begin.

2. While contracting your abdominal muscles, exhale and slowly lift your shoulder blades off the floor. Hold for 1–3 seconds. Don't force yourself to come up higher than is comfortable, and don't use your arms to pull on your neck. Perform this correctly, not quickly.

Inhale and slowly return to starting position, pressing the small of your back into the floor.

Raised-Leg Curl-Ups

This exercise strengthens and conditions the abdominal region.

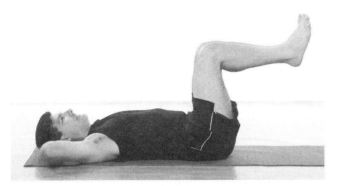

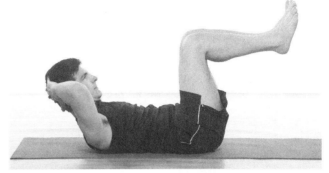

1. Lie on your back, bend your knees 90 degrees, and raise your legs so that your lower legs are parallel to the floor. Find and maintain neutral spine position. Place your hands behind your head to cradle and support your neck. Tuck your chin to your chest and inhale to begin.

2. While contracting your abdominal muscles, exhale and slowly lift your shoulder blades off the floor. Focus on pressing your lower back into the floor. Hold for 1–3 seconds. Don't force yourself to come up higher than is comfortable, and don't use your arms to pull on your neck. Perform this correctly, not quickly.

Inhale and slowly return to starting position, pressing the small of your back into the floor.

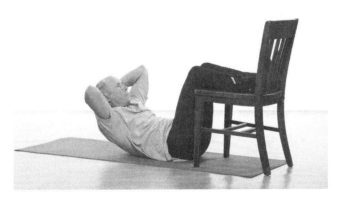

MODIFICATION: You can rest your lower legs on a chair.

Curl-Ups with a Twist

This exercise strengthens and conditions the abdominal region. CAUTION: Do not perform this exercise if rotation aggravates your back.

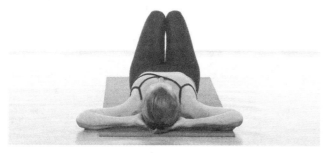

1. Lie on your back with your knees bent and feet flat on the floor; find and maintain neutral spine position. Place your hands behind your head to cradle and support your neck. Tuck your chin to your chest and inhale to begin.

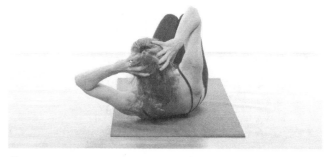

2. While contracting your abdominal muscles, exhale and slowly lift your shoulder blades off the floor, then gently twist your right elbow toward your left knee. Don't force it! Focus on pressing your lower back into the floor. Hold for 1–3 seconds.

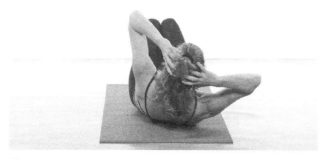

3. Inhale and slowly return to starting position, then repeat on the opposite side.

VARIATION: For an extra challenge, bend your knees 90 degrees and raise your legs so that your lower legs are parallel to the floor.

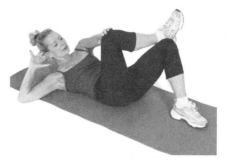

VARIATION: Lie on your back with your feet flat on the floor. Place your right ankle on your left knee, then place your left hand on your right knee. Raise your left shoulder off the floor and push your hand into your knee and your knee into your hand. Hold for 2 seconds.

Opposite Hand-to-Knee Contraction

This exercise strengthens and conditions the abdominal region. CAUTION: Avoid this exercise if you have high blood pressure.

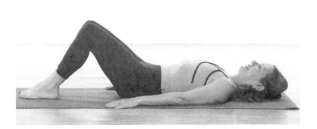

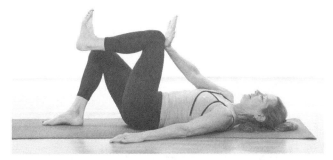

1. Lie on your back with your knees bent and feet flat on the floor; find and maintain neutral spine position.

2. Raise your left knee to 90 degrees and place your right hand on your left knee. Keeping your arm straight, press your hand into your knee while simultaneously pressing your knee into your hand. Release after a count of 2. This is an isometric contraction. Feel the abdominal muscles engage. Do not hold your breath. The focus is on pressing your lower back into the floor.

Repeat and then switch sides.

Unilateral Contraction

This exercise strengthens and conditions the abdominal region. CAUTION: Avoid this exercise if you have high blood pressure.

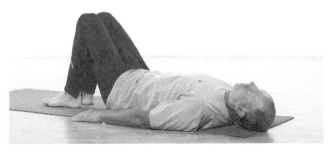

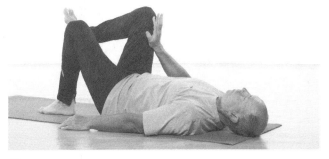

1. Lie on your back with your knees bent and feet flat on the floor; find and maintain neutral spine position.

2. Raise your right knee to 90 degrees and place your right hand on the knee. Keeping your arm straight, press your right hand into your right knee. Release after a count of 2. This is an isometric contraction. Feel the abdominal muscles engage. Do not hold your breath. The focus is on pressing your lower back into the floor.

Repeat and then switch sides.

Figure-4 Half Sit-Ups

This exercise strengthens and conditions the abdominal region. CAUTION: Avoid this exercise if twisting bothers your back.

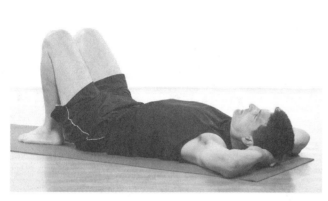

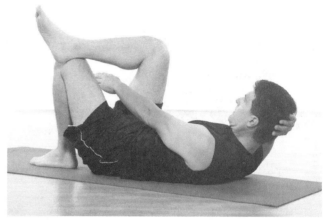

1. Lie on your back with your knees bent and feet flat on the floor. Place your hands behind your head. Find and maintain neutral spine position. Inhale and tuck your chin to your chest.

2. Place your right ankle on your left knee. Exhale and extend your left hand between the open space of your legs while contracting your abdominal muscles to slowly lift your shoulder blades off the floor while gently twisting your torso to the right. Focus on pressing your lower back into the floor. Don't use your arms to pull on your neck. Hold for 1–3 seconds.

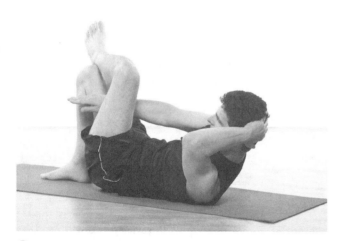

3. Slowly return your shoulders to the floor and repeat on the same side before switching sides.

Supine Double Knee to Chest

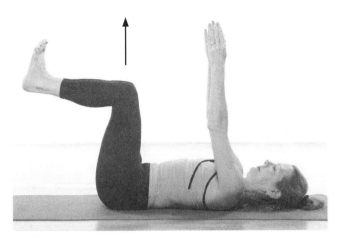

THE POSITION: Lie on your back with your knees bent and feet flat on the floor; find and maintain neutral spine position. Keeping your tailbone down, bring your knees to a 90-degree angle and extend your arms toward the ceiling. Contract the abdominal region to slowly lift your knees 1–3 inches upward. The motion is almost unnoticeable. Do not hold your breath. Relax.

Pelvic Lift

This exercise strengthens the abdominal muscles, buttocks, and lower back. Focus on using your gluteals rather than your hamstrings. CAUTION: Be careful not to perform so many reps that you trigger a hamstring cramp.

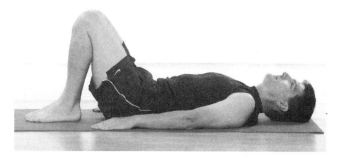

1. Lie on your back with your knees bent and feet flat on the floor; extend your arms alongside your body. Find and maintain neutral spine position.

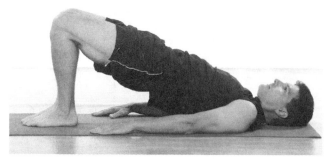

2. Pressing both feet equally into the floor, tuck your tailbone between your legs and squeeze your gluteal muscles to lift your butt off the floor. Do not lift your butt so high that it arches your back. Hold for 3–5 seconds.

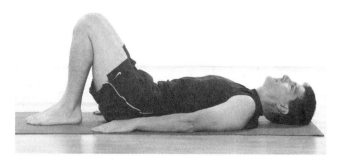

3. Slowly lower to the floor. Realign your spine after each rep.

Pelvic Lift with Arm Lifts

This exercise strengthens the abdominal muscles, buttocks, and lower back. CAUTION: Be careful not to perform so many reps that you trigger a hamstring cramp.

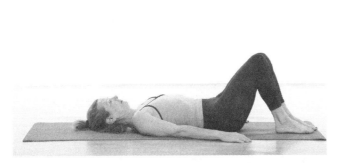

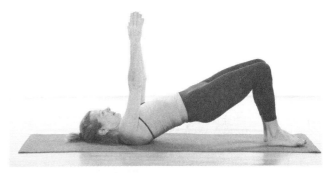

1. Lie on your back with your knees bent and feet flat on the floor. Locate and maintain neutral spine position. Extend your arms along your sides.

2. Pressing both feet equally into the floor, tuck your tailbone between your legs and squeeze your gluteal muscles to lift your butt off the floor. Do not lift your butt so high that it arches your back. Once you're in a comfortable position, raise your arms straight up toward the ceiling with your palms facing each other.

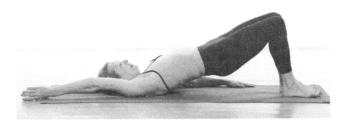

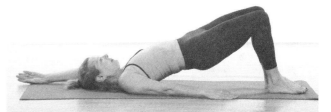

3. Keeping your core engaged and both arms straight, slowly move one arm forward toward the hip and the other hand back toward the ear.

4. Continue alternating arms, making sure to realign your spine after each rep.

Once you've completed the desired number of reps, slowly lower your rear end to the floor.

Pelvic Lift with Leg Extensions

While this exercise may appear to be a leg exercise, it emphasizes lower back muscle engagement and strengthens the abdominal muscles, buttocks, and lower back.

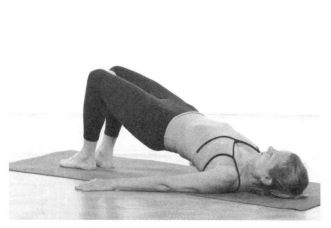

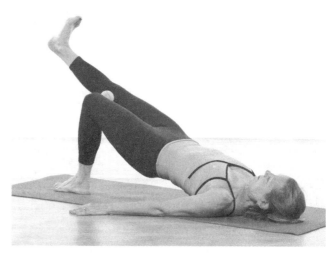

1. Lie on your back with your knees bent and feet flat on the floor. Find and maintain neutral spine position, then place a tennis ball between your knees. Extend your arms alongside your body. Pressing both feet equally into the floor, tuck your tailbone between your legs and squeeze your gluteal muscles to lift your butt off the floor.

2. Keeping the tennis ball in place, slowly and purposefully extend your right leg from the knee joint. Mindfully engage your abdomen and gluteal muscles. Avoid rapid leg motions.

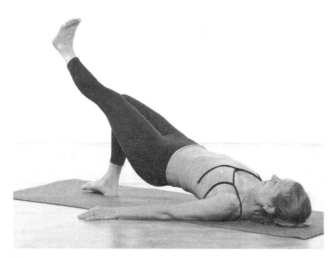

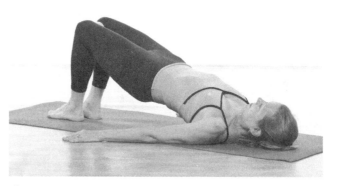

3. Slowly return to starting position and reposition into proper neutral spine position if necessary.

4. Perform with the left leg.

Pelvic Lift with Arm Lift/Leg Extensions

This exercise strengthens the abdominal muscles, buttocks, and lower back. Make sure you can perform Pelvic Lift with Arm Lifts (page 157) and Pelvic Lift with Leg Extensions (page 158) correctly before trying this combination exercise.

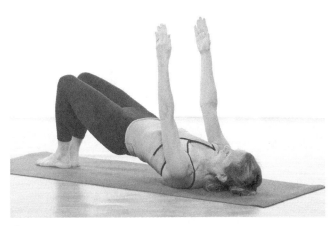

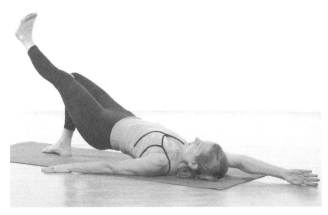

1. Lie on your back with your knees bent and feet flat on the floor. Find and maintain neutral spine position, then place a tennis ball between your knees. Extend both arms straight up to the ceiling, with your palms facing each other. Pressing both feet equally into the floor, tuck your tailbone between your legs and squeeze your gluteal muscles to lift your butt off the floor.

2. Keeping the tennis ball in place, slowly extend your left leg from the knee joint while your left arm moves toward your hip and your right arm moves back toward your ear. Mindfully engage the butt muscles while performing the leg movement.

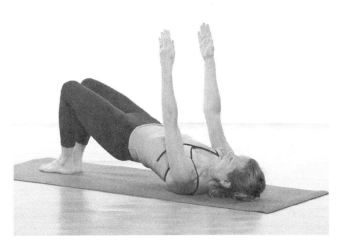

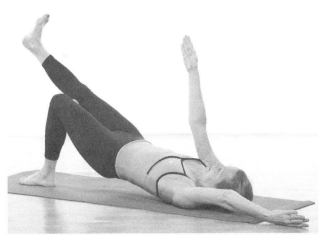

3. Slowly return to starting position.

`4. Reposition into proper neutral spine position and then perform on the other side.

Pelvic Lift with Heel Taps

This exercise strengthens the abdominal muscles, buttocks, and lower back. Periodically touch your butt muscles to make sure that you're engaging them.

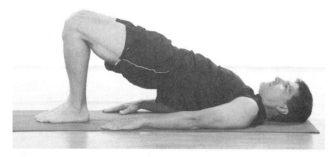

1. Lie on your back with your knees bent and feet flat on the floor. Find and maintain neutral spine position, then extend your arms alongside your body. Pressing both feet equally into the floor, tuck your tailbone under and squeeze your gluteal muscles to lift your butt off the floor. Hold for 3–5 seconds.

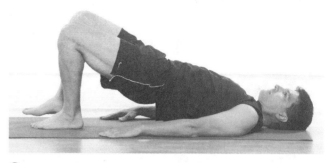

2. Slowly lift your right heel 1–3 inches off the floor.

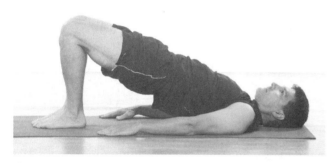

3. Slowly return your heel to the floor and reposition your spine.

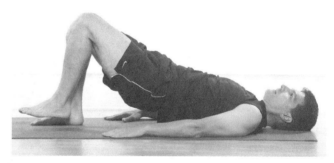

4. Perform with your left heel.

Prone Single-Arm Lifts

This exercise strengthens your lower spine muscles as well as your gluteals. Some people find it more comfortable to place a rolled-up towel or pillow under the hipbones when doing this. Your body will tell you if you need a pillow under your hips. CAUTION: Do not perform this exercise if you find arching your back uncomfortable.

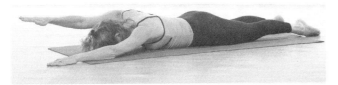

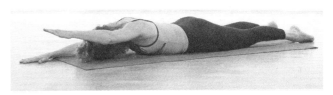

1. Lie face-down with your arms outstretched so that your biceps are next to your ears and your palms are down. Concentrating on maintaining correct alignment (this means no excessive arching of your back), slowly raise one arm to a comfortable height and hold. Do not raise the arm so high that you cause your back to arch! Keep the motion smooth and avoid twisting your body.

2. Lower the arm and raise the other arm and hold.

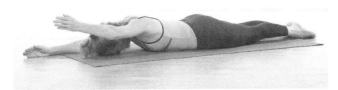

MODIFICATION: If your shoulders are inflexible, place your body or turn your thumbs up while doing this exercise.

Prone Single-Leg Lifts

This exercise strengthens your lower spine muscles as well as your gluteals. Some people find it more comfortable to place a rolled-up towel or pillow under the hipbones when doing this. Your body will tell you if you need a pillow under your hips. CAUTION: If you feel an uncomfortable sensation in your lower back, stop!

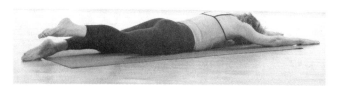

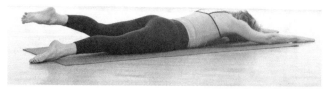

1. Lie face-down with your arms outstretched so that your biceps are next to your ears and your palms are down. Concentrating on maintaining correct alignment (this means no excessive arching of your back), slowly raise one leg a comfortable height and hold for 1–3 seconds. Keep the motion smooth and avoid twisting your body.

MODIFICATION: If your shoulders are inflexible, place your arms alongside your body or turn your thumbs up.

2. Lower the leg, raise the other leg, and hold.

Prone Cross-Body Lifts

This exercise strengthens your lower spine muscles as well as your gluteals. Some people find it more comfortable to place a rolled-up towel or pillow under the hipbones when doing this. Your body will tell you if you need a pillow under your hips. CAUTION: If you feel an uncomfortable sensation in your lower back, stop!

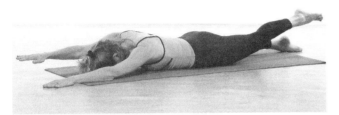 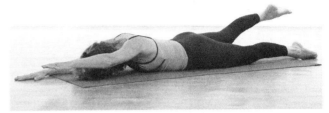

1. Lie face-down with your arms outstretched so that your biceps are next to your ears and your palms are down. Concentrating on maintaining correct alignment (this means no excessive arching of your back), slowly raise your right arm and your left leg a comfortable height and hold for 1–3 seconds. Your foot shouldn't raise up much higher than your rear end. Keep the motion smooth and avoid twisting your body.

MODIFICATION: If your shoulders are inflexible, turn your thumb up while raising your arm.

2. Lower your arm and leg, and then raise the opposite arm and leg. Hold.

Prone Double-Arm Lifts

This advanced exercise strengthens your lower spine muscles as well as your gluteals. Some people find it more comfortable to place a rolled-up towel or pillow under the hipbones when doing this. Your body will tell you if you need a pillow under your hips. CAUTION: If you feel an uncomfortable sensation in your lower back, stop!

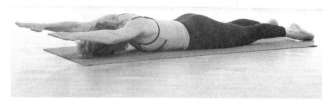

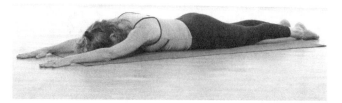

1. Lie face-down with your arms outstretched so that your biceps are next to your ears and your palms are down. Concentrating on maintaining correct alignment (this means no excessive arching of your back), slowly raise both arms and hold for 1–3 seconds. Keep the motion smooth and avoid twisting your body.

2. Lower your arms and relax.

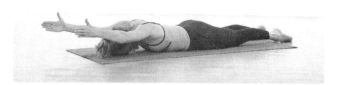

MODIFICATION: If your shoulders are inflexible, turn your thumbs up while raising your arms.

Prone Double-Leg Lifts

This exercise strengthens your lower spine muscles as well as your gluteals. Some people find it more comfortable to place a rolled-up towel or pillow under the hipbones when doing this. Your body will tell you if you need a pillow under your hips. CAUTION: If you feel an uncomfortable sensation in your lower back, stop!

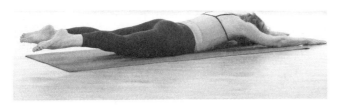

1. Lie face-down with your arms outstretched so that your biceps are next to your ears and your palms are down. Concentrating on maintaining correct alignment (this means no excessive arching of your back), slowly raise both legs and hold for 1–3 seconds. Keep the motion smooth and avoid twisting your body.

MODIFICATION: If your shoulders are inflexible, place your arms alongside your body or turn your thumbs up.

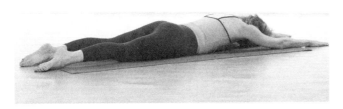

2. Lower your legs and relax.

Prone Double-Double

This exercise strengthens your lower spine muscles as well as your gluteals. Some people find it more comfortable to place a rolled-up towel or pillow under the hipbones when doing this. Your body will tell you if you need a pillow under your hips. CAUTION: If you feel an uncomfortable sensation in your lower back, stop!

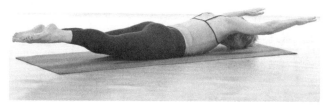

1. Lie face-down with your arms outstretched so that your biceps are next to your ears and your palms are down. Concentrating on maintaining correct alignment (this means no excessive arching of your back), slowly raise both arms and legs and hold for 1–3 seconds. Keep the motion smooth and avoid twisting your body.

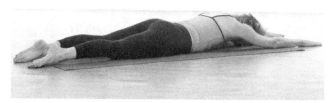

2. Lower your arms and legs and relax.

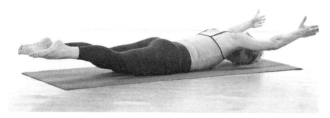

MODIFICATION: If your shoulders are inflexible, turn your thumbs up while raising your arms.

Plank

This exercise tones and conditions the entire core. Additionally, it serves as a foundational exercise and screening tool to let you know if you're ready for the foam roller series that starts on page 174. You need to be able to perform the next two exercises perfectly before moving to the foam roller series. CAUTION: Do not perform this exercise if you have high blood pressure or shoulder joint issues.

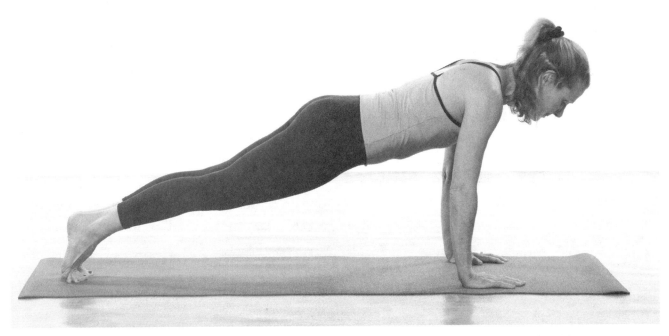

THE POSITION: Assume a traditional push-up position, with your hands under your shoulders, arms extended, and your feet extended behind you. Brace your abs so that your back forms a nice line from head to heels—no "sagging" in the middle or piking your butt to the ceiling. Hold for 3 seconds, working toward the goal of 1 minute. Breathe normally.

MODIFICATION: This can also be performed from your knees.

Side Plank

This exercise works the lateral muscles (the quadratus lumborum) of the torso. CAUTION: Do not perform this exercise if you have high blood pressure or shoulder joint issues.

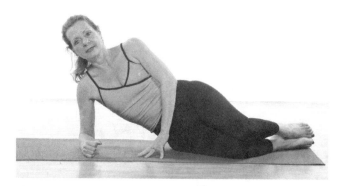

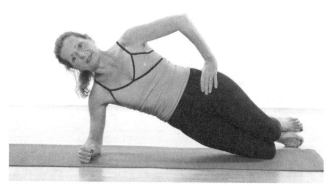

1. Lie on your right side with your knees bent, stacking your shoulders, ankles, knees, and hips atop each other.

2. Balancing on your forearm and lower knee, lift your hips off the floor and straighten yourself up by engaging your entire core. Align your chin, sternum, and mid-pelvic area. Hold. Breathe normally.

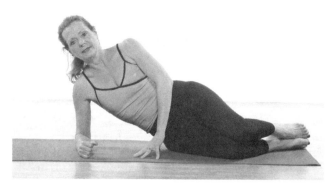

3. Lower to starting position.

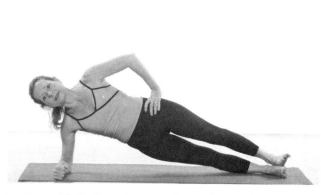

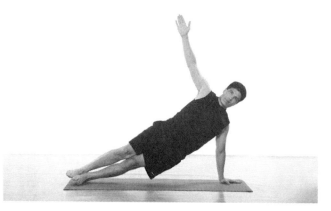

VARIATION: If you're very fit, try balancing yourself on your forearm and lower foot or, if super fit, your hand and lower foot.

Clam Shell

This exercise strengthens your gluteal muscles.

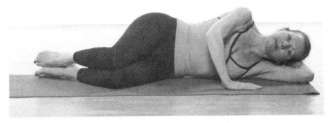

1. Lie on your left side and pull both knees halfway to your chest, stacking your ankles, knees, and hips atop each other.

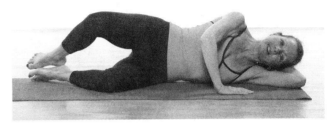

2. Slowly lift your right knee 2–5 inches above the other knee.

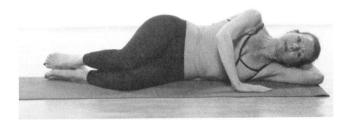

3. Lower and repeat.

Roll over and repeat, lifting the left knee

Tabletop Arm Raises

This exercise strengthens the lower back muscles and teaches body awareness.

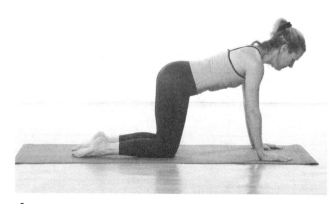

1. Assume proper tabletop position and find neutral spine. Stabilize your lower back by engaging/bracing your abdominal muscles.

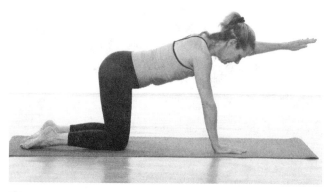

2. Keeping your torso steady and the base of your skull in alignment with your spine, raise your left arm to shoulder height or as high as is comfortable. Hold for 1–5 seconds.

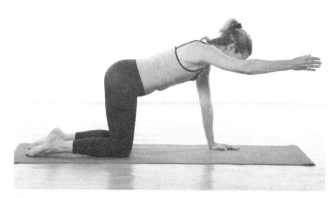

3. Lower to starting position and perform with the other arm.

Continue alternating.

Tabletop Leg Raises

This exercise strengthens the lower back and gluteal muscles and also teaches body awareness.

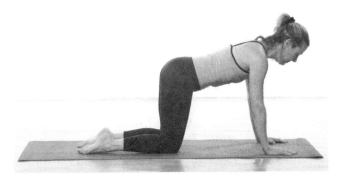

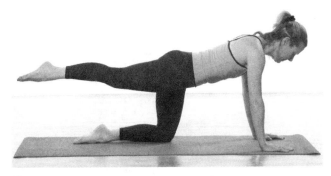

1. Assume proper tabletop position and find neutral spine. Stabilize your lower back by engaging/bracing your abdominal muscles.

2. Keeping your torso steady and the base of your skull in alignment with your spine, raise your right leg. Hold for 1–5 seconds.

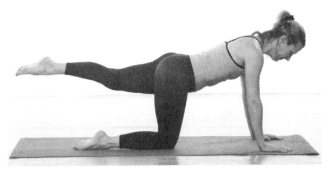

3. Lower to starting position and perform with the other leg.

Continue alternating.

Tabletop Arm & Leg Raises

This exercise strengthens the lower back and gluteal muscles and also teaches body awareness.

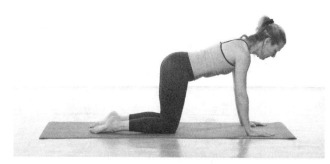

1. Assume proper tabletop position and find neutral spine. Stabilize your lower back by engaging/bracing your abdominal muscles.

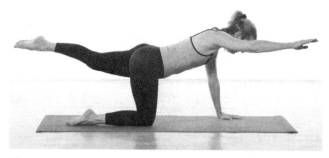

2. Keeping your torso steady and the base of your skull in alignment with your spine, raise your right arm and left leg to a comfortable height. Hold for 1–5 seconds.

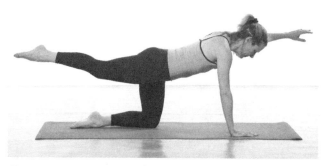

3. Lower to starting position and perform with your right leg and left arm.

Continue alternating.

Tabletop Advanced Combination

This exercise challenges the muscles that maintain core/spinal stabilization. Form and control is critical!

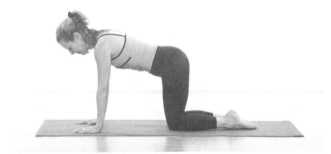

1. Assume proper tabletop position and find neutral spine. Stabilize your lower back by engaging/bracing your abdominal muscles.

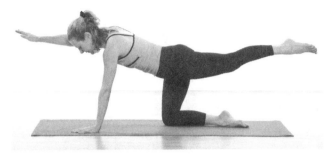

2. Raise your right arm forward, extend your left leg straight behind you, and hold for 1–3 seconds.

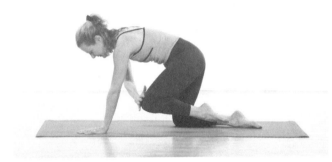

3. Keeping your torso steady and maintaining proper alignment from the base of your skull to your tailbone, bring your right hand toward your left knee and your left knee toward your right hand as they meet under your abdominal region. Hold steady for 1–2 seconds—don't rock!

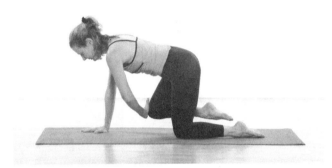

4. Return to starting position, readjust posture, and repeat on the opposite side.

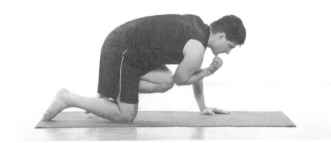

VARIATION: You can also bring your right elbow to your right knee, and then your left elbow to your left knee.

Roller Seated Orientation

This exercise improves lower back range of motion and neutral-spine awareness.

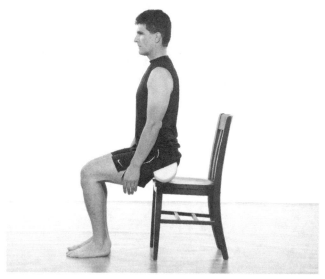

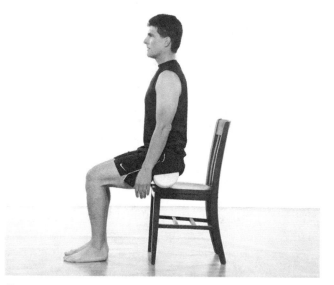

1. Place a full-length half roller flat-side up across a chair. Sit upright on the roller, with your tailbone off the roller. Let your feet rest on the floor.

2. Slowly roll your tailbone under you.

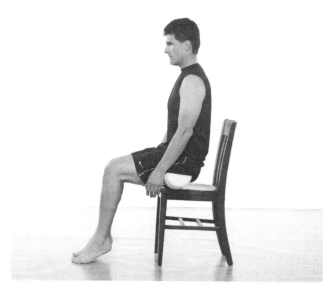

3. Slowly roll your tailbone backward, allowing your back to arch comfortably.

Continue rolling forward and back mindfully, paying attention to the pelvic position that feels best for you.

Roller Supine Orientation

This exercise acquaints you with the roller. This is the starting platform for all foam roller exercises. Once you feel safe and comfortable with this exercise, you're ready for the rest of the foam roller series.

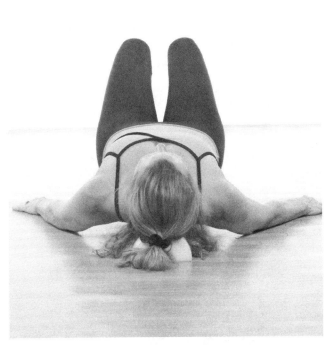

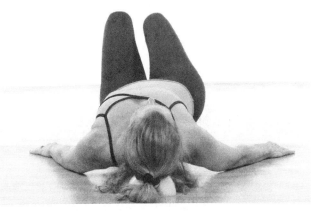

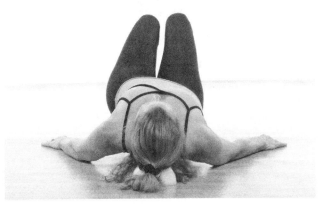

1. Place a full-length roller on the floor and lie on it from head to tailbone. Bend your knees and place your feet on the floor. You may have your arms on the floor to the side for additional stability.

2–3. Once you feel stable, gently rock left and right and recover your balance.

Roller Stabilization—Arms

This exercise helps you improve trunk support.

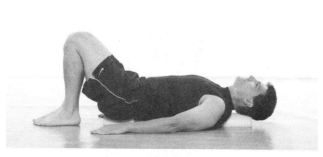

1. Place a full-length roller on the floor and lie on it from head to tailbone. Bend your knees and place your feet on the floor. Position your arms however you need to for support and balance.

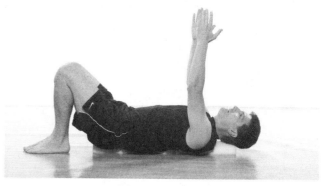

2. Once stable, raise your arms directly above your chest.

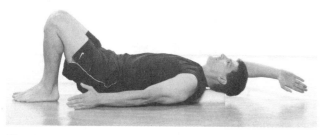

3. Now slowly move one arm forward and the other arm back. Try not to fall off the roller.

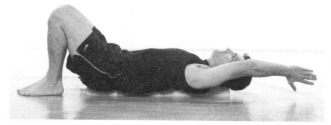

4. Slowly move the arms in the other direction.

Continue alternating arms.

Roller Stabilization—Legs

This exercise helps you gain greater control of your core.

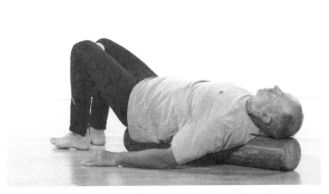

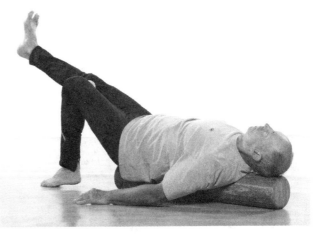

1. Place a full-length roller on the floor and lie on it from head to tailbone. Bend your knees and place your feet on the floor; place a tennis ball between your knees. Position your arms however you need to for support and balance.

2. Once stable, extend your right leg, keeping the ball in place.

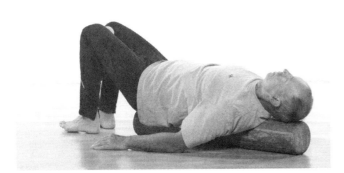

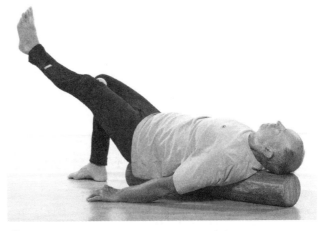

3. Lower your leg, making sure to not let the tennis ball drop.

4. Reposition your body and perform the same movement with the other leg.

Continue alternating.

VARIATION: You can also perform the sequence with your arms lifted off the ground or resting across your chest.

Roller Stabilization Arm/Leg Combination

This extremely challenging exercise fosters core stabilization.

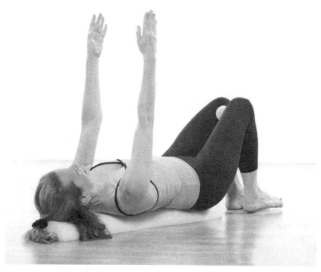

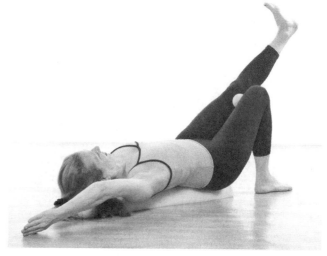

1. Place a full-length roller on the floor and lie on it from head to tailbone. Bend your knees and place your feet on the floor; place a tennis ball between your knees. Once stable, raise your arms above your chest.

2. Keeping the ball in place, lower your left arm toward your left hip and your right arm back toward your ear as you extend your left leg.

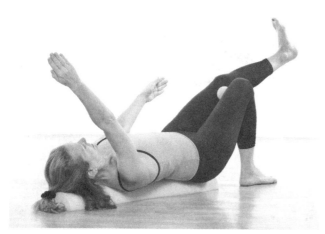

3. Continue alternating.

Supine Marching (Roller)

This exercise improves trunk stabilization and abdominal strength.

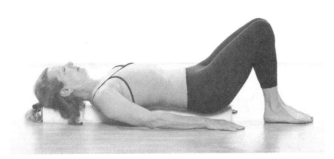

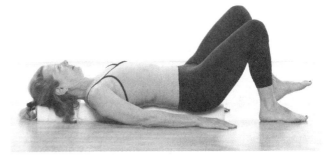

1. Place a full-length roller on the floor and lie on it from head to tailbone. Bend your knees and place your feet on the floor. Extend your arms alongside your body for extra support.

2. Once stable, slowly lift your left foot 1–2 inches off the floor (the less you lift your foot off the floor, the more challenging this exercise is). Hold for 15 seconds. Do not allow your torso or hips to rock.

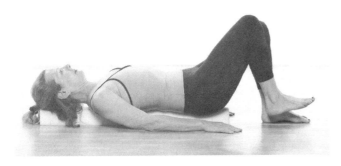

3. Return to starting position and switch legs.

Continue alternating.

Pelvic Lift on Roller

This exercise strengthens the gluteal region and the extensor muscles of the back. CAUTION: Be careful to avoid hamstring cramps.

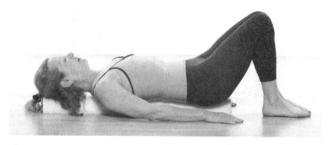 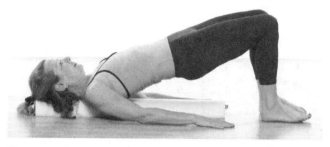

1. Place a full-length roller on the floor and lie on it from head to tailbone. Bend your knees and place your feet on the floor. Extend your arms alongside your body for extra support.

2. Slowly raise your rear end off the roller and hold for 10 seconds. Avoid going too high and arching your back as this can cause cramping of the hamstring muscles.

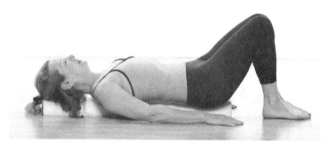

3. Slowly lower yourself to the roller, realign your spine, and repeat.

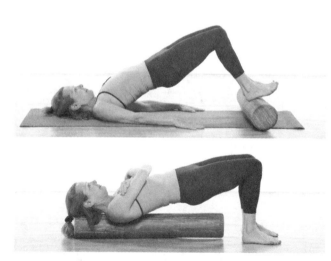

VARIATION: You can also lie on the floor but place the roller or some other unstable object under your feet to perform the movement.

You can also cross your arms over your chest.

Leg Press-Out on Roller

This exercise improves abdominal strength and fosters core stability.

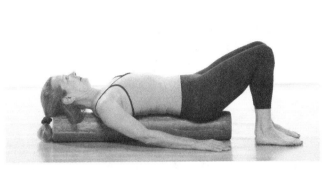

1. Place a full-length roller on the floor and lie on it from head to tailbone. Bend your knees and place your feet on the floor. Extend your arms alongside your body for extra support.

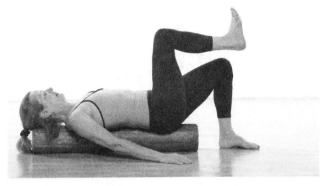

2. Once stable, lift your right leg so that your thigh makes a 90-degree angle with your chest. Hold.

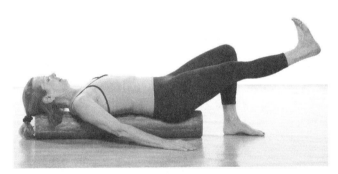

3. Slowly press the leg forward while maintaining proper core stability.

Return to starting position and repeat with the other leg.

Mad Cat on Rollers

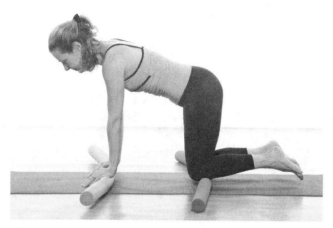

1. Place a full-length roller under your knees and a second one under your hands.

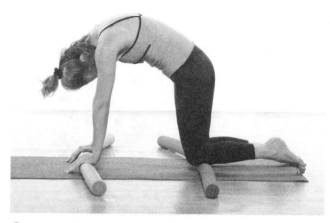

2. Inhale and draw your belly in as you round your back.

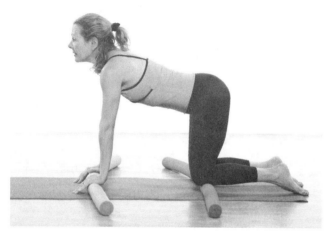

3. Exhale and arch your back slightly if possible.

Pointer Series

This exercise improves core stability and spinal alignment. CAUTION: Do not progress to this exercise until you can maintain core stabilization in the Mad Cat on Rollers (page 182).

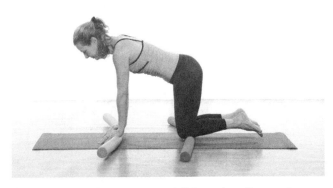

THE POSITION: Place a full-length roller under your knees and a second one under your hands.

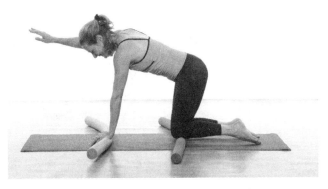

LEVEL 1: Alternate lifting one arm at a time.

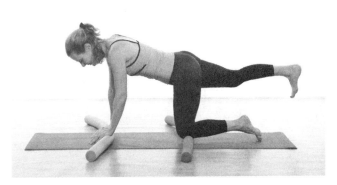

LEVEL 2: Alternate lifting one leg at a time.

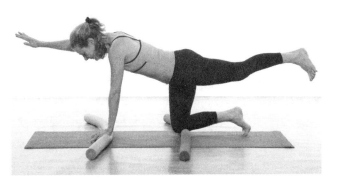

LEVEL 3: Alternate lifting the opposite arm and leg.

VARIATION: You can also try this with your right hand and knee on one roller, and your left hand and knee on another.

Foam Roller Push-Up

This exercise engages the complete kinetic chain. It's about alignment, not how many push-ups you can do.

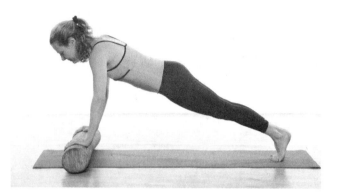

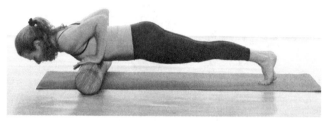

1. Place a full-length roller under your chest and then place your hands shoulder-width apart on top of the roller. Slide your feet back behind you until you're in a high push-up position, with your back forming a straight line from head to heels. Engage your gluteal and abdominal muscles so that you don't sag in the middle.

MODIFICATION: If stability or strength is an issue, you can perform this with your knees on the floor.

2. Keeping your back straight, lower your chest to the roller (or as low as you can) with control.

Press back up to starting position.

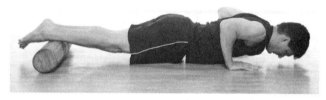

VARIATION: Try this with the roller under your feet.

Plank to Pike

This advanced exercise fosters upper body muscle tone and core stability. Make sure to execute it with proper alignment.

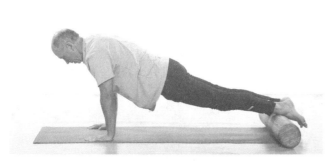 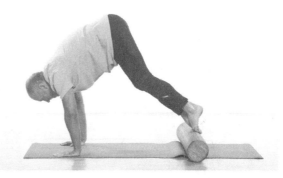

1. Place a full-length roller under your feet and then place your hands shoulder-width apart on the floor. Slide your feet back behind you until you're in a high push-up position, with your back forming a straight line from head to heels. Maintain this position for 15 seconds.

2. Keeping your feet on the roller, roll your feet in toward your hands to lift your rear end up to the ceiling (pike position). Hold.

Plank to Side Salutation

This extremely advanced exercise fosters upper body muscle tone and core stability. CAUTION: Avoid this exercise if you have weak shoulders.

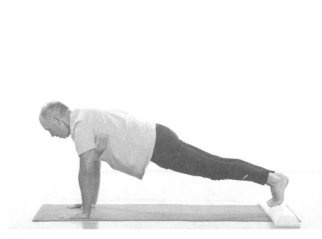 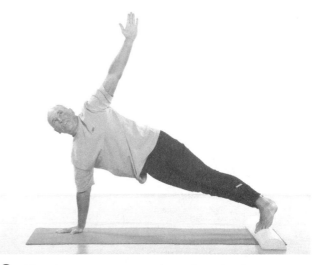

1. Place your toes on a full-length roller and your hands on the floor in a push-up position. Make sure your back forms a straight line from head to heels. Maintain this position for 15 seconds.

2. Keeping your toes on the roller, slowly rotate your body to the left, relying on your right arm to support you. Extend your left arm to the ceiling so that you're in a side plank.

Return to starting position.

Perform on the other side.

Foam Roller Stand

This exercise fosters core stability and balance. If you can't stand on the roller, it's suggested that you return to the seated ball exercises (starting on page 190).

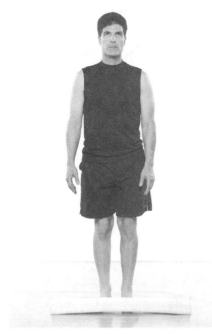

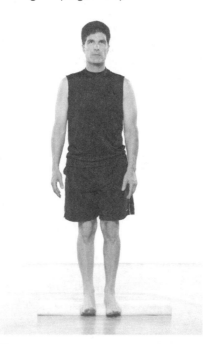

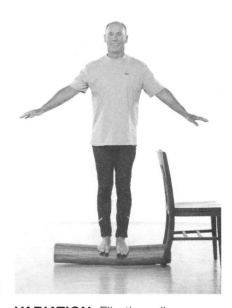

1. Place a full-length half roller horizontally on the floor in front of you with the flat side down.

2. Step onto the roller with your left foot and then your right foot, with your feet comfortably apart. Maintain proper posture and hold.

VARIATION: Flip the roller over and perform the exercise with the flat side up, or stand on a circular roller with a chair or wall nearby for support.

Standing Slide

This exercise improves balance and dynamic core stability. CAUTION: If you can't do the Foam Roller Stand (page 186) with proper posture, do not attempt this exercise.

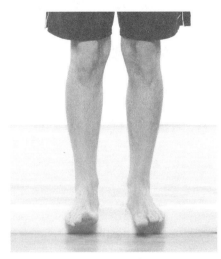

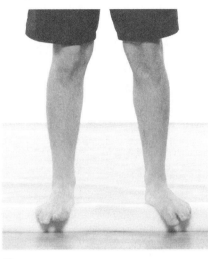

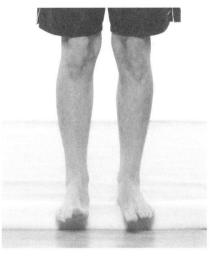

1. Place a full-length half roller horizontally on the floor in front of you with the flat side down. Step onto the roller.

2. Slowly slide your left foot farther to the left and hold.

3. Slowly return your left foot to starting position and hold.

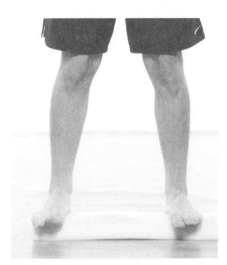

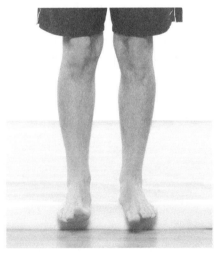

4. Slowly slide your right foot farther to the right and hold.

5. Slowly return your right foot to starting position and hold.

As you advance, move the foot farther toward the end of the roller.

VARIATION: For an extra challenge, try this move with the flat side up.

Standing Foam Roller Mini-Squat

This exercise improves balance and dynamic core stability and stamina.

CAUTION: If you can't do the Foam Roller Stand (page 186) with proper posture, do not attempt this exercise.

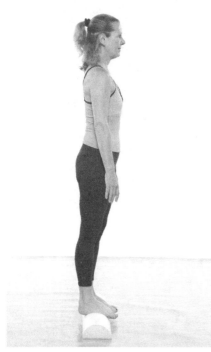 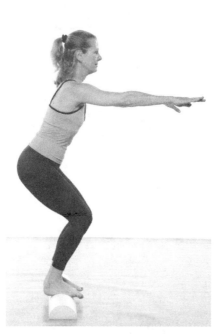 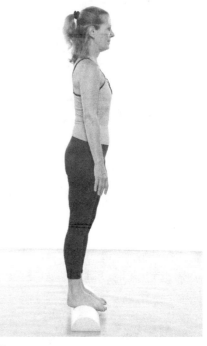

1. Place a full-length half roller horizontally on the floor in front of you with the flat side down. You may position yourself close to a wall for support. Step onto the roller.

2. Using your hands to counterbalance yourself, slowly perform a small squat.

3. Return to starting position.

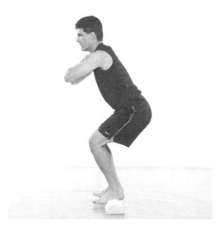

VARIATION: As you improve, try crossing your arms or performing the move with the rounded side down.

Standing Foam Roller Ball Pick-Up

This exercise fosters better balance and core stability.

CAUTION: If you can't do the Foam Roller Stand (page 186) with proper posture, do not attempt this exercise.

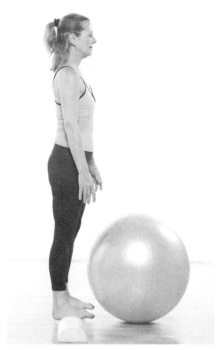 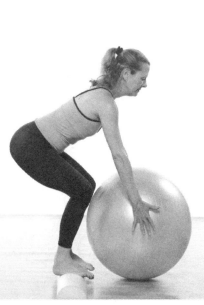 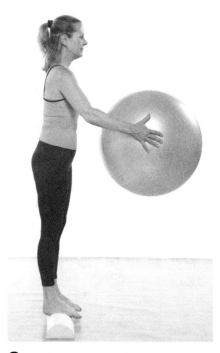

1. Place a full-length half roller horizontally on the floor in front of you with the flat side down. Place a large object such as a big stability ball in front of you. Step onto the roller.

2. Standing in your most stable position, slowly bend down to pick up the object.

3. Return to standing.

Ball Sit

This exercise teaches you how to contract your abdominal wall and maintain neutral spine on an unstable surface. This exercise should become so natural that you perform it anytime when sitting in a chair.

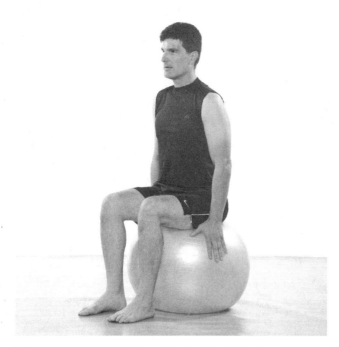

THE POSITION: Sit on the ball and find neutral lumbar spine position. Gently engage your abdominal wall muscles. Focus on proper sitting alignment—imagine your head is being lifted up by a string; keep your chest up and out and your shoulder blades together. Hold, then relax.

Continue performing this, each time trying to increase the duration of the hold up to 1 minute.

Ball Sit with Hip Movement

Do not do the other exercises in this series until you can perform this correctly.

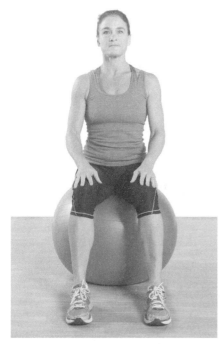

1. Sit on the ball and find neutral lumbar spine position.

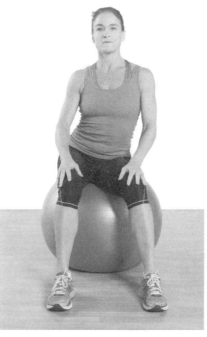

2–3. Using your hips, gently roll the ball from side to side.

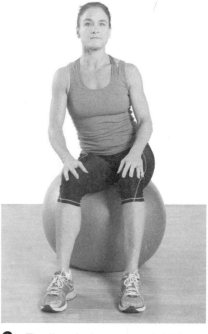

6. Finally, circle your weight in a clockwise direction, then switch directions.

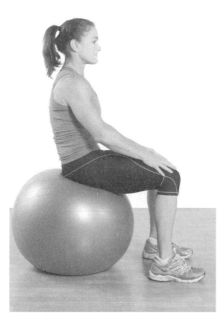

4. Roll your tailbone under you to round your lower back.

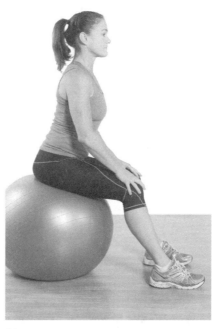

5. Roll your tailbone backward and allow your lower back to curve/arch.

Ball Sit with Foot Lift

This exercise teaches you how to contract the abdominal wall and maintain neutral spine on an unstable surface. It'll also progressively challenge your system.

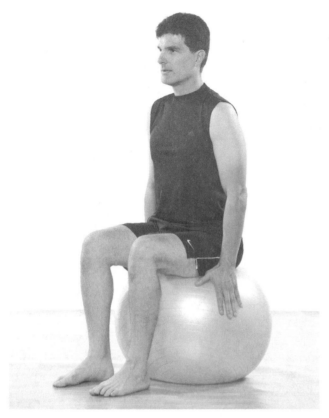 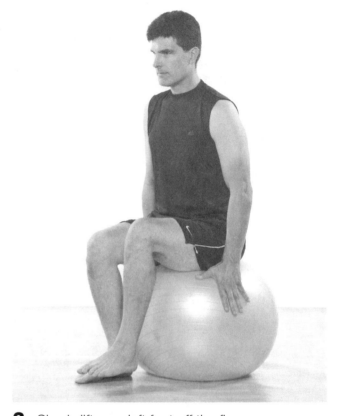

1. Sit on the ball and locate neutral spine position. Gently engage your abdominal wall muscles. Focus on proper sitting alignment—imagine your head is being lifted up by a string; keep your chest up and out and your shoulder blades together.

MODIFICATION: You can try this while sitting in a chair before progressing to an exercise ball.

2. Slowly lift your left foot off the floor approximately 1–3 inches. Hold for 3–5 seconds.

Slowly lower your foot to the floor and then alternate foot lifts.

Ball Sit with Leg Extension

This exercise teaches you how to contract the abdominal wall while maintaining neutral spine on an unstable surface. It'll also progressively challenge your system.

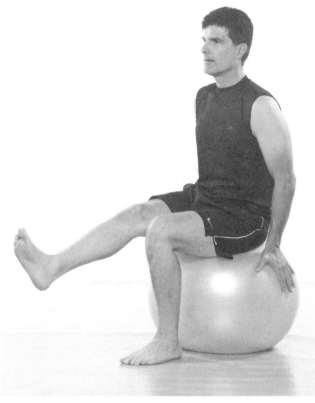 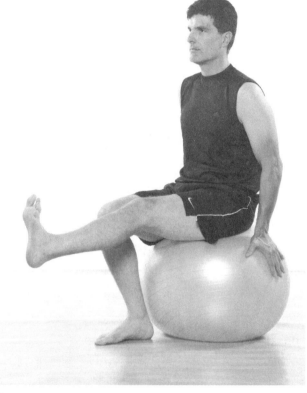

1. Sit on the ball and locate neutral spine position. Gently engage your abdominal wall muscles. Focus on proper sitting alignment—imagine your head is being lifted up by a string; keep your chest up and out and your shoulder blades together.

Slowly lift your right foot off the floor and extend your leg from the knee joint. Avoid rolling or rocking your pelvic joint. Hold for 3–5 seconds

2. Slowly lower your foot to the floor and repeat with your other leg.

Continue alternating.

MODIFICATION: You can try this while sitting in a chair before progressing to an exercise ball.

Ball Sit with Leg Extension & Arm Lift

This exercise teaches you how to contract the abdominal wall while maintaining neutral spine on an unstable surface. It'll also progressively challenge your system.

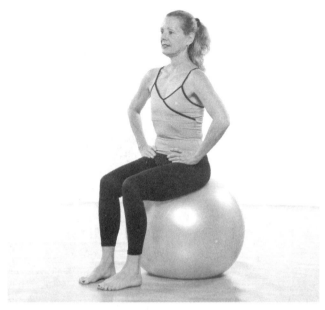

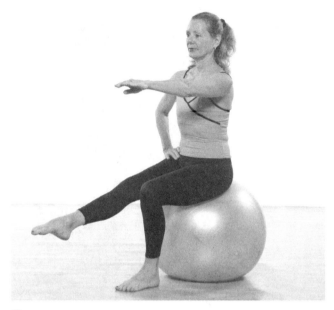

1. Sit on the ball and locate neutral spine position. Gently engage your abdominal wall muscles. Focus on proper sitting alignment—imagine your head is being lifted up by a string; keep your chest up and out and your shoulder blades together.

2. Slowly lift your right foot off the floor, extend your leg from the knee joint, and raise your left arm forward. Avoid rolling or rocking your pelvic joint. Hold for 3–5 seconds.

MODIFICATION: You can try this while sitting in a chair before progressing to an exercise ball.

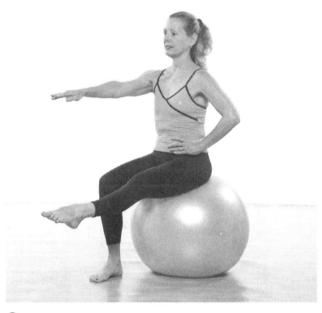

3. Slowly lower your foot to the floor and repeat with your other leg and arm.

Continue alternating.

Supine Base Position on Ball

This exercise teaches you how to contract the abdominal wall and lower back muscles and maintain neutral spine on an unstable surface in a supine position. It'll also progressively challenge your system.

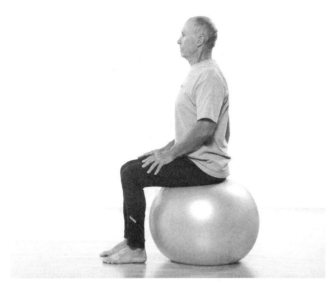

1. Sit on the ball and locate neutral spine position. Gently engage your abdominal wall muscles. Focus on proper sitting alignment—imagine your head is being lifted up by a string; keep your chest up and out and your shoulder blades together.

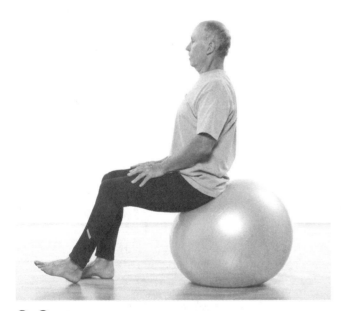

2–3. Slowly walk your feet forward as far as possible, allowing the ball to roll into your mid-back and then the neck region, to form a reverse tabletop position. Hold.

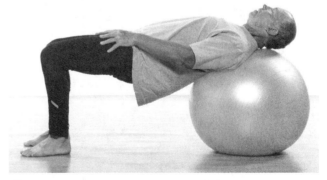

4. Return to starting position and relax.

MODIFICATION: If you don't have enough core control to move back up the ball, just drop your butt to the floor between each repetition.

Ball Crunch

This exercise engages the abdominal muscles as well as the internal and external obliques.

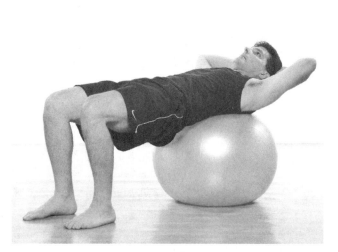

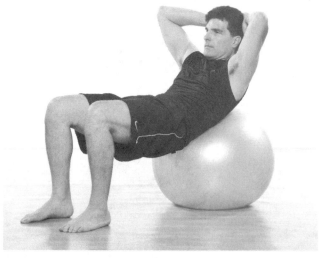

1. Sit on the ball and then slowly walk your feet forward, letting the ball roll beneath you, until you're reclining on the ball with the ball pressed comfortably into your lower back. Locate and maintain neutral spine position and then place your hands behind your head. Your knees should be bent 90 degrees and your feet should be on the floor shoulder-width apart.

2. Slowly perform a half sit-up by bending at your waist to bring your chest toward your knees.

MODIFICATION: For additional stability, move your feet farther away from the ball and spread your feet farther apart.

VARIATION: For an extra balance challenge, place your feet closer together as well as closer to the ball.

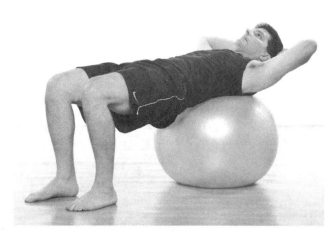

3. Slowly lower to starting position.

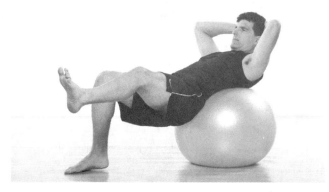

ONE-LEG VARIATION: Try performing the crunch while lifting one leg and extending it.

Twisting Ball Crunch

This exercise engages the internal and external obliques.

CAUTION: Do not perform this exercise if rotation bothers your back.

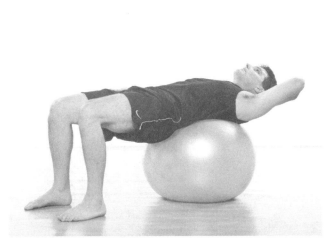

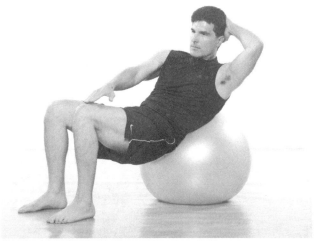

1. Sit on the ball and then slowly walk your feet forward, letting the ball roll beneath your lower back until you're reclining on the ball with the ball pressed comfortably into your lower back. Locate and maintain neutral spine position and then place both hands behind your head. Your knees should be bent approximately 90 degrees and your feet should be on the floor shoulder-width apart. Always keep your knees aligned over your ankles.

2. Keeping your feet on the ground, slowly curl up and gently attempt to touch your right hand to your left knee.

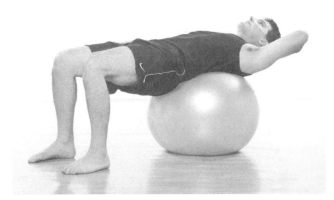

3. Reposition between each rep.

After you've completed your reps on one side, return to starting position, locate neutral spine position, and perform on the opposite side.

Reverse Trunk Curl on Ball

This exercise conditions the abdominal muscles. It's a very advanced exercise—proceed with caution.

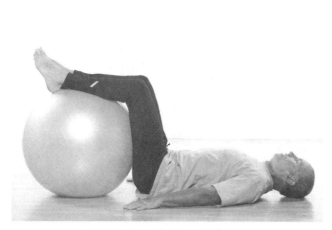

1. Lie on the floor on your back with your lower legs resting on the exercise ball and knees bent 90 degrees. Extend your arms alongside your body.

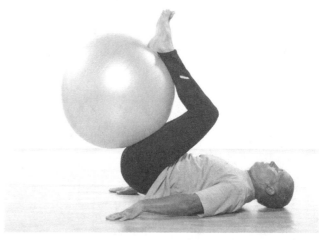

2. Digging your heels into the ball and gripping the ball between your heels and the backs of your thighs, slowly rock/tilt/lift your tailbone off the floor 1–2 inches if possible.

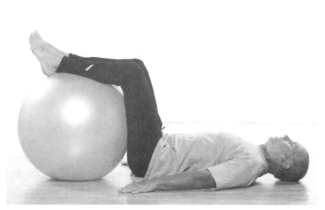

3. Lower to starting position.

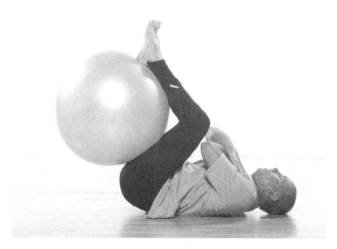

VARIATION: Place your arms across your chest and perform the movement.

Ball Roll-In

This advanced exercise requires good core stabilization. It engages your hamstrings and gluteal muscles.

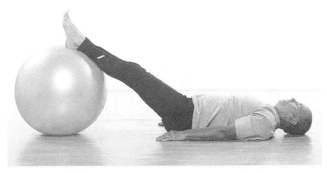

1. Lie on the floor on your back with your legs comfortably extended and lower legs resting on the exercise ball. Rest your arms alongside your body.

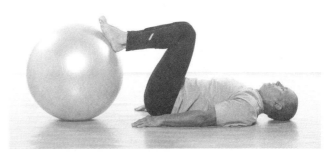

2. Press your heels into the ball while simultaneously rolling the ball toward your butt. Hold.

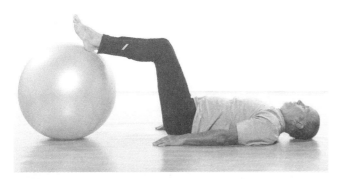

3. Extend your legs back to starting position and realign to neutral position.

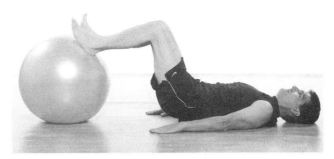

VARIATION: Perform the movement with your butt off the floor, but be careful to avoid getting hamstring cramps.

Ball Pelvic Lift

This exercise engages and strengthens the gluteal and lower back muscles.

CAUTION: Be careful of hamstring cramps.

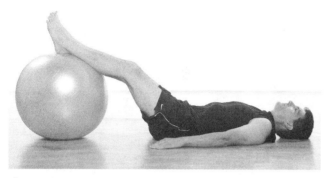

1. Lie on the floor on your back with your lower legs extended and calves resting on the exercise ball. Locate neutral spine. Extend your arms along your sides.

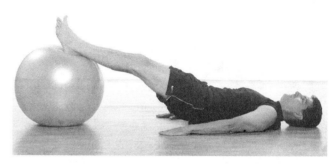

2. Maintaining neutral spine position, press the backs of the legs into the ball, elevating your butt off the floor. Make sure there are no spikes or dips in your posture. Hold.

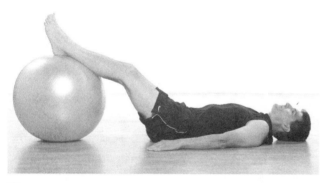

3. Lower to starting position and relocate neutral spine position before performing the next rep.

Prone Arm Raise on Ball

This exercise strengthens the spinal extensor muscle group, gluteus maximus, and shoulders. It also teaches body awareness.

CAUTION: Be alert to any increase in lower back discomfort.

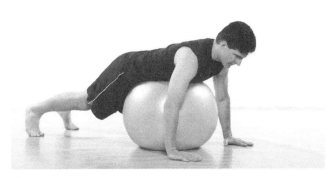

1. Rest your chest or belly on the ball and place your hands on the floor for support. Extend your legs behind you and place your toes on the floor. Stabilize your lower back by engaging your abdominal and lower back muscles.

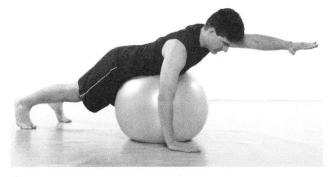

2. Keeping your torso steady and the base of your skull in alignment with your spine, raise your left arm to shoulder height if possible and hold for 3–10 seconds.

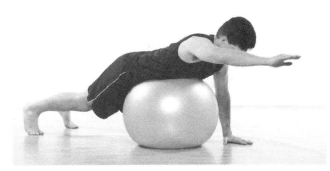

3. Lower your arm to the floor, then raise your other arm.

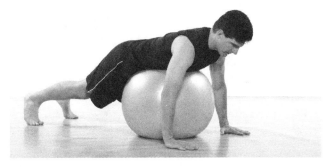

4. Lower your arm to the floor.

MODIFICATION: If your shoulders are inflexible, you can turn your thumbs up and move your arms up slightly to the side.

VARIATION: For an extra challenge, try raising both arms simultaneously.

Prone Leg Raise on Ball

This exercise strengthens the spinal extensor muscle group and gluteal region. It also teaches body awareness.

CAUTION: Be alert to any increase in lower back discomfort.

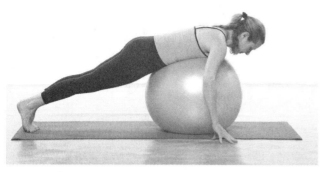

1. Rest your chest on the ball and place your hands on the floor for support. Extend your legs behind you and place your toes on the floor. Stabilize your lower back by engaging your abdominal muscles.

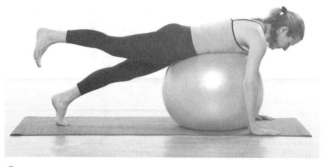

2. Keeping your torso steady and the base of your skull in alignment with your spine, raise your right leg no higher than hip height and hold for 3–10 seconds.

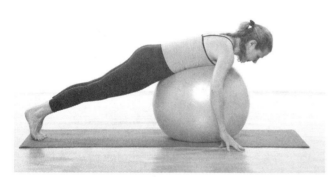

3. Lower your foot to the floor.

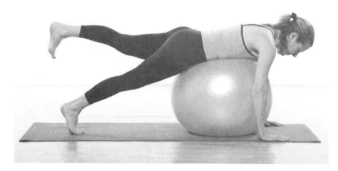

4. Raise your left leg no higher than hip height and hold for 3–10 seconds.

Lower your foot to the floor.

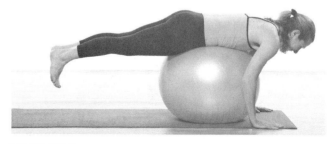

VARIATION: For an extra challenge, try raising both legs simultaneously.

Prone Arm & Leg Raise on Ball

This exercise strengthens the spinal extensor muscle group, gluteus maximus, and shoulders. It also teaches body awareness.

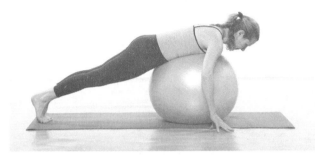

1. Rest your chest on the ball and place your hands on the floor for support. Extend your legs behind you and place your toes on the floor. Stabilize your lower back by engaging your abdominal muscles.

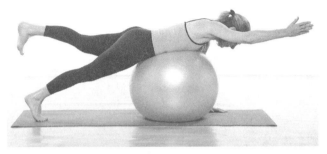

2. Keeping your torso steady and the base of your skull in alignment with your spine, raise your right arm and left leg to a comfortable height.

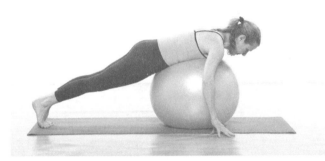

3. Lower to starting position.

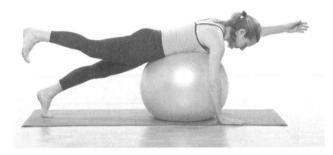

4. Raise your left arm and right leg to a comfortable height.

Lower to starting position.

Prone Torso Extension on Ball

This exercise strengthens the lumbar extensor and gluteal muscle groups.

CAUTION: Do not overdo this exercise as you may trigger a lower back muscle spasm. If you notice any discomfort, cease this move.

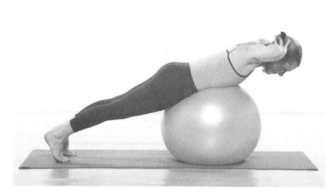

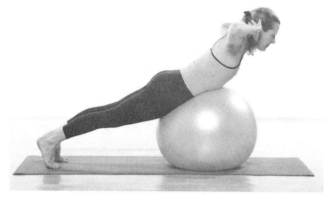

1. Rest your chest or belly on the ball. Extend your legs behind you and place your toes on the floor. Stabilize your lower back by engaging your abdominal muscles. Place your hands behind your head.

2. Slowly contract your lower back muscles and squeeze your gluteal muscles to gently lift your torso a few inches off the ball.

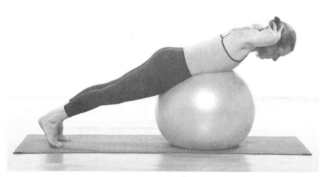

3. Lower yourself to the ball.

Once you've finished your reps, curl your body around the ball to relax your lower back muscles.

MODIFICATION: You can also do this with your hands on the floor, letting them lift as you raise off the ball.

Ball Plank

This is a very advanced exercise that simultaneously engages all the muscles of the core.

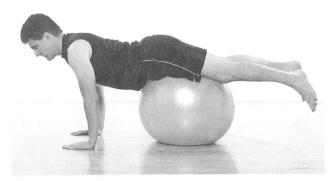

1. Lie face-down on the ball with the ball under your thighs. Place your hands shoulder-width apart on the floor for support.

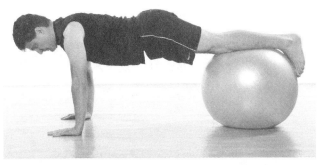

2. Slowly walk your hands forward, allowing the ball to roll down along your legs. Do not allow your back to arch or sag. The farther the ball goes down your legs, the more challenging the exercise becomes.

Slowly and cautiously return to starting position.

Ball Push-Up

This super-advanced exercise simultaneously engages the muscles of the core along with the upper torso.

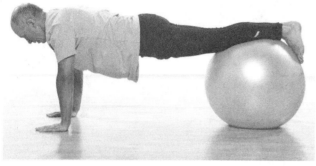

1. Place the ball under your pelvic region and place your hands shoulder-width apart on the floor. Slowly walk your hands forward, allowing the ball to roll down to your shins. Do not allow your back to arch or sag.

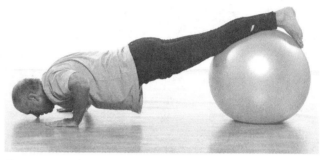

2. Keeping your back straight, bend your elbow to lower your chest toward the floor. Only go as far as you can while still maintaining proper alignment.

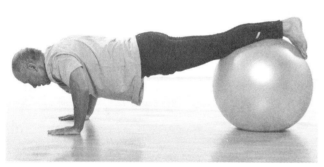

3. Slowly and cautiously press up to starting position.

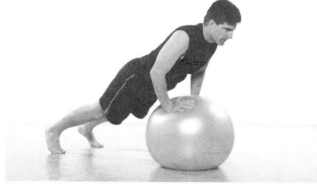

VARIATION: For an extra challenge, perform the push-up by placing your hands in a diamond shape or spreading your hands wide. You can also place your feet on the floor and your hands on the ball.

Ball Wall Slide

This exercise fosters better posture and leg strength.

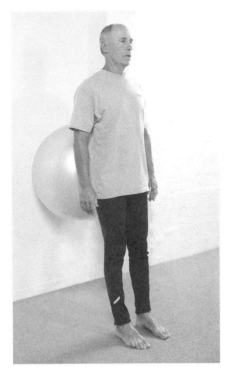

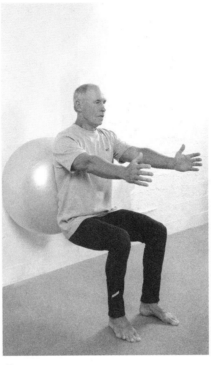

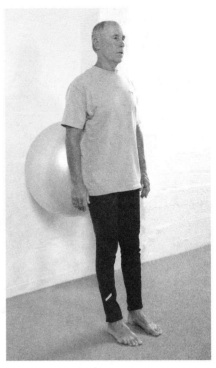

1. Place the ball between your lower back and the wall.

2. Bend your knees and hips and, if possible, lower yourself until your thighs are parallel to the floor. You may raise your arms for balance if necessary. Hold momentarily.

3. Slowly return to upright position.

Medicine Ball Twist

This exercise engages many of the core muscles in a dynamic motion. Any object, including a basketball, tennis ball, or even a book, will suffice.

CAUTION: If rotation bothers your back, avoid this exercise.

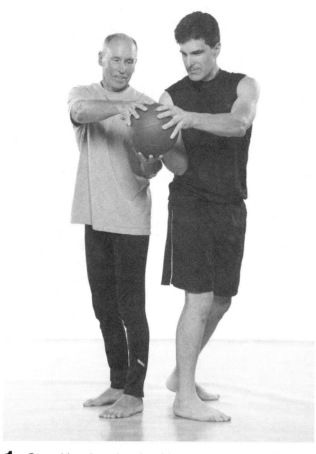

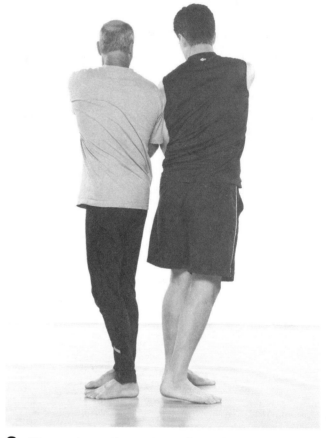

1. Stand back to back with your partner, with one partner holding an object.

The partner with the object twists to the side and passes it to the other partner, who twists to receive the object. The partners pass the object to the same side several times.

2. The partners then repeat the twists to the opposite direction several times.

Plank Clap

This exercise engages the complete kinetic chain of the core and works on spinal stabilization, so don't sacrifice form. Maintain proper alignment at all times. Once one partner either sags or arches his/her back, stop the exercise.

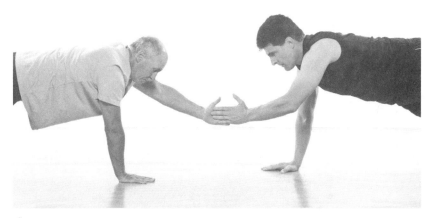

1. Both partners assume a plank position on their hands and toes, about an arm's distance from each other.

While in the plank position, one partner raises his/her right arm while the other partner raises his/her left arm so that you can clap hands.

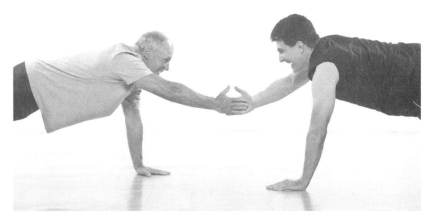

2. After finishing reps on one side, swap positions so that you're now clapping with the other hand.

SUGGESTED STRETCHES FOLLOWING A CORE-STRENGTHENING WORKOUT

PART 3

WEIGHT AND RESISTANCE TRAINING

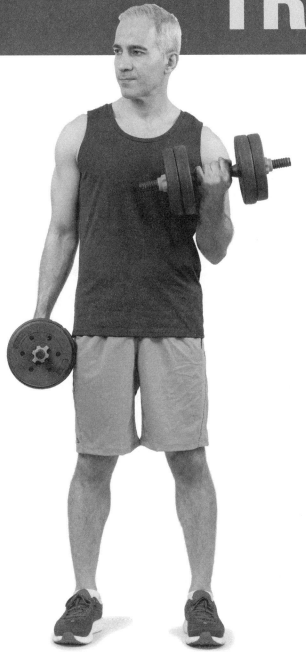

WEIGHT AND RESISTANCE TRAINING PROGRAMS

OVERVIEW

Beyond core strengthening, it is important to exercise and strengthen the full body. This section and the one that follows in this book will help you customize strength-training routines for specific needs as you age. By the time many of us turn 50, we may be suffering from twinges in our hinges. The joints affected most frequently are the knees, hips, and shoulders, as well as the joints of the lower back. Often these joint issues are the result of abusing or misusing our bodies in our younger days and, unfortunately, may affect our ability to perform daily movements as well as pursue leisure activities. In addition, as we age, our chances of having some type of chronic condition increases.

In the US, millions of people over 50 years of age have a chronic condition such as diabetes, cancer, heart disease, stroke, hypertension, or arthritis. This section provides strength-training programs to help improve many chronic conditions seen in the 50-plus group, as well as make recreational pursuits easier.

GENERAL GUIDELINES

- Always consult your health professional about suggestions regarding exercise and your condition. Information in this section is not a substitute for medical advice.
- Perform your exercise program when you are having the least amount of pain/discomfort. Avoid exercising on days when you are experiencing a flare-up.

- If you are exercising alone, carry ID and medical information with you.
- Be mindful of doing the movement with the best pain-free technique you can do. If it hurts—STOP! Also stop if the amount of pain you experience increases both during and after. Exercise should be pain-free.
- Never hold your breath.
- If you exercise alone, keep a phone handy.
- Don't forget to warm up first and cool down after a workout.

ARTHRITIS

There are more than 100 forms of arthritis. Stiffness and chronic pain are common characteristics. The phrase "use it or lose it" really applies to arthritis: If you don't move that joint, it will become stiffer and weaker. Unfortunately, many people with arthritis are afraid to exercise for fear that they will make the condition worse. Thus the downward spiral begins: As the person with arthritis starts to do less, the muscles weaken, which in turn puts more load and strain on an already compromised joint.

A mild to moderate strength-training routine can go a long way in preventing further atrophy of the muscle that supports the joint. It also increases muscle tone and strength, which adds integrity to the joint, and helps maintain or increases bone strength. The goal of this program is to maximize benefits and minimize risks, so always consult with your doctor or therapist before starting a routine. Learn what kind of arthritis you have and what kind of exercise is best for your condition.

No matter what type of arthritis you have, it is critical that you do not cause any further harm to the joint—train the muscles, don't strain the joints. Also, do everything you can to prevent additional pain, but do not increase your medications to cover up pain. I've suggested some stretches to increase range of motion.

Guidelines

- Avoid extremes in motion of flexion and extension.
- Avoid jarring and twisting motions.

ARTHRITIS

Kneeling Wrist Stretch	page 77	Quad Setting	page 238
Elbow Touches	page 73	Seated Leg Extensions	page 233
Rear Calf Stretch	page 116	Leg Curls	page 242
Hold/Relax Turtle	page 59	Biceps Curls	page 273
Seated Knee to Chest	page 88	Shrugs	page 264

BACK PAIN

Lower back pain is caused by a variety of sources: weak abdominal muscles, improper body mechanics, poor posture, overuse, and facet and joint problems along with herniated discs. Since there are many causes, always consult a health professional for a proper diagnosis.

It is also a good idea to have a physical therapist show you how to stand properly and teach you proper body mechanics for daily life activities so as not to exacerbate your condition any further. Core training stabilizes and supports the spine by strengthening the muscles that surround the spine and torso, commonly called the "core." It's much like building your own internal back brace. Think of your body as a sunflower: Develop a solid stem to hold the flower tall. See pages 22–24 for a brief lesson on how to stand and sit properly.

Most back issues can be improved with a sound exercise program using proper body mechanics. However, avoid overdoing it and performing questionable moves. Once a person has had a back problem, it is likely to occur again.

BACK PAIN			
Bicycle	page 249	Shoulder Retractions	page 262
Curl-Ups (Weights)	page 248	Triceps Band Extensions	page 284
Buttocks Lifts	page 251	Sit & Reach	page 99
Pointer	page 252	Seated Knee to Chest	page 88
Incline Presses	page 257	Figure 4	page 104
Military Presses Variation	page 267	Rock 'n' Roll on Roller	page 93

Guidelines

- If you notice an increase in pain and/or numbness in your legs or feet, stop and see your health professional.
- Avoid movements that increase the load on your spine, such as the Military Press and bending over at the waist.

BREATHING CONDITIONS

Chronic obstructive pulmonary disease (COPD) is a progressive disorder of the lungs characterized by the destruction of the alveoli, retention of mucus secretions, and so on. Common conditions grouped under this heading include bronchitis, asthma, emphysema, and sometimes, allergies—all of which make breathing difficult. It is common to see individuals who have COPD not engage in much activity. Research shows that a slow, progressive overall fitness program often leads to better aerobic fitness, which in turn leads to a better quality of life.

A gentle strength-training program with several rest breaks is the first step toward reversing the downward spiral often associated with COPD. The goal of strength training is to improve the muscles of the legs that make getting up and down from a chair easier, as well as being able to move around without getting short of breath. This program will also improve ventilation, improve strength and endurance of respiratory muscles, maintain and improve chest and back mobility, improve leg strength to make activities of daily living easier, and teach effective breathing patterns.

Guidelines

- Start very, very slow. Avoid getting out of breath.
- Never overextend yourself. It is better to do 1–2 minutes of exercise, rest, and then repeat your bout of exercise than it is to try to work up to 10–15 minutes of non-stop exercise.
- Learn how to do "pursed-lip breathing" from your health care provider and follow their recommendations. If you use an inhaler, consult your doctor about exercising and the use of the device.

BREATHING CONDITIONS

Shoulder Retractions	page 262	Seated Leg Extensions	page 233
Bow & Arrow	page 263	Elbow Touches	page 73
Shrugs	page 264	Long Body Stretch	page 122
Sit to Stand	page 232		

DIABETES

There are two types of diabetes mellitus: juvenile diabetes, or type 1 diabetes, and adult-onset diabetes, or type 2 diabetes. When a person has diabetes, the body does not provide enough of the hormone insulin, which helps regulate the amount of sugar in the bloodstream.

Regular exercise can help a person with diabetes stabilize the condition. Having diabetes or being at risk for developing diabetes is not an excuse not to exercise but rather a reason to exercise. As with any other chronic condition, prior to starting an exercise program, consult your health professional for any special recommendations and precautions specific to you.

Flexibility training is another important aspect of training for someone with diabetes.

Guidelines

- Set a goal of performing at least 30 minutes of aerobic exercise most days of the week at a comfortable pace. If you are unable to do 30 minutes of non-stop exercise, it is okay to break it up into three bouts of 10 minutes each.
- Avoid activities that are stressful to your feet.

- Extended warm-up and cool-down periods are important for diabetics when transitioning from moderate exercise to rest.
- Perform strength-training loads that are not strenuous. Do 10–15 reps with a light to moderate load. If you have diabetic retinopathy, avoid intense exercise such as lifting heavy weights.
- Train at a heart rate that is less than someone who does not have diabetes. Train, don't strain.
- Consult your health professional about which insulin level and glucose level is right for you. Keep some hard candy or easily digestible carbohydrate available should you need it.
- Exercise at predictable times to minimize blood sugar fluctuations.
- Be alert to signs of hypoglycemia and diabetic coma.
- Drink fluids regularly.
- Monitor your blood pressure levels (consult your doctor regarding this matter).
- If you are injecting insulin, be mindful of where the injection is and what set of muscles you are planning to use. Discuss with your health professional about appropriate injection sites when exercising. A general tip is not to inject the area that you will be exercising that day.

Don't exercise if you have:

- Retinal hemorrhages
- Fever or infection
- Very low or very high blood glucose levels (consult your doctor for specific details).

DIABETES

Hold/Relax Turtle	page 59	Shrugs	page 264
Kneeling Wrist Stretch	page 77	Seated Leg Extensions	page 233
Lunges (Weights)	page 236	Biceps Curls	page 273
Pull-Downs	page 261	Rear Calf Stretch	page 116

HEART ISSUES

Heart disease, the leading cause of death for both men and women in the United States, includes such things as high blood pressure, arteriosclerosis, coronary artery disease, angina, and congestive heart disease. Fit people have less heart disease than do less-fit individuals. A sensible and medically approved exercise program, along with modifications in diet and stress levels, will improve the quality of life. If you have had a heart attack or stroke, it is prudent to attend a medically supervised exercise program before exercising on your own.

Many people who have suffered a heart attack are afraid to live for fear of dying. This can often be more devastating than the heart attack itself, which is why a regular fitness routine is so critical to the person who wants to fully engage in the mainstream of life once more. Strength training should only be added after a baseline of fitness has been achieved and your doctor has given you permission to do so. Strength training can help activities of daily living become less strenuous. In addition to engaging in a sensible exercise program, a healthy lifestyle must be adopted: Stop smoking; eat right and eat lean; reduce stress; exercise aerobically; follow your doctor's recommendations, and take your medications as directed.

Guidelines

- If you are on a beta-blocker or similar medication to "cap" your heart rate, use the "talk test" to determine your intensity: If you can't talk easily, then you are working too hard—slow down.
- Slow and steady wins the race: Avoid exercising hard and fast. You are exercising for your life—don't put it at risk while exercising.

HEART ISSUES

Hold/Relax Turtle	page 59	Leg Presses	page 237
Kneeling Wrist Stretch	page 77	Leg Curls	page 242
Chair Push-Ups	page 254	Biceps Curls	page 273
Sit to Stand	page 232	Triceps Band Extensions	page 284

HIGH BLOOD PRESSURE

It is believed that high blood pressure (hypertension) is the third most common chronic condition in the United States, right behind sinusitis and arthritis. Your blood pressure fluctuates from moment to moment and is affected by everything from stress and environmental stimulation to physical exertion. High blood pressure is a major risk factor in developing a stroke, heart disease, and several other health issues. High blood pressure is often called the silent killer since it does not manifest any outward symptoms until either you die, have a stroke, or have a heart attack. Always monitor your blood pressure! It is wise to ask your doctor if resistance training is okay for you before starting.

The first approach to improving blood pressure is lifestyle changes that include diet, stress management, and regular exercise. Numerous studies have shown that aerobic exercise has a positive influence on lowering blood pressure. Use caution if you choose to strength train. Strength training can elevate your blood pressure to dangerous levels; therefore, consult your doctor before doing any strength-training moves.

Guidelines

- Avoid heavy strength training. Performing higher reps with light weights is a better way to go.
- If your blood pressure is above 160/90, check with your doctor before lifting weights.

- Be careful of overhead lifts.

- Always adequately warm up and cool down. People with vascular issues such as high or low blood pressure can get into trouble if they start out too hard and stop exercising abruptly.

- Emphasize muscular endurance over strength and power. The goal should be to do a higher number of reps rather than fewer reps with a heavier load.

HIGH BLOOD PRESSURE

Chair Push-Ups	page 254	Biceps Curls	page 273
Sit to Stand	page 232	Triceps Band Extensions	page 284
Leg Presses	page 237	Outer Thigh Stretch	page 115
Leg Curls	page 242		

KNEE PROBLEMS

Chronic knee problems can be the result of poor anatomical design. For example, being knock-kneed or bowlegged can set you up for injury. Simple activities such as jogging or even walking can increase the load on the knee joint three to five times the person's body weight. In addition, sports injuries from soccer, football, or even biking with poor form can harm your knees. The causes of knee problems are many and range from arthritis to misuse and abuse. See your doctor to get a proper diagnosis and corrective suggestions. To reduce knee pain, strengthen all the muscles of your quads, and remember that exercise should not increase pain or swelling.

Guidelines

- Always point your toes and knees in the same direction.
- Never go past your safe range of motion.
- Avoid over-straightening your legs.
- If you are told to wear a brace when exercising, be sure to follow all recommendations.
- Ice your knee after exercise, if recommended.
- Wear good supportive shoes and replace them every 500 miles or three to six months.

KNEE PROBLEMS

Quad Setting	page 238	Seated Leg Extensions	page 233
Prone Quad Stretch	page 111	Lunges (Weights)	page 236
Wall Squats	page 241	Leg Curls	page 242
Leg Presses	page 237	Rear Calf Stretch	page 116

OSTEOPOROSIS

Osteoporosis is a significant loss of bone mass that leads to increased porosity, making the bone more at risk for a fracture. One of the leading risk factors is lack of regular weight-bearing exercise. Osteoporosis is a silent disease; the first sign of it is often a fracture. A turn can cause the hip joint to snap; a simple fall can result in a fracture of the wrist or, even worse, a broken hip.

Fortunately, osteoporosis is not inevitable. It is never too late for action. Your bones are living structures that are re-modeling themselves every day. Along with sound lifestyle choices, resistance-training exercise can minimize the weakening of your bones. Wolfe's law says that "the robustness of the bone is directly related to the forces applied to it." In other words, your bones are what you make of them. If you lead a sedentary life, you will have bones designed for easy living; if, on the other hand, you challenge your bones, you will have bones better prepared for an occasional tumble. Additionally, if you make your muscles stronger, the research shows that the bones will get stronger too. Also, if you get stronger, maybe you will be strong enough to catch your balance and not fall. If you only have osteopenia now, by beginning strength training right now you may be able to prevent yourself from ever developing full-blown osteoporosis.

Strength-training exercises have been shown to improve balance and gait, improve flexibility, and reverse muscle atrophy, which can prevent falls. Strength training also places good stresses on bones that will stimulate density of the bones and improve their density.

Exercise Contraindications

While exercise has been proven to improve bone density, certain exercises could cause a compression fracture. Therefore, avoid the following moves:

- Bent over rowing
- Overhead lifts with weights
- Twisting moves
- Squats with a load placed on your shoulders or any exercise that places a load down on your spine
- Heavy-impact moves

OSTEOPOROSIS

Heel Raises	page 246	Single-Arm Rows	page 259
Sit to Stand	page 232	Back Flatteners	page 251
Leg Presses	page 237	Buttocks Lifts	page 251
Shoulder Retractions	page 262	Outer Thigh Stretch	page 115

SHOULDER PROBLEMS

The design of the shoulder is remarkable, allowing a baseball pitcher to throw a ball 90 mph or allowing a person to rock a baby to sleep. The shoulder is a ball and socket joint that gets its support from muscles, ligaments, and tendons. Some experts believe that when you move your arm, as many as 26 muscles are engaged at some time in the movement. The more active you are, the greater the risk of injuring your shoulder. It is common to see adults over 50 years of age suffer from a shoulder condition as they get older. Shoulder problems can be the result of many things, including bursitis and tendinitis; or they can be idiopathic (i.e., no known cause).

Many times the corrective exercises will be the same regardless of the cause. But it is still wise to have a medical doctor provide you with a proper diagnosis and have a physical therapist give you corrective exercises. Some of the common conditions seen in the older adult population are rotator cuff injury and frozen shoulder. Stretching is very important for people with shoulder problems—I've included some in this workout.

Exercise Contraindications: Avoid overhead arm exercises or any moves that increase pain and/or limit your range of motion.

SHOULDER PROBLEMS

Internal Rotations	page 271	Pull-Downs	page 261
External Rotations	page 272	Soup Can Pours	page 65
Reverse Band Flyes	page 260	Bow & Arrow	page 263
Shrugs	page 264	Choker	page 70
Sword Fighters (Band)	page 269	Over the Top	page 69
Reverse Sword Fighters	page 270	Seated Inner Thigh Stretch	page 96

***

Many sports and recreational pursuits require the body to perform the same movement over and over again, causing overuse syndrome and the adaptive shortening of a muscle. Strength training for recreational pursuits has several functions. It reverses the muscle imbalances caused by repetitive movements, and it strengthens the muscle so that it can handle the stress placed on it when training. In this sense, strength training prevents possible injuries. A well-conditioned muscle easily outperforms a weak or unconditioned muscle. Here are some workouts for popular activities.

BIKING

More than just a lower body activity, biking impacts overall posture. In addition, it places much of your weight on your wrists and hands. While biking does primarily engage the lower body, requiring muscular endurance and strength of the legs and stamina of the lower back, a person needs enough strength to support the upper body and head.

A fitness program for cycling conditions all the muscles of the leg in addition to correcting the muscles of the body that are fostering poor posture. The bottom line is to increase the strength and endurance of the lower extremities by performing higher reps, as well as condition the upper body to counteract any muscular imbalances caused by cycling.

BIKING

Squeezer	page 79	Reverse Band Flyes	page 260
Inverted Figure 4	page 103	Shoulder Retractions	page 262
Lunges (Weights)	page 236	Curl-Ups (Weights)	page 248
Hands and Knees Leg Curls	page 244	Side Quad Stretch	page 110
Single-Leg Squats	page 239	Buttocks Lifts	page 251
Standing Leg Extensions	page 234	Rear Calf Stretch	page 116
Lateral Arm Raises	page 265	Pec Stretch	page 75
Prone Reverse Flyes (Weights)	page 258	Double Knee to Chest	page 90

ADVANCED ADDITIONS

Band Push-Ups	page 256	Chair Dips 2	page 283
Chair Dips 1	page 282		

BOWLING

Many people don't think of bowling as a sport, yet it can be very hard on the lower back, hips, and shoulders. Bowling is a one-sided activity that requires you to throw a heavy ball with significant force to knock over the pins. This can cause muscle imbalances, which can lead to injury. Strength training can help to correct many of these issues by strengthening the total body as well as improving flexibility. Since bowling is an activity that requires strength and power, you should work toward improving both. Therefore, once you establish a baseline of muscular strength and endurance, start focusing on doing moves more quickly. However, keep in mind that explosive moves put you at more risk for injury, so train smart, not hard.

GOLF

Many people compete at golf, either against others or themselves. Golf is a tough game on the body, requiring twisting of the knees and lower back. This asymmetrical sport, with moves repeated sometimes up to 90 times, presents a whole set of problems. Ironically, the worse you are at the game, the harder it is on your body because you take more swings—with biomechanically incorrect form.

A golfer does not require big muscles or a lot of strength, but the game requires controlled power. Therefore, your exercise program should try to replicate the moves and the speed used on the course. But for your health, a sound fitness program should be aimed at undoing the unilateral movement. Work all the muscles of the body and keep the body fluid. Stretch what is tight and inflexible, and strengthen what is weak. After you develop a baseline of strength, increase your power by doing the moves more quickly. However, be careful—ballistic moves can cause injuries.

JOGGING/WALKING

Walking and jogging are excellent aerobic activities that, unfortunately, stress the lower limbs by placing three to five times your body weight on your knees. However, the muscles of the torso are engaged as well, so when designing your routine, place most of your focus on upper body conditioning and stretching the muscles of the lower body and back. Focus on muscular endurance more than strength and power. A strength program for a walker/jogger will be aimed at higher reps with lighter load.

JOGGING/WALKING

Bent-Over Toe Touch	page 100	Wall Squats	page 241
Inverted Figure 4	page 103	Heel Raises	page 246
Shrugs	page 264	Rear Calf Stretch	page 116
Sword Fighters (Band)	page 269	Sit & Reach	page 99
Seated Rows	page 263	Squeezer	page 79
Incline Presses	page 257	Elbow Touches	page 73
Hammer Curls	page 274	Pretzel	page 114
Side-Lying Triceps Extensions	page 279	Seated Inner Thigh Stretch	page 96
Curl-Ups (Weights)	page 248	Side Quad Stretch	page 110
Buttocks Lifts	page 251	Prone Quad Stretch	page 111
Straight-Leg Lifts	page 235	Kneeling Quad Stretch	page 112

ADVANCED ADDITIONS

Band Push-Ups	page 256	Chair Dips 2	page 283
Chair Dips 1	page 282		

SWIMMING

Although swimming does not provide much challenge for the bones of the body, it is an excellent way to improve cardiovascular fitness. However, people mistakenly believe that swimming is a gentle way to get fit. In fact, swimming can be hard on the shoulders and even the neck and lower back if your form is faulty. Another problem arises if you don't vary your strokes—all the muscles on the front of your body get worked (and consequently get tight) while your upper back becomes hunched over.

If you are a competitive swimmer, you need to focus on improving your muscular endurance. If you are swimming for health and fitness, you'll want to improve muscular strength, challenge the bones of the body by doing weight-bearing exercises, and reverse hunched-over posture. When designing your routine, the bottom line is to stretch what is tight and inflexible and strengthen what is weak.

SWIMMING

Hold/Relax Turtle	page 59	Sit to Stand	page 232
Kneeling Wrist Stretch	page 77	Leg Curls	page 242
Squeezer	page 79	Lunges (Weights)	page 236
Bent-Over Triceps Extensions with Chair	page 280	Prone Quad Stretch	page 111
Frontal Arm Raises	page 266	Soup Can Pours	page 65
Upright Rows	page 268	Elbow Touches	page 73
Reverse Sword Fighters	page 270	Pec Stretch	page 75
Pull-Downs	page 261	The Zipper	page 71
Incline Presses	page 257	Rock 'n' Roll on Roller	page 93
Reverse Band Flyes	page 260		

SKIING

Skiing requires good lower body strength and endurance. You also have to contend with cold weather and high altitudes—generally, the muscles, tendons, and ligaments of people over 50 often gel up under these circumstances. Skiing is a total-body sport that can be hard on the shoulders and the knees.

Downhill skiing is explosive, asking you to work hard for short periods of time, whereas cross-country skiing requires good muscular endurance. Both forms of skiing also place high demands on the upper body when using your poles either to plant for a turn or pull. This sport insists that you be in fine shape if you plan to ski aggressively, and demands that you be well conditioned before you make your trek up the mountain, so your training routine should start long before you plan to ski. Specificity of training is required in this sport. The routine for cross-country skiing is much different than downhill skiing. However, both require a baseline of cardiovascular fitness and an OK by the doctor before heading to the mountains. The purpose of this strength-training program is to give you a total-body workout that addresses muscular power and endurance.

DOWNHILL SKIING

CROSS-COUNTRY SKIING

TENNIS/PICKLEBALL

Tennis and pickleball are fun but can take their toll on the lower body, shoulders, and elbows. The knees take a pounding and also make quick turns and twists. The shoulders reach and stretch in all directions and respond with speed and power. The load placed upon the back, not to mention the cardiovascular system, is tremendous. Additionally, for most people tennis and pickleball are one-sided sports, further contributing to physical problems. Many people over 50 find that a singles game of tennis is more than they want to engage in and opt for a friendly game of doubles.

The following strength program gives you enough strength to continue playing. Since tennis and pickleball are explosive sports that require bursts of speed and power, once you establish a baseline of muscular strength and endurance, your program should start focusing on developing power by doing moves more quickly. However, keep in mind that explosive moves put you at more risk for injury, so train smart, not hard. But most important and critical for the health of your body is a total comprehensive fitness program that includes exercising all the muscles of the body, regular stretching, and aerobic work.

TENNIS/PICKLEBALL

WEIGHT AND RESISTANCE TRAINING EXERCISES

Standing Leg Raises

Target: outer thighs

If you find this exercise too difficult, try it without weights.

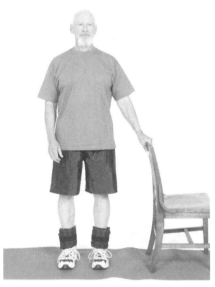 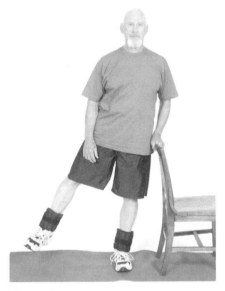 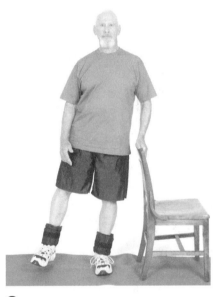

1. Strap an ankle weight around each ankle and stand with proper posture. Place your left hand on a stable chair for balance. Inhale to begin.

2. Keeping your foot pointed forward, exhale and slowly raise the outside leg out to the side as high as is comfortable and hold.

3. Inhale and slowly return to starting position with control.

Repeat, then switch sides.

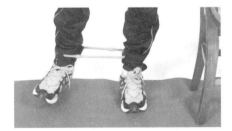

VARIATION: To perform this with an exercise band, tie the ends of the band together and loop it around both ankles.

Leg Squeeze & Spread

Target: inner & outer thighs

Do not apply too much resistance in either of these steps.

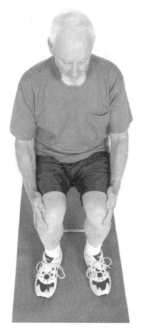 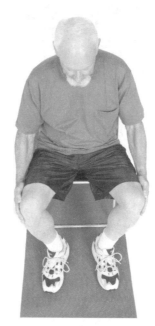 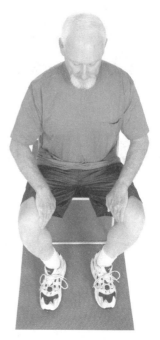

1. Sit toward the front of a chair with both feet flat on the floor. Place your hands on the outsides of your thighs near your knees. Breathe comfortably.

2. Spread your legs a comfortable width as you resist the motion with your hands.

3. Now place your hands on the insides of your thighs and resist the motion as you squeeze your legs together.

Side Lunges

This is a very advanced move and requires excellent balance. Beginners can hold onto a chair for balance or try this without weights.

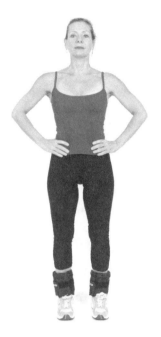

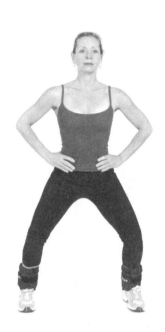

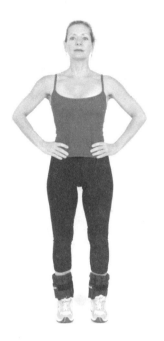

1. Strap an ankle weight around each ankle and stand with proper posture, hands on your hips. Inhale to begin.

2. Exhale and slowly step out to the left side, making sure your knees don't go past your toes.

3. Inhale to return to starting position.

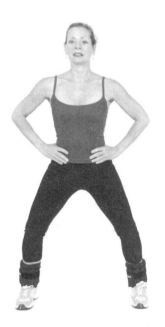

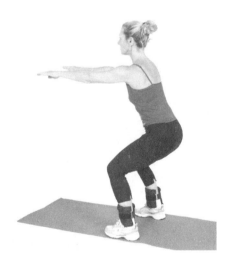

4. Exhale and slowly step out to the right side. Inhale to return to starting position.

VARIATION: As this move becomes easy, you can step out to the side and perform a quarter squat.

Side-Lying Leg Raises

Target: outer thighs

If you find this exercise too difficult, try it without weights.

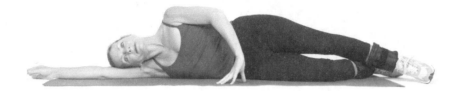

1. Strap an ankle weight around each ankle and lie on the right side of your body, positioning your body in a comfortable position so as to not hurt your back. You can bend your lower leg to reduce stress on your back. Rest your head on your right upper arm and straighten the top leg. Inhale to begin.

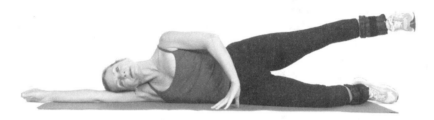

2. Keeping your left leg straight, exhale and lift it up to shoulder height.

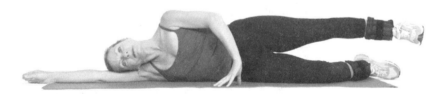

3. Inhale and slowly return to starting position.

Repeat, then switch sides.

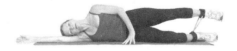

VARIATION: To perform this with an exercise band, tie the ends of the band together and loop it around both ankles.

Reverse Side-Lying Leg Raises

Target: inner thighs

If you find this exercise too difficult, try it without weights.

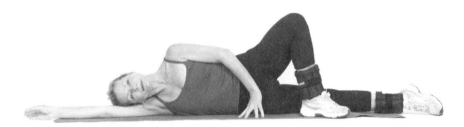

1. Strap an ankle weight around each ankle and lie on the right side of your body. Rest your head on your right upper arm and straighten the lower leg. Bend your top leg and place the foot over and in front of your other leg; try to keep this foot flat on the floor. Place your other hand on the floor in front of your pelvis for support. Inhale to begin.

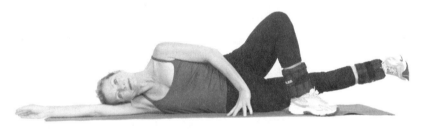

2. Keeping your lower leg straight, exhale and lift it as high as is comfortable and hold.

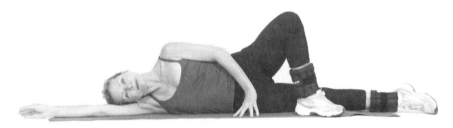

3. Inhale and lower to starting position.

Repeat, then switch sides.

Sit to Stand

If you find this exercise too difficult, try it without weights.

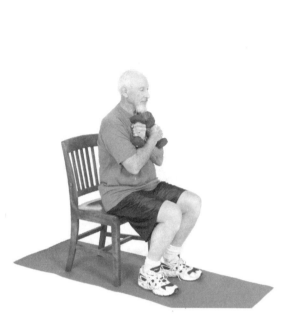 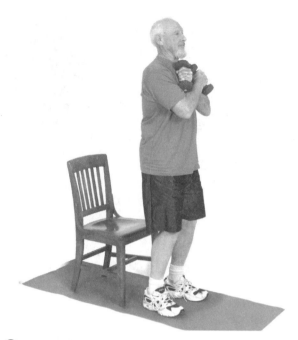

1. Sit toward the front of a sturdy chair, placing your feet flat on the floor, just slightly behind your knees. Hold a dumbbell in each hand and cross your arms in front of your chest. Lean slightly forward and keep your torso firm as you perform this exercise. Inhale to begin.

2. Exhale and slowly stand up without using your hands, if possible.

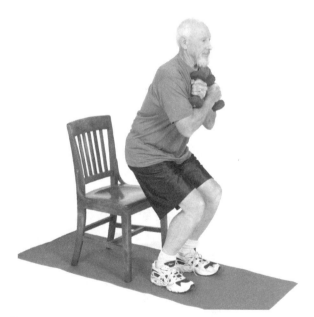

3. Inhale and lower yourself slowly into the chair.

Seated Leg Extensions

Target: quadriceps

If you have long legs, roll up a towel and place it under your knees to raise them. If you find this exercise too difficult, try it without weights.

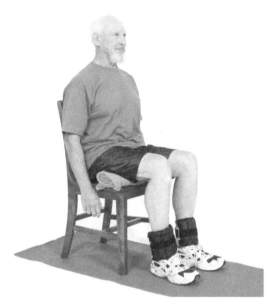

1. Strap an ankle weight to each ankle and sit with your back against the back of the chair. Place your hands in a comfortable position. Inhale to begin.

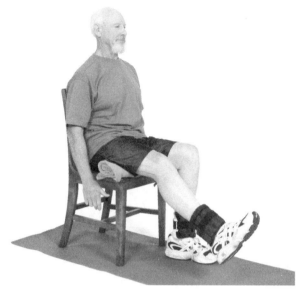

2. Exhale and slowly extend your right leg until it's straight, but not hyperextended. Hold for a count of 1-2.

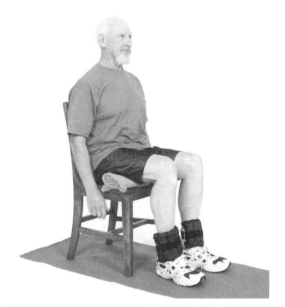

3. Inhale and slowly return your leg to starting position.

Repeat, then switch sides.

Standing Leg Extensions

If you find this exercise too difficult, try it without weights.

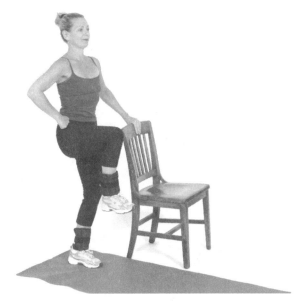

1. Strap an ankle weight to each ankle and stand with proper posture next to a sturdy chair. Lift your right thigh in front of you as high as is comfortable (but no higher than parallel with the floor). Inhale to begin.

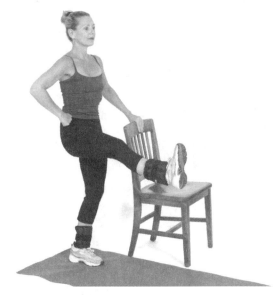

2. Exhale and slowly extend (kick) your right foot forward until it is fully extended. Hold for a count of 1-2.

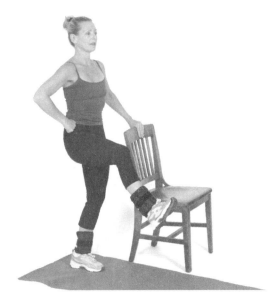

3. Inhale and slowly return your leg to starting position.

Repeat, then switch sides.

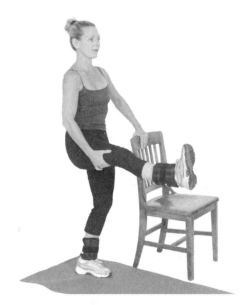

MODIFICATION: If you are not strong enough to hold the leg up unsupported, it is okay to use your hands to help keep the leg up.

Straight-Leg Lifts

Target: quadriceps

If you find this exercise too difficult, try it without weights.

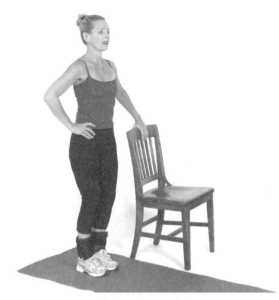

1. Strap an ankle weight to each ankle and stand next to a sturdy chair. Maintain proper posture throughout the movement. Inhale to begin.

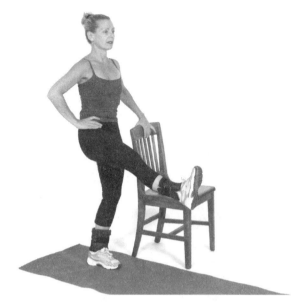

2. Exhale and straighten your outside leg and move it forward as high as is comfortable. Make sure you don't lean back while you raise your leg.

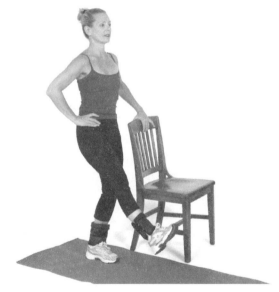

3. Inhale and slowly return to starting position.

Repeat, then switch sides.

Lunges (Weights)

If you find this too difficult, do a bodyweight lunge; do the movement without weights and place your hands on your hips instead.

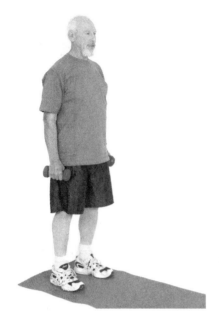 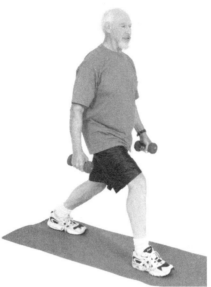 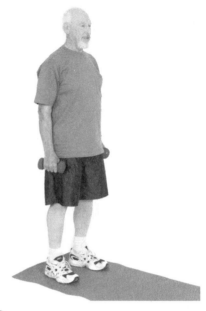

1. Stand with proper posture and hold a dumbbell in each hand by your sides. Inhale to begin.

2. Keeping your left leg in place, exhale and lunge forward with your right leg as far as is comfortable, but keeping your knee in line with your ankle.

3. Inhale as you step back to starting position.

Repeat, then switch sides.

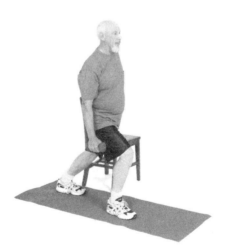

MODIFICATION: If balance is an issue, hold a dumbbell in one hand and hold onto a chair with your free hand.

VARIATION: As your balance and strength improve, alternate legs with each lunge rather than doing all reps on one side.

Leg Presses

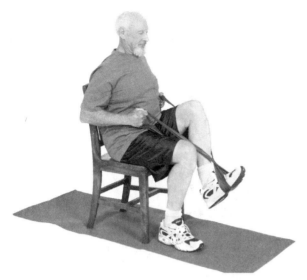

1. Sit with proper posture in the middle of the chair. Wrap the exercise band around your left foot once and hold onto the ends of the band. Inhale to begin.

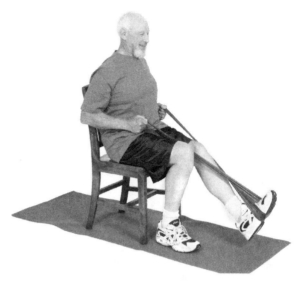

2. Exhale and slowly extend your left leg forward, but do not lock your knee.

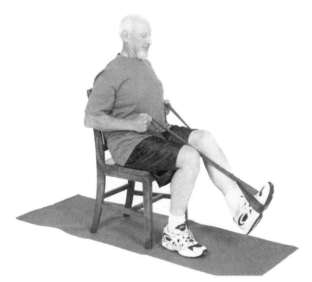

3. Inhale and slowly return to starting position.

Repeat, then switch sides.

Quad Setting

If you find this exercise too difficult, try it without weights.

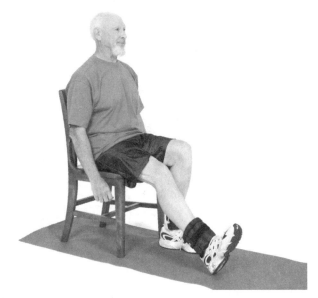

1. Strap an ankle weight to each ankle and sit in a chair with proper posture. Straighten your right leg by tightening the upper leg muscles. Inhale to begin.

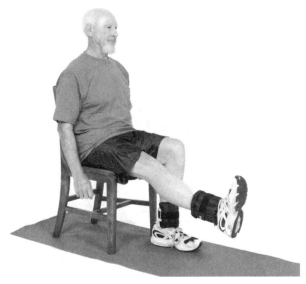

2. Keep your right leg straight as you exhale and lift it up so that it's parallel with the floor. Do not lean back as you lift your leg.

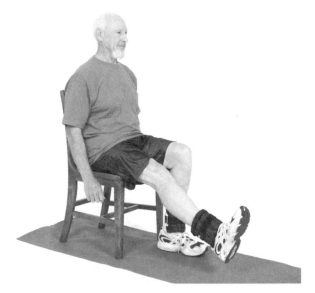

3. Inhale and slowly return the leg to the floor.

Repeat, then switch sides.

Single-Leg Squats

If you find this exercise too difficult, try it without weights.

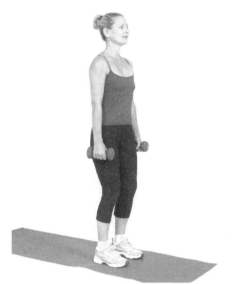 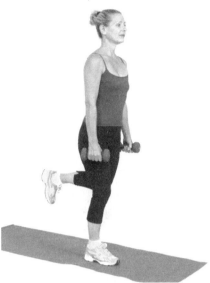 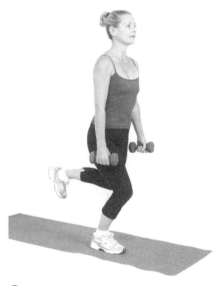

1. Stand with proper posture and hold a dumbbell in each hand.

2. Inhale and bring your left heel up halfway toward your buttocks or as high as is comfortable.

3. Exhale and slowly squat down as low as you can on your other leg, keeping your foot flat on the floor.

Inhale and slowly return to full standing position.

Repeat, then switch sides.

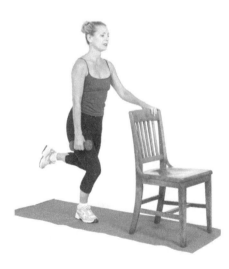

MODIFICATION: If balance is an issue, hold one weight and hold onto a chair or wall with your free hand for support.

Downhill Skier

If you find this exercise too difficult, try it without weights.

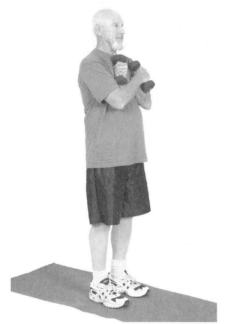 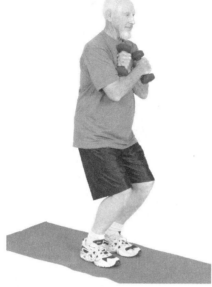 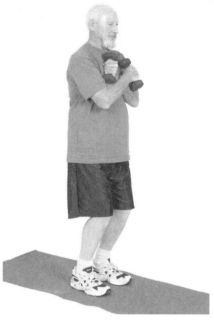

1. Stand with both feet as close together as is comfortable. Hold a dumbbell in each hand and cross your arms over your chest. Inhale to begin.

2. Exhale and squat down a quarter of the way, keeping your feet flat on the floor and your knees over your toes. Do not allow your knees to turn in or out. Hold for a count of 1-2-3-4-5.

3. Inhale and slowly return to starting position.

MODIFICATION: If balance is an issue, try the movement without weights and hold onto a chair for support.

Wall Squats

CAUTION: If you have heart or blood-pressure issues, avoid this exercise.

If you find this exercise too difficult, try it without weights.

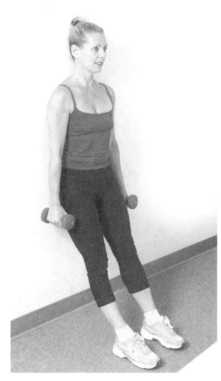 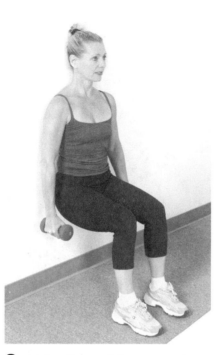 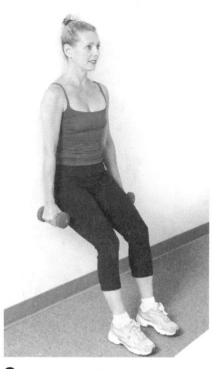

1. Stand with your back against the wall and your feet approximately 12–18 inches from the wall. Hold a dumbbell in each hand. Inhale to begin.

2. Using the wall for support, exhale and lower yourself as low as is comfortable or until your thighs are parallel with the floor. Do not allow your knees to extend past your toes. Hold for a count of 1-2-3-4-5, breathing comfortably. As your strength improves, hold the position up to 30 or 60 seconds.

3. Inhale and slowly return to starting position.

Leg Curls

CAUTION: Avoid this exercise if you have lower back issues.

If you find this exercise too difficult, try it without weights.

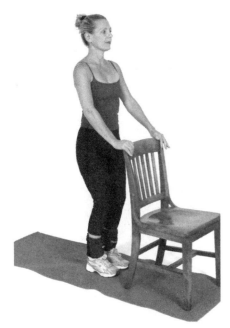 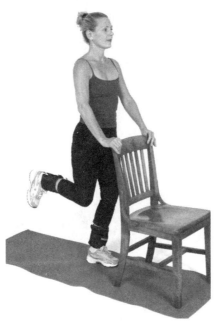 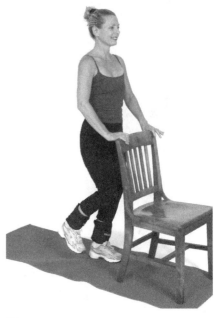

1. Strap an ankle weight to each ankle and stand with proper posture, both feet together. Hold onto the back of a stable chair for balance. Inhale to begin.

2. Slowly exhale as you curl your right leg up toward your buttocks. Stop when your leg is parallel to the ground.

3. Hold for a moment, then inhale as you slowly return the leg to starting position.

Repeat, then switch sides.

Prone Leg Curls

CAUTION: Avoid this exercise if lying on your stomach is uncomfortable. However, placing a pillow or rolled-up towel under your hips does help most people.

If you find this exercise too difficult, try it without weights.

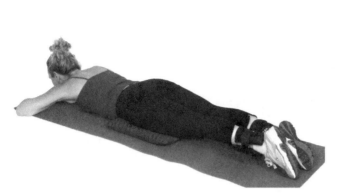

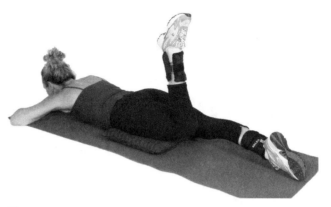

1. Strap an ankle weight to each ankle and lie face-down on the floor. If necessary, position a pillow beneath your hips so that your back is in a comfortable neutral position. Rest your head on your forearms. Inhale to begin.

2. Exhale and slowly bring your left heel up toward your buttock, stopping when it reaches 90 degrees.

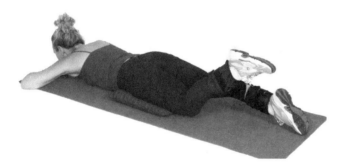

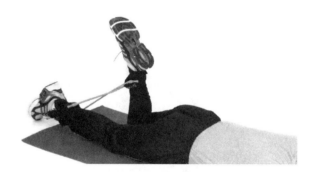

3. Inhale as you to slowly return your foot to starting position.

Repeat, then switch sides.

VARIATION: To perform this with an exercise band, tie the ends together and loop it around both ankles.

Hands and Knees Leg Curls

Target: hamstrings

If you find this exercise too difficult, try it without weights.

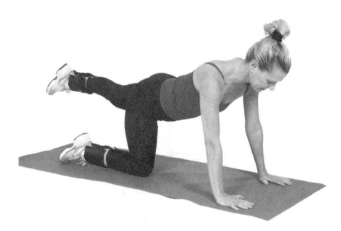

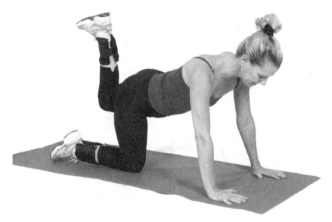

1. Strap an ankle weight to each ankle and get down on your hands and knees. Keeping your back straight, extend your left leg straight back and lift it up parallel to the floor; make sure your upper leg is parallel to the floor throughout the exercise. Inhale to begin.

2. Exhale as you bend your left knee and pull your heel toward your buttocks, stopping when you reach 90 degrees. Hold for a moment. If you feel a cramp coming on, stop and stretch your leg.

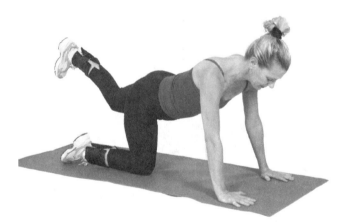

3. Inhale and extend your leg back to starting position.

Repeat, then switch sides.

Gas Pedals (Band)

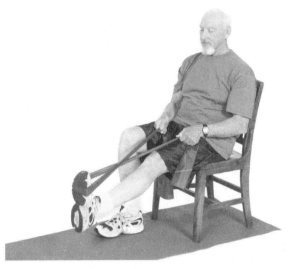

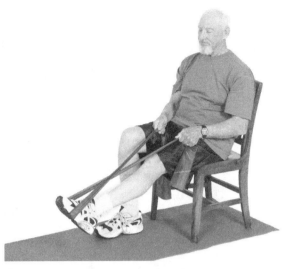

1. Sit in a chair with proper posture. Extend your left leg and loop a band around your foot, crossing the band above your shin for safety. Keep your leg straight and your toes pointing straight up. Inhale to begin.

2. Exhale and point your foot away from you, against the band's resistance. Hold for a moment.

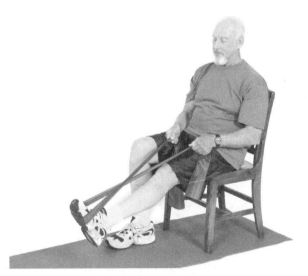

3. Inhale and return to starting position.

Repeat, then switch sides.

Heel Raises

If you find this exercise too difficult, try it without weights.

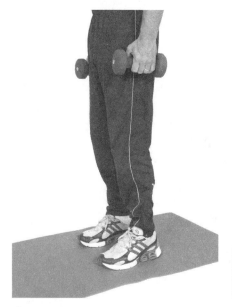

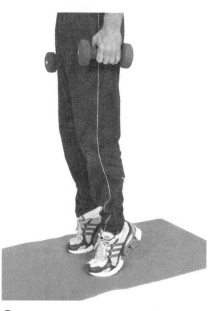

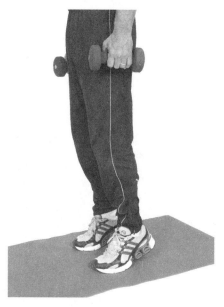

1. Stand with your feet hip-width apart and parallel to each other. Hold a dumbbell in each hand. Inhale to begin.

2. Exhale and slowly rise up onto the balls of your feet, lifting your heels off the floor. Hold for a moment.

3. Inhale to slowly return to starting position.

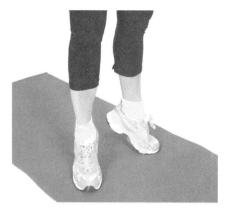

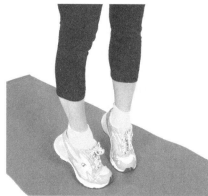

VARIATION 1: Point your toes out slightly and perform the heel raise.

VARIATION 2: Perform the move with the toes pointed slightly in.

MODIFICATION: If balance is an issue, use a chair to help steady yourself.

One-Leg Heel Raises

Target: calves

If you don't have a yoga block, you can use a 2x4 or some other solid, flat object like a telephone book.

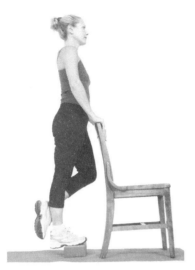

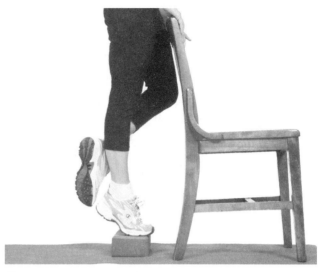

1. Place a yoga block on the floor behind a chair. Stand with the balls of your feet on the block and hold onto the chair for balance. Place your left foot behind your right heel. Inhale to begin.

2. Exhale as you rise up on the ball of your right foot as high as is comfortable. Do not perform this movement to an extreme range of motion. Hold for a moment.

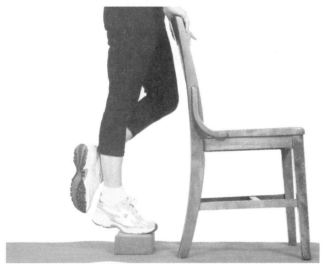

3. Inhale as you return to starting position.

Repeat, then switch sides. Stretch your calf muscle after completing a set.

Curl-Ups (Weights)

Target: abdominals

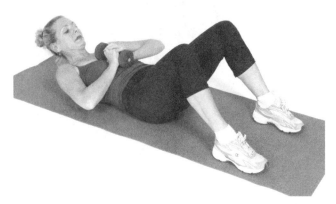

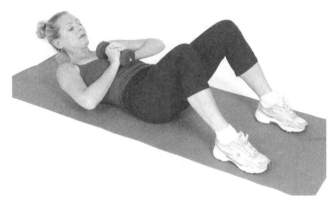

1. Lie on your back with your feet flat on the floor. Hold a dumbbell in your hands on top of your chest. Tuck your chin toward your chest. Inhale to begin.

2. Exhale as you lift your shoulders off the floor. Hold for a moment.

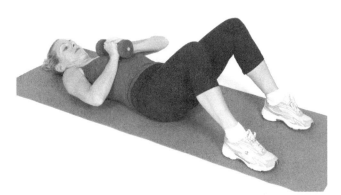

3. Inhale and slowly return to starting position.

MODIFICATION: To reduce the intensity, you can try this without weights. Place your hands lightly behind your head but be careful not to pull hard on your head.

Bicycle

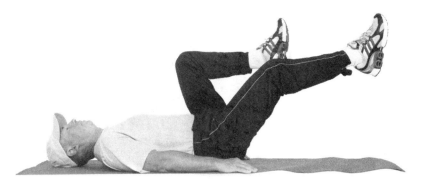

1. Lie on your back with your feet flat on the floor and your arms alongside your body. Keeping your lower back neutral throughout the exercise, lift both legs off the floor as if resting them on an imaginary chair. Keep control of your core. Inhale to begin.

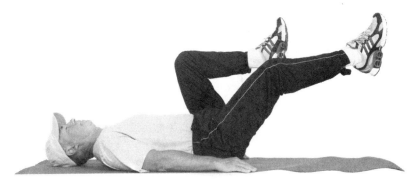

2. Without allowing your pelvis to rock or roll, exhale and contract your abdominal muscles as you press one leg forward and pull the other toward your chest.

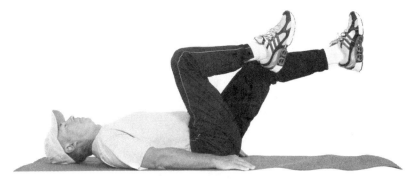

3. Inhale and switch sides, pressing the other leg forward as you pull the forward leg back.

Marching

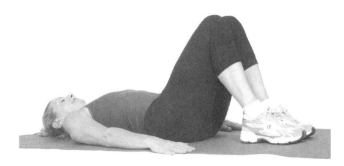

1. Lie on your back with your feet flat on the floor and your arms alongside your body. Keep your core contracted and your lower back in neutral throughout the movement.

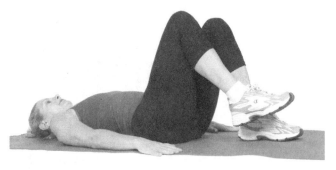

2. Imagining that a wire is pulling your knee upward, inhale and slowly lift your right foot an inch or two off the floor. The smaller the distance you lift the foot off the floor (such as leaving just enough space to slip a piece of paper under), the more challenging the move.

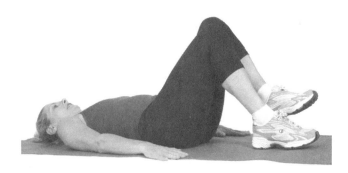

3. Exhale and slowly raise your left foot off the floor as you lower your right.

Back Flatteners

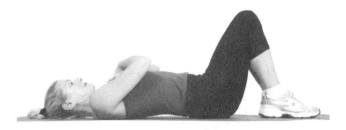 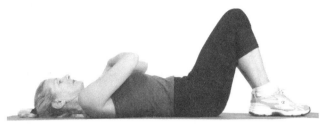

1. Lie on your back with your feet flat on the floor and your arms crossed over your chest. Inhale to begin.

2. Exhale and press your lower back into the floor (the normal curve of your spine should be lying flat so not even a piece of paper can slide between your back and the floor). Hold for a count of 1-2-3 and then relax.

Buttocks Lifts

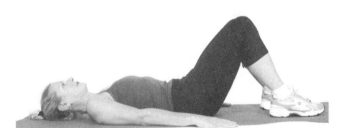 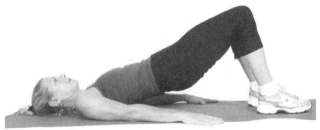

1. Lie on your back with your feet flat on the floor and your arms along your sides. Press the small of your back into the floor as you tighten your core muscles. Find your neutral spine position and maintain this position throughout the exercise. Inhale to begin.

2. Exhale and lift your hips and lower back off the floor. Hold this position for a moment, keeping your pelvic area stationary.

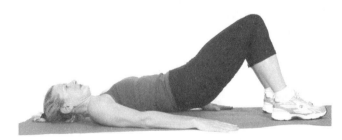 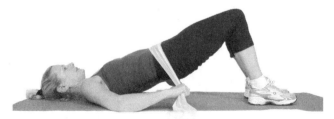

3. Inhale and lower yourself to the floor.

VARIATION: Perform the exercise after you've placed a band over your pelvis and secured the band in each hand at a position for ideal resistance.

Pointer

This can be very challenging. It is better to perform only a few perfectly than many with poor form. Try this without the weights if you find that they compromise your form.

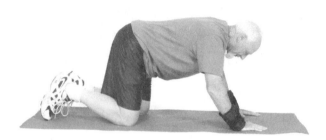

1. Start on your hands and knees, an ankle weight around each wrist. Pull in your abdominal muscles. Keep your back flat throughout the exercise. Breathe comfortably.

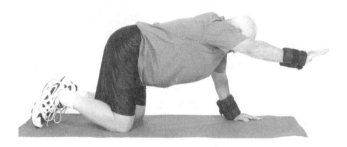

2. Lift your right arm slowly to shoulder height but no higher.

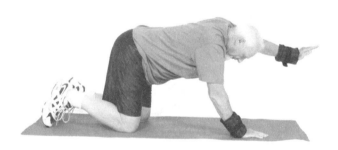

3. Return your right hand on the floor and raise your left arm.

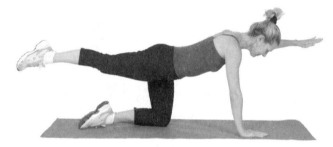

VARIATION: As your core strength improves, progress to raising your left arm and your right leg, then alternating with your right arm and your left leg. As you get stronger, you can also incorporate ankle weights.

Dumbbell Presses

Target: pectorals, front shoulders, triceps

This can also be done on a sturdy bench, but do not allow your elbows to drop below your torso.

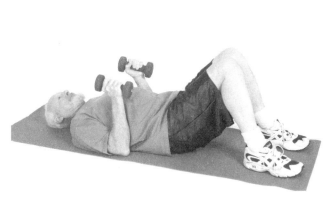 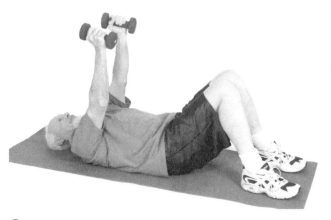

1. Lie on your back with your feet flat on the floor. Hold a dumbbell in each hand with your palms facing each other, your elbows resting on the ground, and your forearms perpendicular to the floor. Inhale to begin.

2. Exhale as you slowly press the dumbbells toward the ceiling, keeping your elbows close to your sides and your arms perpendicular to the ground. Don't allow your lower back to arch, and don't lock your elbows.

Inhale as you return to starting position.

Dumbbell Flyes

Target: pectorals

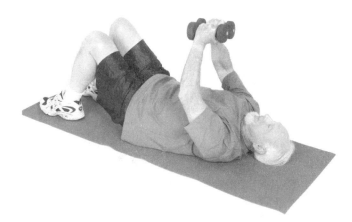 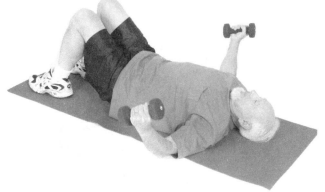

1. Lie on your back with your feet flat on the floor. Hold a dumbbell in each hand with your arms extended toward the ceiling and palms facing each other. Keep your elbows slightly bent, as if you were hugging a large barrel. Inhale to begin.

2. Exhale as you lower your arms out toward the floor to form a T; do not let your upper arms touch the ground. As you perform this move, keep your lower back flat on the floor.

Inhale as you return to starting position.

Chair Push-Ups

Target: pectorals, front shoulders, triceps

Caution: Be careful not to tip over the chair.

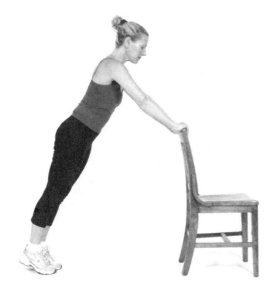
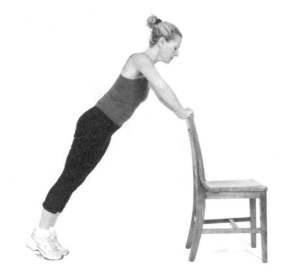

1. Stand with proper posture next to a sturdy surface such as a chair, table, or countertop. Lean forward and place your hands shoulder-width apart on the surface. Keep your arms fully extended while you walk your legs back until your body is at approximately a 45-degree angle. Your legs should be straight but not locked. Inhale to begin.

2. Exhale as you slowly lower your chest to the chair, trying to keep your elbows close to your body. Remember to keep your torso in a straight line with your legs.

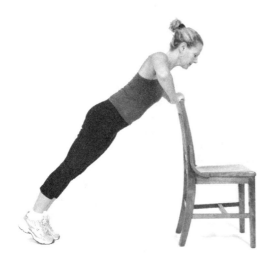
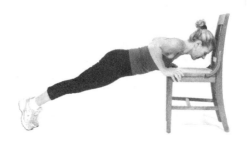

3. Inhale as you press your body away until your arms are fully extended without being locked.

ADVANCED VARIATION: To increase the resistance, use a sturdy surface, such as a coffee table or seat of a chair, that is closer to the ground. Once these become easy, progress to Baby Boomer Push-Ups.

Baby Boomer Push-Ups

Target: pectorals, front shoulders, triceps

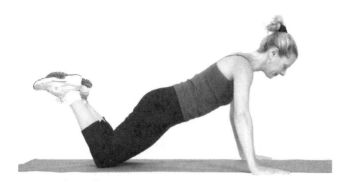

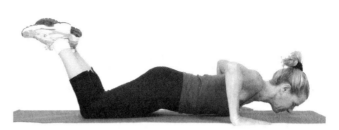

1. Start on your hands and knees, moving your hands forward so that your torso is slanted yet at a comfortable angle. Keep your back straight and pull your abdominal muscles in. Inhale to begin.

2. Exhale as you bend your elbows to lower your chest toward the floor. Keep your elbows close to your body and go down only as far as is comfortable. As you improve, try to get as close to the floor as possible without resting on it.

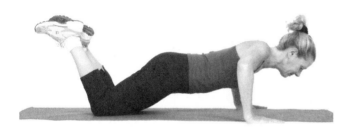

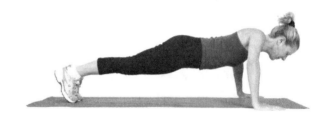

3. Inhale as you return to starting position.

ADVANCED VARIATION: As you become stronger, straighten your legs and perform the push-up from your hands and toes.

Band Push-Ups

Target: pectorals, front shoulders, triceps

The exercise band provides additional resistance in this challenging variation of the standard push-up.

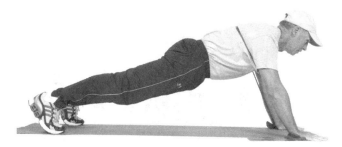

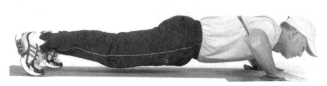

1. Assume a push-up position (your body should form one plane from head to heels) and position the band around your upper back and under your arms. Keeping your arms extended, secure the ends of the bands under your hands. Spread your legs about hip-width apart. Inhale to begin.

2. Exhale as you slowly lower your body to the floor, trying to keep your elbows close to your body. Only go as low as you feel comfortable.

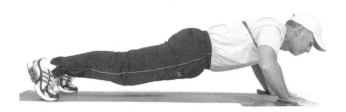

3. Inhale as you extend your arms to starting position. Once you start to sag in the middle or lift your butt, you have lost proper form—stop!

Incline Presses

Target: pectorals, front shoulders, triceps

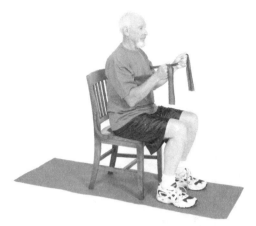 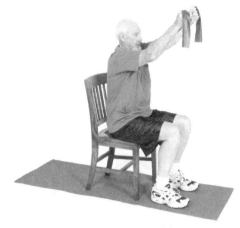

1. Sit with proper posture in a stable chair with your feet flat on the floor. Wrap the exercise band around your back and under your arms. Grasp the band in each hand at a length that provides adequate resistance. Position your hands close to your torso, palms facing in and elbows by your sides. Inhale to begin.

2. Exhale as you press your arms up at a 45-degree angle. Keep the movement controlled.

Inhale and resist the band as you return to starting position.

High Flyes

Target: pectorals, front shoulders

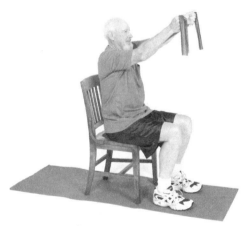 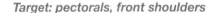 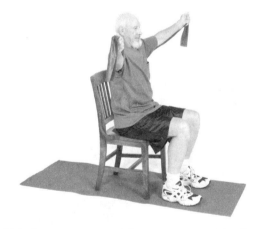

1. Sit with proper posture in a stable chair with your feet flat on the floor. Wrap the exercise band around your back and under your arms. Grasp the band in each hand at a length that provides adequate resistance. Position your hands close to your torso, palms facing in and elbows by your sides. Straighten your arms upward at a 45-degree angle. Inhale to begin.

2. Exhale as you spread your arms out to the side to form a "T," keeping your elbows slightly bent. Don't spread your arms so far as to hurt your shoulders. Focus on feeling the chest muscles contract.

Inhale and bring your arms back to starting position.

Prone Reverse Flyes (Weights)

Target: upper back, rear shoulders

CAUTION: Do not perform this move if you have lower back issues—do Reverse Band Flyes instead. This exercise can also be done on a sturdy bench or weight bench, but do not do so if you have poor balance.

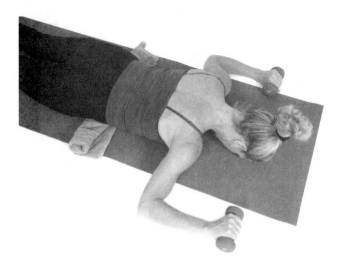

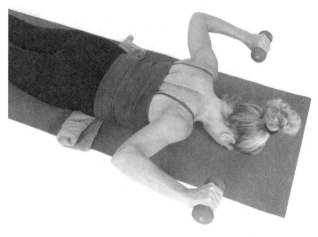

1. Lie face-down on the floor, keeping your head in line with your spine. Position a rolled-up towel under your hips so that your back is comfortable. Grasp a dumbbell in each hand and position your legs to provide the most support and balance possible.

2. Inhale and, while squeezing your shoulder blades together, slowly lift your arms toward the ceiling until they are parallel to the floor. Do not lift your arms higher than your shoulders.

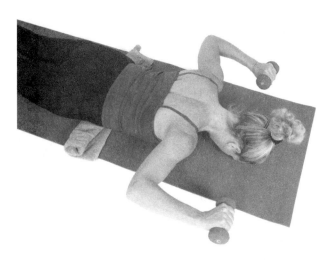

3. Exhale and slowly lower your arms to starting position.

Single-Arm Rows

Target: upper back, rear shoulders

CAUTION: Do not do this exercise if you have back issues.

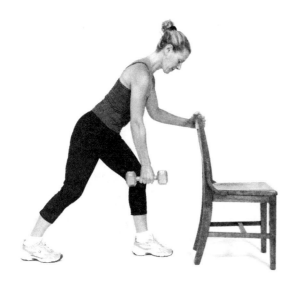 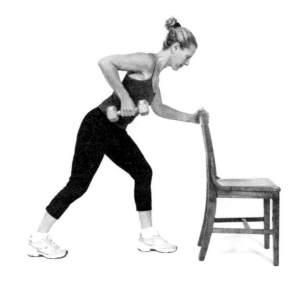

1. Stand behind a stable chair and place your left hand on the chair's back. Position your left leg forward and right leg back a comfortable distance apart, keeping your knees slightly bent and upper body angled forward. Grasp a dumbbell in your right hand with your elbow slightly bent, as if you are about to start a lawnmower. Tighten your core muscles to protect your back. Inhale to begin.

2. Exhale as you slowly pull your right hand in toward your right armpit, pinching your shoulder blades together. Do not twist your torso.

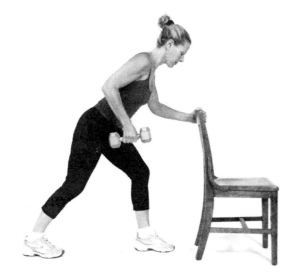

3. Inhale and slowly return to starting position.

Repeat, then switch sides.

Reverse Band Flyes

CAUTION: If you feel discomfort in your shoulders, STOP!

This can be done while standing or sitting.

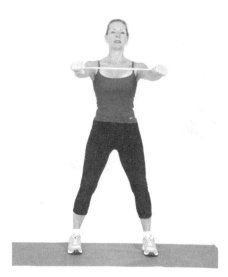 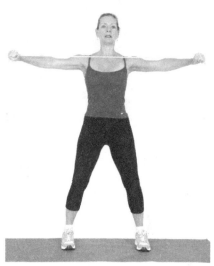 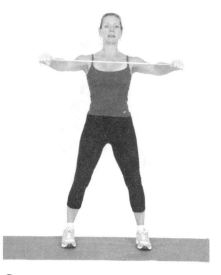

1. Stand with proper posture. Hold an exercise band in front of you with your palms facing down, shoulder-width apart. Grasp the band at a place that provides adequate resistance. Raise your arms to shoulder height, keeping them straight but not locked. Inhale to begin.

2. Exhale and slowly spread your arms to the side. Only go as far apart as you can still see your hands. Don't allow your shoulders to shrug and don't arch your back.

3. Inhale and slowly return to starting position.

Pull-Downs

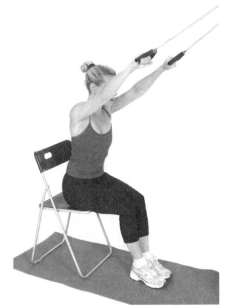

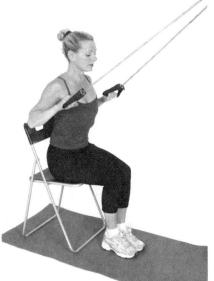

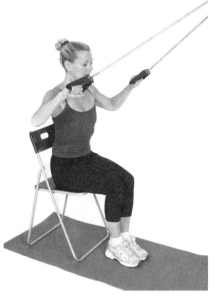

1. Attach an exercise band to a solid overhead item (loops are available at sporting goods stores). Sit in a chair and lean slightly forward toward the band's attachment. Reach up and grasp the band at a place that provides adequate resistance. Keep your torso firm to protect your back. Inhale to begin.

2. Exhale and, while squeezing your shoulder blades together, slowly pull your hands down toward your shoulders.

3. Inhale and return slowly to the starting position.

Y Pull-Downs

Target: upper back

This exercise can be done while standing or sitting. You can also alternate arms.

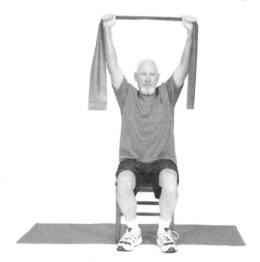
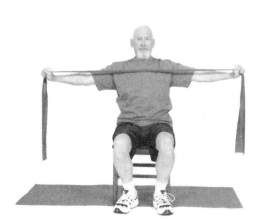

1. Sit in a chair with proper posture. With your palms forward, shoulder-width apart, grasp an end of the band in each hand at a place that provides adequate resistance. Raise your arms overhead. Inhale to begin.

2. Exhale and slowly lower your arms to the sides, stopping at shoulder level. Don't arch your back.

Inhale and return to starting position.

Shoulder Retractions

Target: upper back, rear shoulders

This exercise can be done while standing or sitting. If standing, place one leg forward and the other back for support and balance. You can also alternate arms.

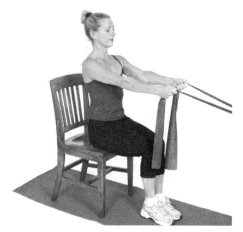
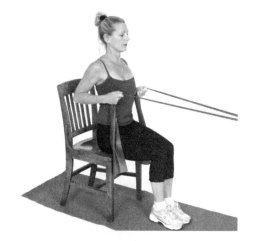

1. Sit in a chair with proper posture. Securely attach a band to the doorknob of a closed door or similar stable object. Grasp an end of the band in each hand at a place that provides adequate resistance. Keep your core firm to protect your back. Inhale to begin.

2. Exhale as you slowly pull your hands toward your shoulders. Keep your shoulder blades together at all times, moving only your arms.

Inhale as you slowly return to starting position.

Bow & Arrow

This exercise can be done while standing or sitting.

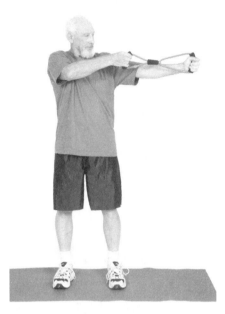 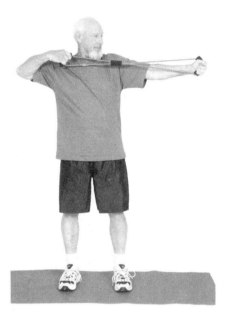

1. Stand with proper posture. Grasp one end of the band with your left hand, then extend the arm out to the side at shoulder height. With your right hand, reach across your body and grasp the band near your left elbow.

2. Inhale as you pull the band across your chest toward your right shoulder, as if pulling a bow.

Exhale as you return to starting position.

Repeat, then switch sides.

Seated Rows

This exercise can also be done while sitting in a chair.

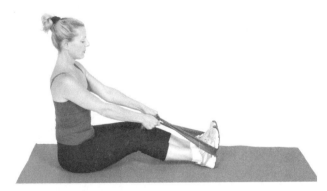 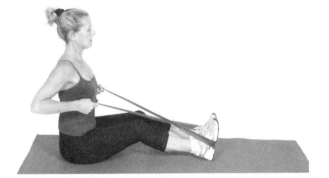

1. Sit on the floor and extend your legs out in front of you. Loop an exercise band around your feet, crossing the band over your shins to provide better safety. With your palms facing each other, grasp the band at a position for ideal resistance. Inhale to begin.

2. Exhale as you slowly pull your hands toward your chest, trying to keep your arms close to your body. Focus on keeping your shoulder blades together throughout the movement and move only your arms.

Inhale as you slowly return to starting position.

Shrugs

Target: shoulders, upper back

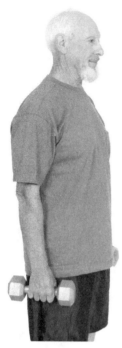 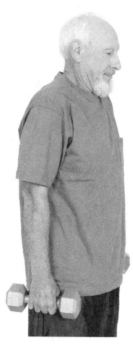 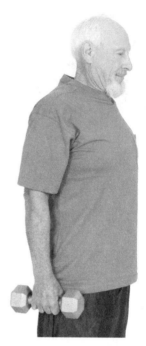

1. Stand with proper posture and hold a dumbbell in each hand. Extend your arms straight alongside your body.

2. Inhale as you slowly "shrug" your shoulders up toward your ears.

3. Exhale and roll your shoulders back, slowly lowering your shoulders to starting position.

Lateral Arm Raises

Target: shoulders, upper back

CAUTION: If you feel clicking in the shoulder area while doing this exercise, STOP!

If you feel any discomfort in your lower back, readjust your posture and try the exercise by alternating your arms.

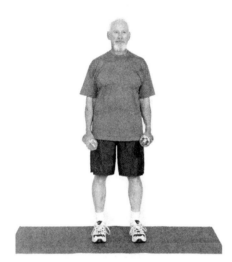 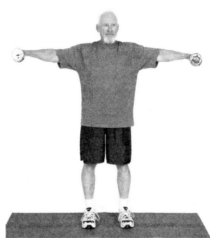 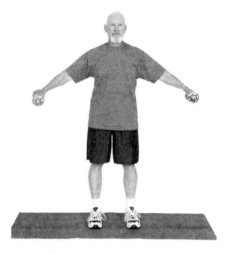

1. Stand with proper posture with your arms straight alongside your body and hold a dumbbell in each hand. Keep your torso firm to protect your lower back.

2. Inhale as you slowly lift your arms out to the side, no higher than shoulder level.

3. Exhale as you slowly return to starting position.

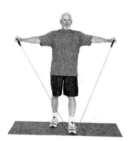 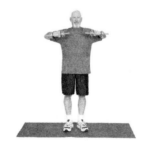

VARIATION: Stand on the exercise band and with both hands grasp the band at a position that provides adequate resistance.

MODIFICATIONS: If doing this exercise with straight arms is too difficult, flare your elbows out like a chicken. If your arms feel uncomfortable going out to the side, try moving them slightly forward to see if the motion feels better.

Frontal Arm Raises

Target: front shoulders, upper back

If you feel any discomfort in your lower back, readjust your posture and don't go as high.

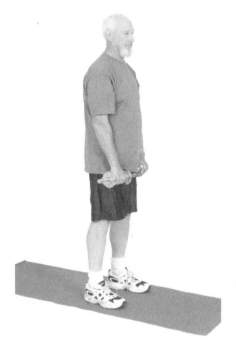 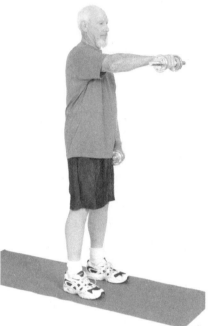 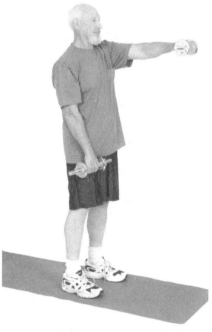

1. Stand with proper posture. Hold a dumbbell in each hand with your arms straight, but not locked, and your palms facing your thighs. Keep your torso firm to protect your lower back.

2. Inhale and slowly raise your right arm forward to shoulder height but no higher.

3. Exhale as you lower your arm to the starting position more slowly than when you lifted it. Alternate arms.

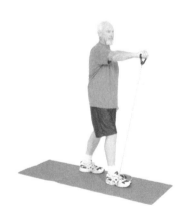

VARIATION: Stand on one end of the exercise band then grasp the band at a position that provides adequate resistance.

Military Presses

Target: shoulders, upper back, triceps

CAUTION: Avoid this exercise if you have a history of shoulder or lower back complaints or have osteoporosis/osteopenia.

This exercise can be done while standing or sitting. If done from a standing position, don't arch your back—maintain proper neutral spine at all times.

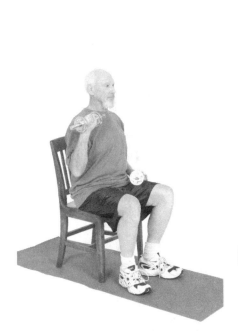
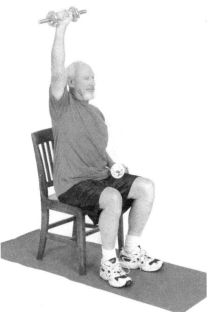
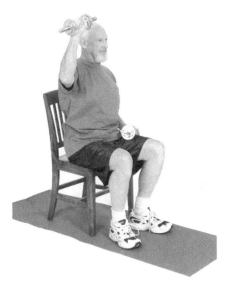

1. Sit with proper posture on a stable chair. Hold a dumbbell in your right hand next to your right shoulder with your palm facing forward. Make sure you are balanced and keep your back in its neutral position. Inhale to begin.

2. Exhale as you press your right arm to the ceiling. Your arm doesn't need to extend directly above your shoulder—slightly forward is acceptable.

3. Inhale as you lower the dumbbell slowly to starting position.

Repeat then switch sides.

VARIATION 1: Wrap an exercise band around your back and under your arms. Hold an end of the band in each hand, adjusting the band length to regulate the resistance.

VARIATION 2: Try positioning your palms inward and perform the same movement. See which feels most comfortable to you.

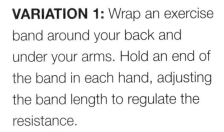
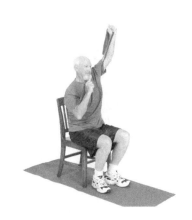

Upright Rows

Target: shoulders, arms, upper back, core

CAUTION: If you have a history of shoulder problems, avoid this exercise.

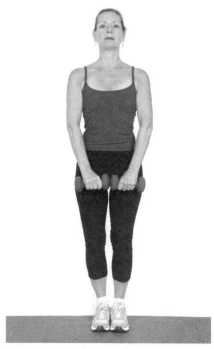 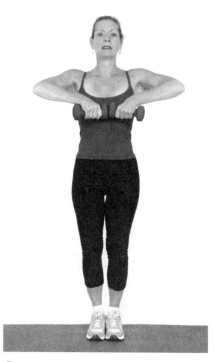 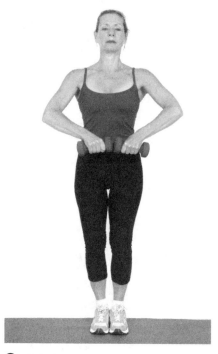

1. Stand with proper posture. Hold a dumbbell in each hand with your arms in front of your body and your palms facing your thighs. Inhale to begin.

2. Keeping your hands close to your body, bend your elbows and exhale as you pull the dumbbells up to chest level. Don't allow your wrists to go higher than your elbows or your elbows to go higher than your shoulders, and don't arch your back.

3. Inhale as you slowly lower the dumbbells to starting position, resisting the force of gravity by keeping your muscles tense.

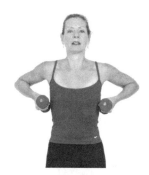

MODIFICATION: If your shoulders feel uncomfortable, try pulling the dumbbells up alongside your body until they reach your armpits. If you still feel discomfort, avoid this exercise.

THE STRENGTH TRAINING BIBLE FOR SENIORS

Sword Fighters (Band)

Target: shoulders, upper back, rotator cuff

This can also be done while sitting.

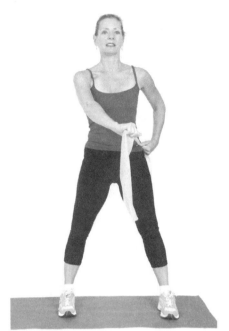 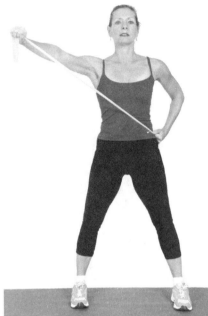 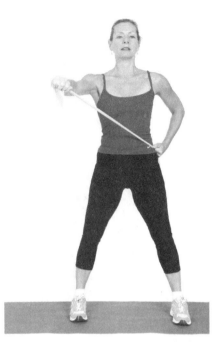

1. Stand with proper posture. Hold an end of the band on your left hip with your left hand then grasp the band with your right hand, thumb down, at the point that will provide adequate resistance. Keep your right arm straight but not locked. Inhale to begin.

2. Exhale as you slowly pull the band diagonally across your body as if pulling out a sword.

3. Inhale as you return to starting position.

Repeat, then switch sides.

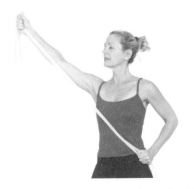

VARIATION: Grab the band with your thumb up to activate the front deltoid.

Reverse Sword Fighters

This exercise can be done while standing or sitting.

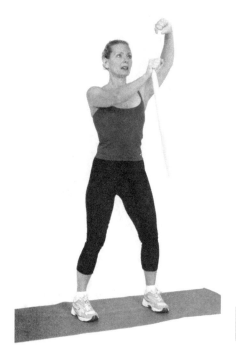 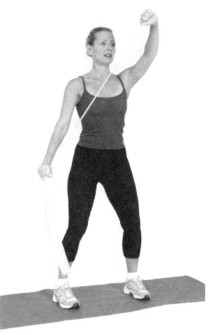 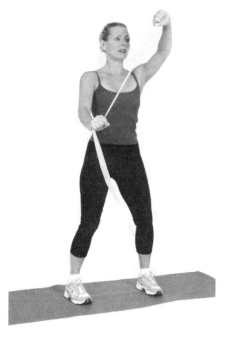

1. Stand with proper posture. Hold an end of the band in your left hand then extend your left arm out and above your left shoulder, pointing your thumb down. With your right hand, thumb up, grasp the other end of the band at a point that provides adequate resistance. Keep your left arm stationary. Inhale to begin.

2. Exhale and slowly pull the right arm down alongside the right side of your body.

3. Inhale as you return to starting position.

Repeat, then switch sides.

Internal Rotations

Target: rotator cuff

Caution: Do not perform this exercise quickly as you may harm yourself.

You can also use a doorknob instead of a chair (door attachment devices are commercially available). To reinforce proper positioning, you may want to place a towel between your elbow and torso.

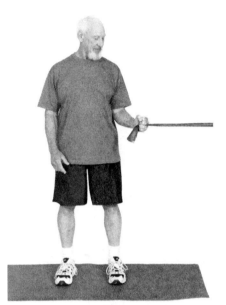 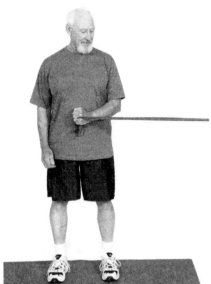 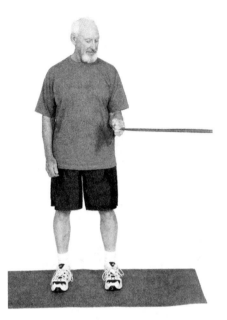

1. Attach the band securely to a stable chair so that you'll be pulling the band at belly button height. Stand with the left side of your body next to the chair. Grasp the band with your left hand, thumb up and palm facing in. Bend your left elbow 90 degrees and keep it close to your body. Stay mindful of engaging the deep muscles of the shoulder area. Inhale to begin.

2. Moving only your forearm, exhale as you slowly bring your left hand toward your belly button.

3. Inhale as you slowly return to starting position.

Repeat, then switch sides.

External Rotations

Caution: Do not perform this exercise quickly as you may harm yourself.

You can also use a doorknob instead of a chair (door attachment devices are commercially available).

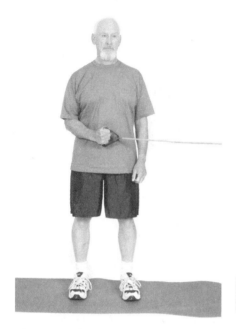 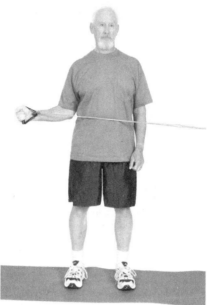 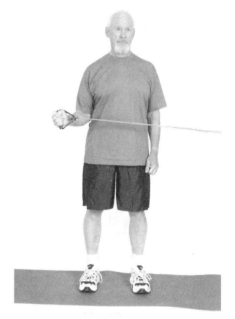

1. Attach the band securely to a sturdy chair so that you'll be pulling the band at belly button height. Stand with the left side of your body a band's distance away from the chair. Reach across your body to grasp the band with your right hand, thumb facing up. Bend your right elbow 90 degrees and keep it next to your body. Stay mindful of engaging the deep muscles of the shoulder area. Resistance is not important in this exercise. Inhale to begin.

2. With your right elbow next to your body and moving only your lower arm, exhale and slowly move your right hand away from your body, leading with your knuckles. Do not twist your torso.

3. Inhale and slowly return to starting position.

Repeat, then switch sides.

Biceps Curls

Target: biceps, forearms

These curls can be done using both arms simultaneously or alternately; they can also be done while standing or sitting.

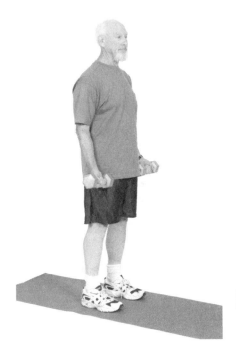

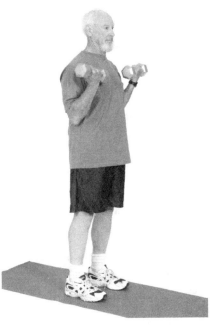

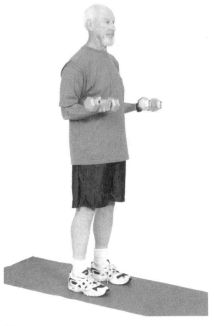

1. Stand with proper posture, feet hip-width apart. Hold a dumbbell in each hand with your palms facing up, keeping your elbows tucked against your torso. Keep your torso firm to protect your lower back. Inhale to begin.

2. Exhale as you slowly curl the dumbbells toward your shoulders.

3. Inhale and slowly lower your arms to starting position.

VARIATION: Place your left foot in the center of the band and grasp the ends in each hand at a place that allows the band to be taut and provide adequate resistance. (To increase the workload, grab lower on the band.) Keep your torso firm and your elbow close to your body. Perform the curl from here.

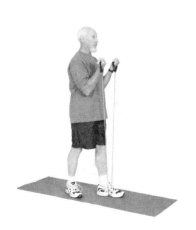

Hammer Curls

These curls can be done using both arms simultaneously or alternately; they can also be done while standing or sitting.

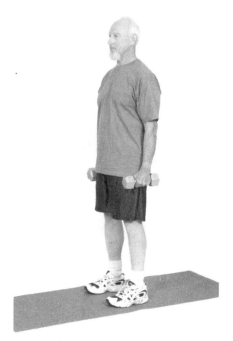

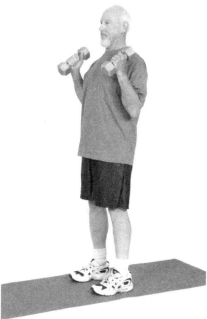

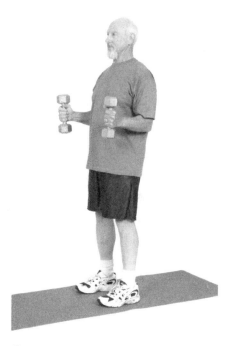

1. Stand with proper posture, feet hip-width apart. Hold a dumbbell in each hand with your thumbs forward, keeping your elbows tucked against your torso. Keep your torso firm to protect your lower back. Inhale to begin.

2. Exhale as you slowly curl the dumbbells toward your shoulders.

3. Inhale and slowly lower your arms to starting position.

VARIATION: Place your left foot on the center of the band and grasp the ends with your left hand at a place that allows the band to be taut and provide adequate resistance. (To increase the workload, grab lower on the band.) Keep your torso firm and your elbow close to your body. Perform the curl from here.

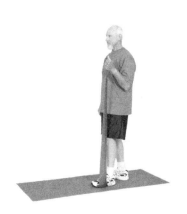

Cross-Your-Heart Curls

These curls can be done using both arms simultaneously or alternately; they can also be done while standing or sitting.

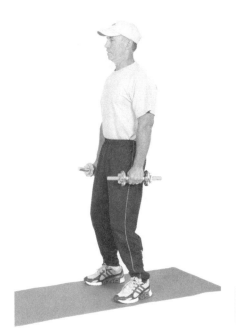 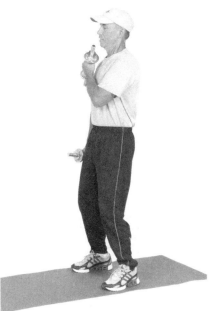 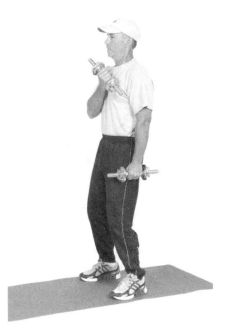

1. Stand with proper posture, feet hip-width apart. Hold a dumbbell in each hand with your palms facing your legs, keeping your elbows tucked against your torso. Keep your torso firm to protect your lower back. Inhale to begin.

2. Exhale as you slowly curl your hand across your body to take your left hand to your right shoulder.

3. Inhale and slowly lower your left arm to starting position. Now exhale and slowly curl your right hand to your left shoulder. Inhale and return to starting position.

Concentration Curls

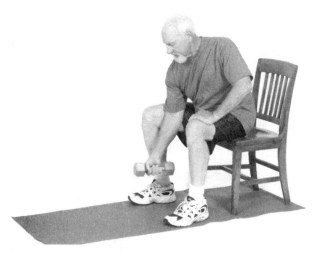 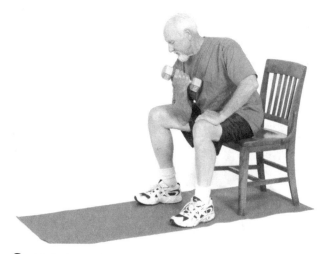

1. Sit at the end of a bench or chair and lean slightly forward. Place your left hand on your left thigh for support and place your right elbow on the inside of your right thigh. Grasp a dumbbell with your right hand, palm up. Start with your arm straight but not locked and keep your elbow pressed against your thigh. Inhale to begin.

2. Exhale and curl your right hand toward your right shoulder.

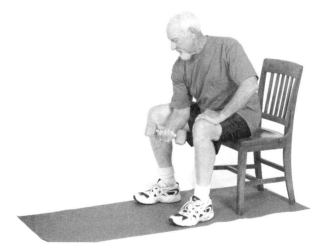

3. Inhale and slowly return to starting position.

Repeat, then switch arms.

VARIATION: You can also grasp the dumbbell with your thumb up.

276   THE STRENGTH TRAINING BIBLE FOR SENIORS

Reverse Curls

These curls can be done using both arms simultaneously or alternately; they can also be done while standing or sitting.

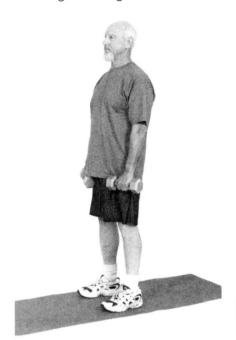 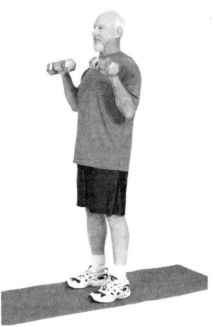 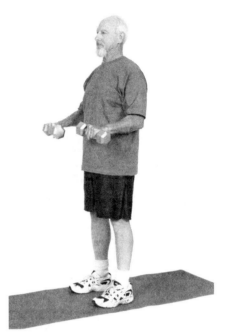

1. Stand with proper posture, feet hip-width apart. Hold a dumbbell in each hand, with your knuckles facing forward. Keep your elbows tucked against your torso. Inhale to begin.

2. Exhale as you slowly curl your arms up, bringing your knuckles toward your shoulders.

3. Inhale as you slowly lower your arms to starting position.

Wrist Curls

Target: forearms

CAUTION: If you have arthritis of the wrist, consult your doctor before doing this.

Keep the weights light and work up to higher repetitions. You can also do this exercise one arm at a time.

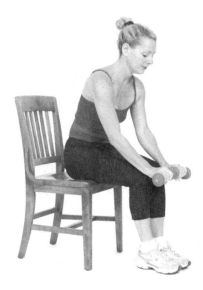

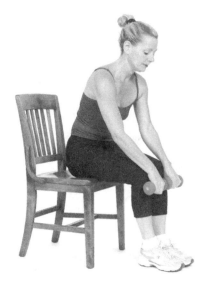

1. Sit in a stable chair. Hold a dumbbell in each hand and rest your forearms on your thighs so that your hands extend over your knees. Breathe in a comfortable manner.

2. Allow your wrists to relax (flex) downward.

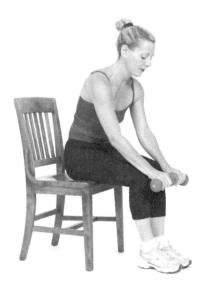

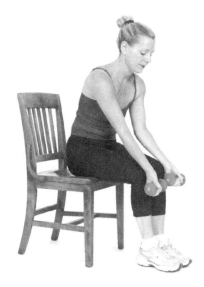

3. Slowly bring your knuckles upward to return to starting position.

VARIATION: Perform the same exercise except turn your palms upward.

THE STRENGTH TRAINING BIBLE FOR SENIORS

Side-Lying Triceps Extensions

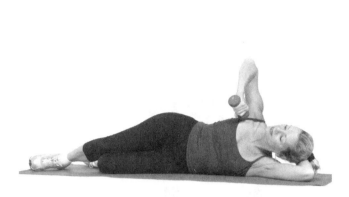

1. Lie on the left side of your body in a comfortable and stable position. Hold a dumbbell in your right hand close to your right shoulder, with your elbow up and your thumb down. Inhale to begin.

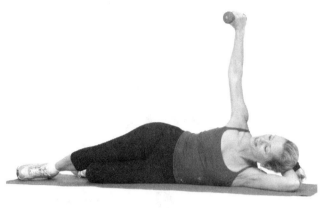

2. Exhale and, hinging slowly from your elbow, extend your right hand up toward the ceiling.

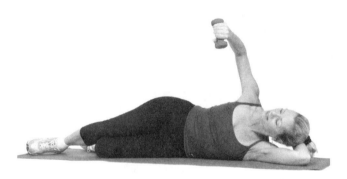

3. Inhale and slowly return to starting position.

Repeat, then switch sides.

Bent-Over Triceps Extensions with Chair

Target: triceps, upper back

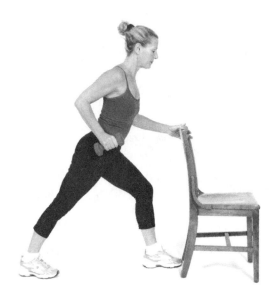

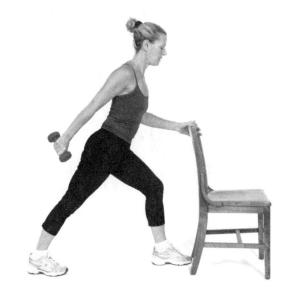

1. Standing with one foot in front of the other for stability, bend over at the waist and rest your left hand on a chair. Grasp a dumbbell in your right hand, keeping your right elbow close to your torso so that your upper arm is at a 45-degree angle with the floor. Inhale to begin.

2. Exhale, keeping your right upper arm stationary and at a 45-degree angle with the floor, as you slowly extend your arm at the elbow to full extension, but avoid locking your elbow and don't let your arm swing up.

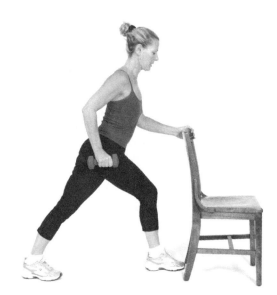

3. Inhale as you return to starting position.

Repeat, then switch sides.

Supine Triceps Extensions

CAUTION: If you feel any discomfort in your elbow or shoulder, stop.

This exercise can be performed by alternating arms or using them simultaneously.

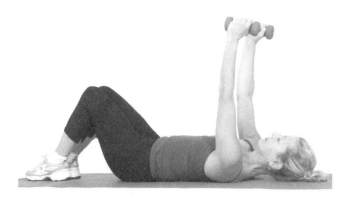

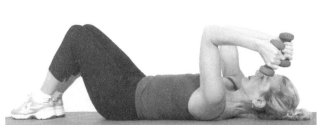

1. Lie on your back with your feet flat on the floor. Hold a dumbbell in each hand with your palms facing each other and your arms extended above your shoulders. Inhale to begin.

2. Exhale and, hinging only at the elbows, lower the dumbbells toward your shoulders, stopping when your elbows make 90-degree angles. Keep your elbows pointed toward the ceiling.

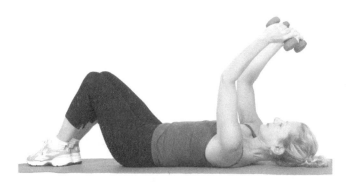

3. Inhale as you slowly return to starting position.

Chair Dips 1

Target: triceps

CAUTION: Be careful the chair does not tip over.

You can also do this on a countertop or a coffee table.

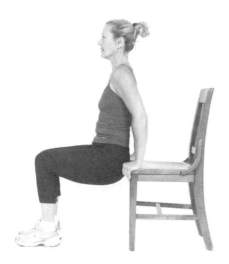

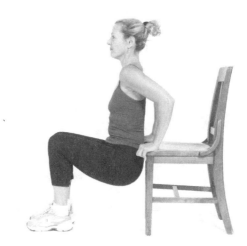

1. Sit in a solid and stable chair. Place your hands flat on the seat, fingers pointing toward the edge, and slide forward until your bottom is just off the seat. Inhale to begin.

2. Exhale as you slowly bend your elbows, trying to keep them close to your torso as you lower your bottom toward the floor.

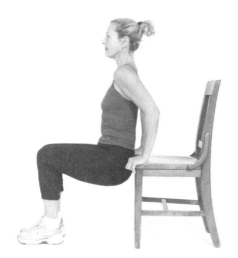

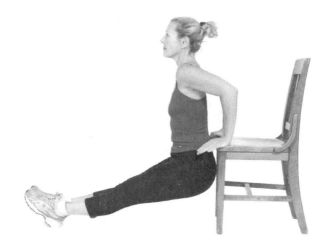

3. Inhale as you return to starting position.

ADVANCED VARIATION: As you get stronger, extend your legs out farther from the chair.

Chair Dips 2

Caution: Be careful the chairs do not tip over.

This is a challenging move. If needed, rest your feet lightly on the floor behind you.

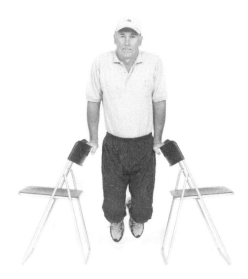

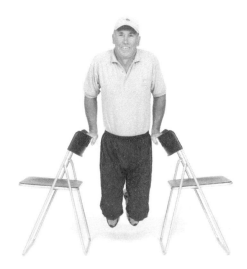

1. Position two sturdy chairs with their backs parallel to each other. Space them apart so that you can stand between them and place your hands on the tops.

2. Inhale as you slowly bend your elbows and lower your bottom toward the floor.

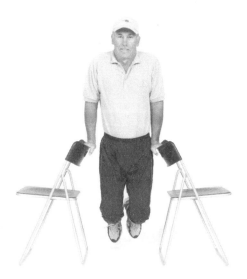

3. Exhale as you return to starting position.

Triceps Band Extensions

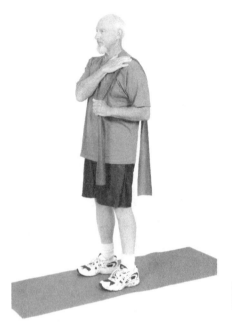 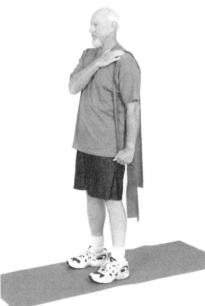 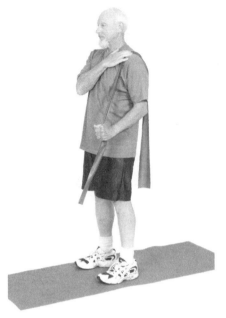

1. Stand with proper posture and drape the exercise band over your left shoulder and place your right hand on your left shoulder to secure it. Keep your left elbow next to your body and grasp the band with your left hand to make a 90-degree angle with your arm; make sure the band is taut at all times. Keep your right and left hands lined up. Inhale to begin.

2. Without using momentum, Exhale as you slowly extend your left arm downward.

3. Inhale and even more slowly return to starting position.

Repeat, then switch sides.

Horizontal Triceps Extensions

This can also be done with both arms simultaneously, or while sitting.

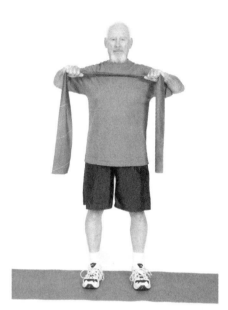 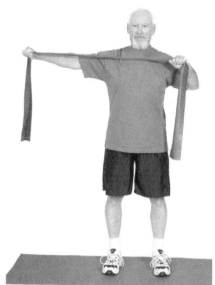 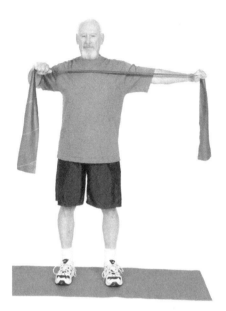

1. Stand with proper posture and grasp the band with both hands, palms down. The closer you position your hands toward the middle of the band, the more resistance you will have. Lift your elbows up and away from your body so that everything is at shoulder height. Keep your torso firm to protect your lower back. Inhale to begin.

2. Exhale as you slowly extend your right arm out to the side.

3. Inhale and return to starting position even more slowly.

Alternate sides.

SUGGESTED STRETCHES FOLLOWING A WEIGHT TRAINING WORKOUT WORKOUT

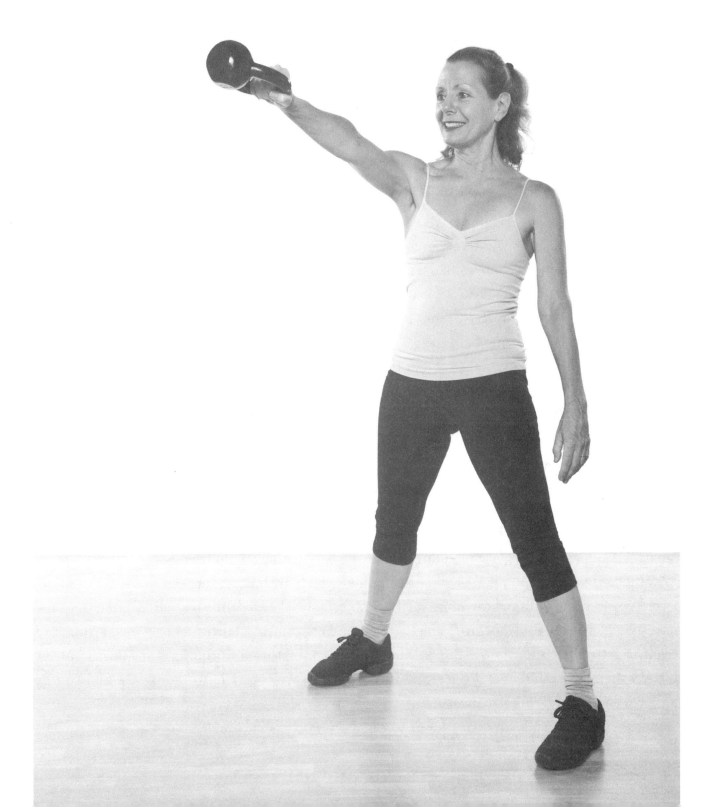

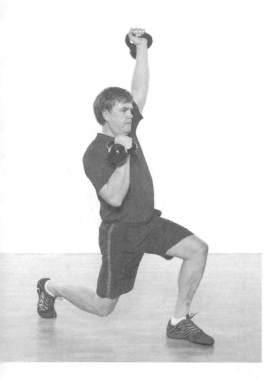

THE POPULARITY OF KETTLEBELL WORKOUTS

The kettlebell, or *girya* in Russian, is a cast-iron weight that looks like a cannonball with a teapot handle (personally, I think the name should be "kettle*ball*" because of its shape). It's believed to have originated in the eastern European countries in the late 1800s, originally used an activity to pass the time and as circus stunts by big burly men displaying feats of strength. As time progressed, people started to use the kettlebell as a method to improve strength and fitness. In the former Soviet Union, Olympic weightlifting coaches used kettlebells as a training device.

The kettlebell arrived in the United States in the early 1900s and was used by immigrants and, along with the medicine ball, was slowly introduced into boxing clubs as a training device. The kettlebell lost favor in the '70s when the fitness industry moved toward selectorized weight machines. It was at this time that Nautilus equipment became the rage and old-time medicine balls, club bells, dumbbells, barbells, and kettlebells were replaced with shiny, cambered, belt-driven resistance-training equipment.

After this brief period of interruption, "old-school" training devices have steadily come back into vogue. Today we see boot-camp training programs and shadow boxing put to music. Many personal trainers new to fitness think that push-ups, jumping jacks, squat thrusts, and kettlebells are something very innovative but most of us 50+ folks can say, "Been there, done that." For some of us, reintroducing kettlebells into our lives may be like visiting an old friend.

Kettlebells are part of the plyometric family, which includes exercises such as jumping, bounding, and throwing and catching weighted objects such as medicine balls or kettlebells. These movements involve rapid eccentric (lengthening) and concentric (shortening) actions. Plyometric exercises have their roots in the 1960s, when they were first used in the Eastern Bloc countries to train their weightlifters and track-and-field athletes. A plyometric workout was, and still is, designed to improve explosive muscular power.

The reason the kettlebell is gaining favor again is that the motions involved in a kettlebell workout mimic activities of daily living much more than the unidirectional exercise machines seen in most gyms today. The kettlebell is used to perform dynamic exercises that foster power, agility, strength, flexibility, and even aerobic fitness. The shape of the kettlebell places the center of gravity beyond the handle, which allows the bell to be thrown about easily, facilitating swing movements. Some versions of kettlebells include bags filled with steel shot, sand, or adjustable weight plates. When used properly, kettlebells are a challenging and enjoyable adjunct to a standard total-body fitness program.

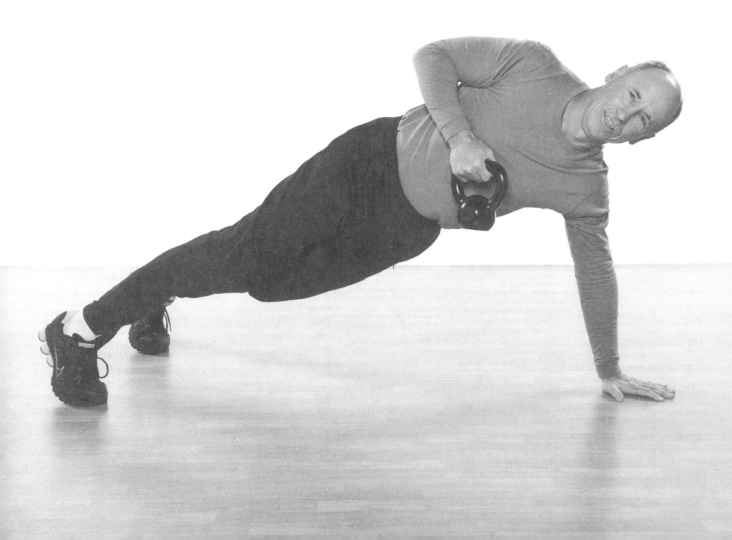

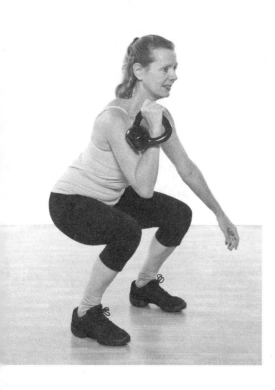

WHY USE KETTLEBELLS?

Anyone who has exercised for any period of time has probably gotten stale, bored, or burnt out with the same old routine. Kettlebells aren't a be-all and end-all piece of equipment, but they do offer a fabulous diversion and can be used alone in an exercise routine or integrated into an existing strength-training program. They can provide you with a comprehensive total-body workout that addresses strength, power, core stabilization, agility, and hand-to-hand coordination as well as hand-eye coordination.

Kettlebells are basically odd-shaped weights with handles. The handle placement in relation to the weighted ball off-balances the load, creating an additional dynamic force when used. With this design, you can move in several planes and develop strength and power in the legs, lower back, grip, and shoulders. We need to think of our body as a total kinetic chain unit, which means that what happens at one point affects something else down the chain. Just gripping the bell handle engages the forearm muscles; swinging the bell from the floor to overhead engages the calf muscles, the butt muscles (gluteals), the back muscles, and the shoulder muscles (deltoids), as well as many deep-lying muscles. To engage all those same muscles on an exercise machine would require at least three different machines.

Most traditional exercise programs performed with free weights or machines generally focus on one set of muscles at a time. Kettlebell movements often target not only primary muscles but also the supporting muscle groups. Moves that involve momentum (such as swings) incorporate both acceleration and deceleration, but kettlebells can be used in a slow, controlled manner much like free weights. In this regard, when used correctly, the kettlebell is an ideal training device for all levels.

Most beginners need to start at the slow, controlled level and then progress to the more dynamic and advanced moves.

What are the advantages of kettlebells? They:

- are reasonably priced and last forever.
- are small and easy to store.
- are very adaptable—you can move them slowly, quickly, and in almost any conceivable direction.
- are an efficient way to get a total-body workout in a shorter period of time.
- often better replicate functional activities of life and sport than exercise machines because of the incorporation of acceleration and deceleration.
- are a creative way to improve power and challenge the body.
- improve neuromuscular proprioception.
- improve body awareness and coordination.
- foster improved joint stabilization.
- are a fun and challenging diversion from the same old push-and-pull weight machines.

But the real beauty of a kettlebell workout is that it can replicate activities of daily living. The key to aging successfully is to be able to perform the tasks necessary to live a functionally independent life. The kettlebell helps you to attain that goal by personalizing your routine for your particular needs. However, a kettlebell program requires practice and patience to learn the correct body mechanics. As with any exercise tool, kettlebells can cause injury if you proceed too quickly or perform moves incorrectly. Too often seniors have the mindset that more is better, but proper execution and engaging the mind and the body are the key to a successful kettlebell workout.

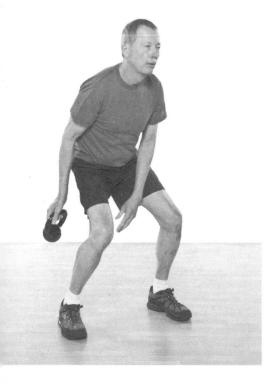

KETTLEBELLS
FOR 50+ FOLKS

The exercises in this section are practical and functional, and they have been tested and selected for the 50+ person based on years of experience. Some have been adapted from their original form to better serve the aging body. These movements will provide a complete and comprehensive workout of both the major and minor muscles of the body in a short amount of time. While more kettlebell exercises exist, many have been eliminated from this book to offer you the safest kettlebell approach possible.

The 50+ population runs the gamut from extremely fit to very frail. Some exercises in this book may be too difficult for some and too easy for others, but again this book is written for the middle group. Please seriously consider the movements and the size of the kettlebell you select with regard to your health status before you jump fully into a kettlebell workout. If you're an exercise novice, you should do well following the progression outlined in the kettlebell programs starting on page 299. As with any exercise program, check with your doctor before proceeding.

Most exercises performed with weight machines or free weights are done in a slow, controlled manner, whereas many kettlebell exercises can be done with momentum and in a freestyle manner. Note, however, that many of the exercises in this book utilize slower, controlled movements that are similar to using a dumbbell because they're considered more appropriate for the 50+ age group or someone starting a kettlebell program.

As you begin your workout, you'll find the exercises are more challenging than a basic dumbbell or conventional gym machine workout. Faster movements such as swings and catch-and-release exercises are more appropriate for stronger, well-conditioned exercisers who have a substantial foundation of strength training.

To train well, your mission is to train smart, not hard, and to not harm yourself. Please do not perform any movement beyond your skill set or fitness level. Too often as people age they are in a hurry to get fit, but before they ever get fit they get hurt and quit. That might be okay for a 30-something who can recover quickly, but this could be devastating for a 50-something. Just getting up in the morning can be hazardous to your health, and any exercise program can be harmful as well if not performed correctly. So use caution when selecting any exercise method to gain fitness, especially if you have back or shoulder concerns.

KETTLEBELL CAUTIONS

Plyometric exercises are safe if used with common sense. The National Strength and Conditioning Association suggests the following safety guidelines:

- Don't do kettlebell exercises when distracted or fatigued.
- Wear proper footwear and choose proper flooring.
- Warm up properly.
- Follow proper progressions: Learn less-intense and less-complex moves before trying more complex ones.

PLEASE NOTE: Kettlebell exercise can be a more strenuous form of exercise. Therefore, it is highly recommended that you consult your health professional prior to engaging in a kettlebell workout.

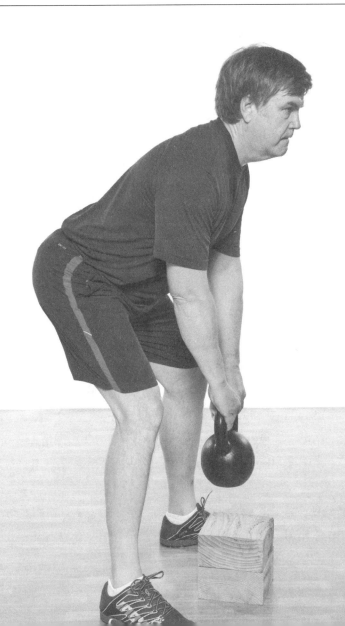

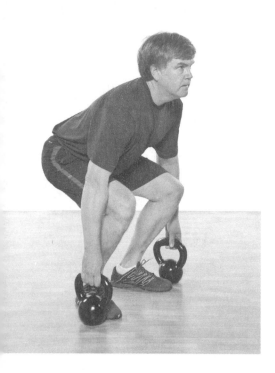

GETTING STARTED WITH KETTLEBELLS

Performing kettlebell exercises is like hitting a tennis ball with a racquet. There's a big difference between hitting the ball in the sweet spot and just hitting the ball anywhere. If you perform the kettlebell move correctly, it just "feels" right. The exercises in the section are about fluidity and grace, not grunt power. To achieve this, you'll need to find the right kettlebell (or two) for your workout.

Kettlebells by design are very different from dumbbells. You may notice that a 5-pound kettlebell feels very different from a 5-pound dumbbell. The influence of momentum is a major factor. It's critical to be comfortable with your particular range of motion. I often ask students to test out just the movement of the kettlebell exercise they'll be performing before even touching a kettlebell. Once they learn their safe range of motion, I have them use a light kettlebell to see how the element of momentum makes the movement feel different. Learning to accelerate and decelerate the kettlebell before you select a training kettlebell load is critical.

SELECTING YOUR KETTLEBELL

In the olden days, kettlebells were only available in black, and weights ranged from heavy to very heavy. Today, kettlebells come in a variety of weights, styles, and colors. Some kettlebells have rounded handles, others have more rectangular ones. Some are polished and smooth, others are rough. Traditionalists may prefer the black cast-iron version while others may prefer colorful, rubber-coated bells. Some trainers suggest that the unpainted handle version provides better control, but the selection of a kettlebell is a personal issue. Find one that fits your hands and your training objectives.

Old-time kettlebell users refer to the weight in terms of *pood*, which is roughly 16 kilograms or 35 pounds. Nowadays, you'll find kettlebells weighing as little as 2 pounds or as much as 165 pounds (75 kilograms). The weight you select depends on numerous variables, from the type of exercise you plan to perform, to your level of strength, to any underlying joint issues.

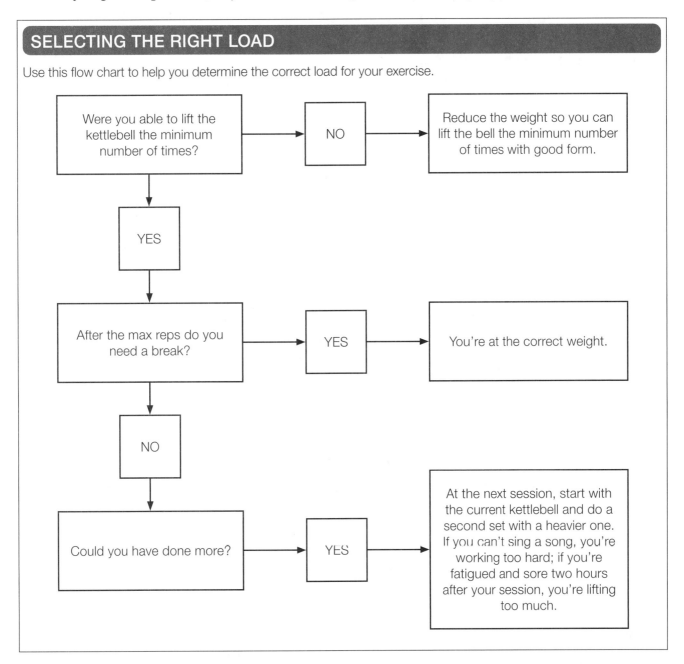

SELECTING THE RIGHT LOAD

Use this flow chart to help you determine the correct load for your exercise.

Were you able to lift the kettlebell the minimum number of times?

NO → Reduce the weight so you can lift the bell the minimum number of times with good form.

YES

After the max reps do you need a break?

YES → You're at the correct weight.

NO

Could you have done more?

YES → At the next session, start with the current kettlebell and do a second set with a heavier one. If you can't sing a song, you're working too hard; if you're fatigued and sore two hours after your session, you're lifting too much.

In general, I strongly suggest you start with a light kettlebell and increase the resistance slowly after seeing how your joints respond. Going heavier encourages you to compromise form and thus "cheat" to overcompensate for lack of strength and technique. In addition, the heavier you go, the more you increase your risk of injury. Don't let anyone say you should go heavier—listen to your inner trainer. If you plan to train regularly with kettlebells, you may need several different kettlebells to accommodate different types of moves (e.g., heavier for deadlifts, lighter for kneeling get-ups).

Some of my clients, before they purchase any kettlebells, try some of the basic kettlebell moves with standard dumbbells they already have. Many kettlebell exercises can be easily performed with a standard dumbbell. As you progress into the swing exercises, you'll know what size kettlebells to purchase. The cost of kettlebells has dropped significantly, with some sporting goods stores, department stores, and online retailers now selling sets in various ranges of weights.

STANCES AND GRIPS

Before you start your kettlebell workout, you should familiarize yourself with a few standard foot and handgrip positions. The way you grasp the kettlebell influences the types of motions you can perform. You should practice getting the feel of it before you commence a full-blown workout.

I'm a fanatic about proper body mechanics and posture, but your common sense will be a good determinant of what grip feels best for you for each

> ### DOUBLE GRIPS
>
> Most double grips are used to start a grab-and-release move, but they're also ideal for swing moves if you prefer a better grip. Slight adjustments of hand position can often take the strain off a 50+ shoulder joint.

exercise. Some authors tell you that there's only one way to grip the kettlebell for a specific exercise, but it's okay to adapt the position for your body. Remember, these are *adapted* kettlebell exercises, so as long as you're enjoying the motions and they're not causing discomfort, go for it! This is your kettlebell program. However, it's extremely important that you have a solid grip of the kettlebell because once it gets moving, it's hard to hold on to!

It might be wise to invest in gloves or lifting chalk to improve your grip (gloves may prevent calluses, too). Switching grips mid-air is an option and requires good grip strength and hand-eye coordination, but it's not recommended until you're advanced. Note that hand switching is not necessary to improve strength and power.

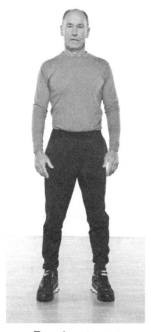
Regular stance

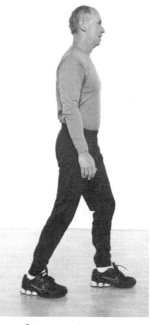
Staggered stance

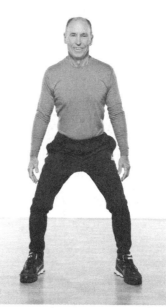
Athletic stance

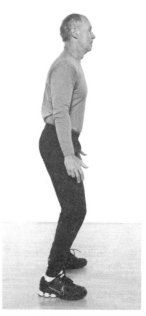
Athletic stance

Foot Positions

Wear shoes that provide you feedback with the ground and protect your foot should the kettlebell drop. Running shoes are not ideal for kettlebell training. A walking shoe, or some other flat footwear that provides lateral support and won't slip would be a better choice.

Regular Stance: Stand erect with your feet shoulder-width apart and weight evenly distributed over both feet, shoulders relaxed, chest open, and shoulder blades retracted (pulled back and down).

Staggered Stance: Step one foot forward and the other foot back, with your feet slightly wider than hip-distance apart in a well-balanced lunge position. The knees should be slightly bent to provide stability and mobility. Engage your core. When performing exercises in this position, it's recommended that you perform one set with one leg forward and then switch sides in order to help maintain symmetry.

Athletic Stance (Shortstop): Stand with your feet a little wider than your shoulders and keep your back slightly rounded and ready for action.

Handgrips

Overhand (Palm Down): Place one hand on top of the handle as if you were grabbing a dumbbell to perform an exercise. This grip is often used when performing swings.

Underhand (Palm Up): Grab the handle from beneath (with your palm up). This grip is often used in arm curl movements.

Thumb Up: Grab the handle with an overhand grip then rotate the hand so the thumb is up. For people with shoulder concerns, this grip is more comfortable when performing overhead presses.

Side by Side (Double Hand): Place your hands side by side on top of the handle with an overhand (palm-down) grip. This grip is often used when doing upright rowing motions, heavy deadlifts, swings, or as a start grip for grab-and-release moves. You can also try a side-by-side grip with palms facing each other.

Hand Over/On Hand: Place one hand on top of the handle and then the other hand on top of that hand. This grip is often used for heavy swings and grab-and-release moves. It's also preferred by those with hand issues.

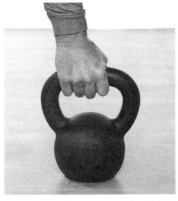
Overhand (palm-down) grip.

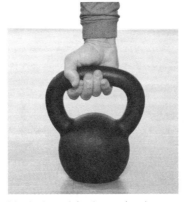
Underhand (palm-up) grip.

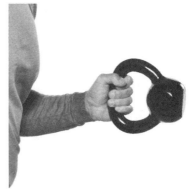
Thumb-up grip.

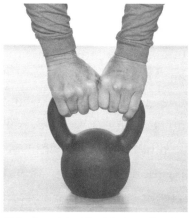
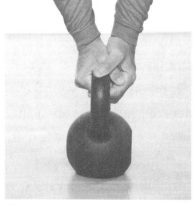

Side-by-side (double-hand) grip.   Hand-over/on-hand grip.

Rack Position: The rack position is where the kettlebell move either ends or begins. In the rack position, the kettlebell rests against the outside of your forearm, with your elbow as close to your ribs as possible. The handle of the bell should be slightly above the belly of the kettlebell. To get to rack position, you can perform a clean or, if the kettlebell is light, an arm curl.

The "clean" (page 355) is the hallmark move of kettlebell training. This move is much like what's seen in Olympic lifting, except in kettlebell training it's one-handed in most cases. This is a ballistic move used to get a heavy kettlebell to the rack position.

Overhead Lockout Position: The top position of an overhead press or a snatch is often referred to as the "lockout." The hand is turned slightly toward the body and is directly over the shoulder; the kettlebell handle rests diagonally across the palm, and the fingers are often just slightly bent to hold onto the handle.

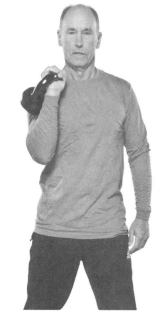

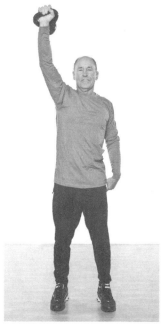

Rack position   Overhead lockout position

KETTLEBELL PROGRAMS

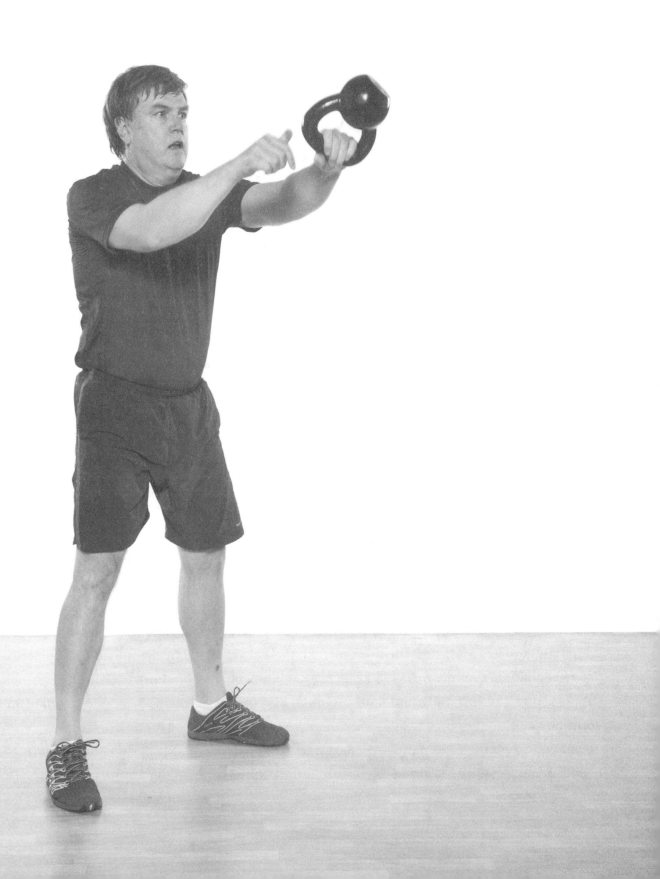

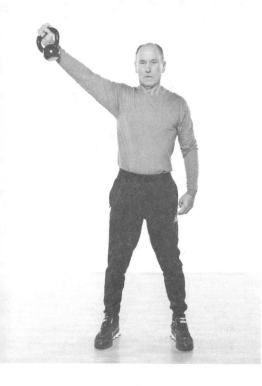

KETTLEBELL WORKOUT BASICS

A well-designed kettlebell program will help you function better in activities of daily living as well as in sports. The beauty of a kettlebell is that it can be used to meet a number of fitness goals. If the routines starting on page 303 aren't quite what you're looking for, you can personalize your own workout.

An important concept in fitness training today is "functional training." The philosophy behind this is to train the muscles to "function" in a variety of ways that mimic the movements engaged in daily living or when participating in a sport. Unfortunately, today we're finding that many older adults can't perform "normal" functional activities of daily life. It's not uncommon to find a 65-year-old having a hard time getting up easily from the floor because their leg strength has deteriorated. The term *sarcopenia* is what scientists call atrophy caused by a sedentary lifestyle. More simply put (and as I have said before in this book): Move it or lose it!

Functional training is usually based on a progression of movements, graduated from simple to complex and from slow to fast. Functional training routines generally begin with isolation-type exercises that work one or two muscles around a single joint, working up to compound movements, such as on page 344. This principle applies whether you're a world-class athlete, post-rehab person, or senior looking to build strength, and this book takes the same approach.

When you design a functional fitness program using kettlebells, every effort should be placed on making the program real. Include movements that have practical applications, fostering sound postural alignment and always following a good biomechanical pattern; maintain a proper base of support, improve flexibility and joint mobility, and balance strength versus dynamic stability. In addition, coordinate proper sequencing of movement with proper motor control.

A sound, functional, progressive-resistance kettlebell exercise program should have a balance between progressions of strength, speed, agility, and power. A balanced program should also address eccentric versus concentric moves and closed-kinetic-chain and open-kinetic-chain exercises. Let's use the Sumo Squats (page 320) to illustrate eccentric versus concentric movements: Lifting the kettlebell up is the concentric portion of the movement, while lowering the kettlebell to the floor is the eccentric portion. The lunge (page 328) is an example of a closed-kinetic-chain exercise for the legs when the feet are planted on the floor. The basic arm curl (page 344) is a common example of an open-kinetic-chain exercise. For a comprehensive exercise program, be sure to include some cardiovascular exercises such as walking, biking, and swimming.

The key to a successful kettlebell experience is knowing how and when to incorporate the above training principles into your routine. To prevent an injury, understand how to incorporate intensity, duration, frequency, and mode in a safe and sane manner. You have two options: Train hard and make improvements quickly but get hurt and quit; or train smart, lessen your risk of getting injured, and stay motivated to continue. Don't focus on being better than someone else. Instead, focus on being healthier and better tomorrow. Slow and steady wins the fitness race.

Here are several elements you should include in your individualized kettlebell workout: a warm-up, exercises that address your goals, and a cool-down/stretch. Other elements that should be included in your overall fitness routine are regular 20- to 30-minute bouts of comfortably paced aerobic exercise most days of the week, as well as proper nutrition.

WARMING UP

Since exercising with a kettlebell is a total-body exercise, it's recommended that you perform an active thermal warm-up, perhaps by going for a light jog for 5–10 minutes, jogging/jumping in place, skipping rope, or riding a stationary bike. You can also do bodyweight exercises such as jumping jacks, squats, lunges, arm circles, arm swings, and planks. The purpose of the warm-up is to enhance core temperature and ready the muscles and joints for an exercise session. Don't confuse warming up and stretching. Warming up increases the temperature of the muscles, much like warming up the old '57 Chevy before a drive. Stretching is a passive activity.

Once your body is warmed up, perform your favorite full-body kettlebell exercises at a slow speed or with a light weight to prepare your body for the more engaging movements. This warm-up concept is the same as when you prepare for a round of tennis by hitting the ball back and forth before playing the actual game. Once your body is warmed up, you can start your workout. Failure to adequately warm up can set you up for an injury. Other warm-up approaches involve sitting in a sauna, taking a warm shower or bath, or even putting a heat pack on a stubborn body part (shoulder, back).

TRAINING FOR YOUR GOAL

An effective kettlebell program for a 50+ person needs to be unique to the individual. Pick moves that best meet your particular needs and mood. As stated earlier in the book, kettlebell training for 50+ folks is not about a prescriptive routine designed for you but rather a routine designed by you and for you. You're the captain of your fitness ship! Adapt and modify your kettlebell program by tweaking each session. Include exercises that allow you to move in manners that respect your 50+ frame and are enjoyable to you without causing you any discomfort.

Keep in mind that age-related muscle loss (sarcopenia) and bone loss (osteoporosis) are becoming major health concerns for 50+ folks. Therefore, improving muscle mass needs to be a goal for the 50+ person who desires to grow well, not old.

Kettlebells are also an excellent tool to foster improved sports performance. To effectively use kettlebells to improve performance, learn to understand the demands and skills of your sport—this is the key. A sport may even have several positions that require different skills. When designing this kind of workout, consider the following:

- What are the physical requirements of your sport (e.g., strength, power, flexibility, agility, speed, quickness, coordination)?
- Does your sport rely on raw athletic traits or precision?
- Does your sport require greater upper body strength or leg strength?

The "FITT" concept is an excellent model to follow when designing your special program.

F stands for Frequency, or the number of times something is done. To obtain optimal results, you should perform your kettlebell workout one to two times a week. The more frequently you can exercise, the better the results.

I stands for Intensity, or how heavy a weight you lift. The intensity is determined by your goals. When building strength, go heavy and do the move six to eight times. For general fitness, aim for 10 times. As you become more fit, increase the intensity.

T stands for Time, or the length/duration of each training session. To gain physical results, you should train long enough that mild muscle fatigue occurs—10 reps is a good rule of thumb for general fitness—and then rest long enough to feel refreshed (usually after a 30-second rest). As you become more fit, increase the time on task and reduce recovery time.

T stands for Type, or the mode of activity that you perform to produce the desired results. In this case it's kettlebells.

COOLING DOWN & STRETCHING

After you're done with your kettlebell workout, spend 5–10 minutes stretching the major joints and muscles of the body, such as shoulders, hamstrings, calves, back, neck, and hands. See stretches on page 358. If you have a problem area, spend extra time at that location and consider using ice on the area. Stretching after an exercise session, while the muscles are warm and more receptive, is ideal. Post-exercise stretching helps maintain mobility of the joints. As a person gets older, a daily dose of flexibility works wonders in warding off stiffness.

INTRODUCTION TO KETTLEBELLS

This general-fitness kettlebell workout is geared toward those who are new to lifting weights or kettlebell training. Perform all motions without a kettlebell several times until you're familiar with the motions and how your body reacts to them. Then practice gripping the kettlebell. Start with a kettlebell weight that you can lift at least 5 times then progress to 15 reps.

Perform this program for at least two weeks before progressing to the next level. If you display any discomfort, back off or eliminate any exercise that produces that discomfort. Always perform a thermal warm-up for at least 10 minutes to prepare your body for exercise. Post-workout stretches have been included to facilitate flexibility and reduce injury.

INTRODUCTION TO KETTLEBELLS

Warm up for at least 10 minutes.

EXERCISE	SETS	REPS/TIME	REST
Double-Bell Squats, page 322	1	5–10	30 sec
Deadlifts, page 326	1	5–10	30 sec
Overhead Presses, page 331	1	5–10	30 sec
Sword Fighters, page 336	1	5–10	30 sec
Picture Frame, page 70	1	30 sec	30 sec
Soup Can Pours, page 65	1	30 sec	30 sec
Double Knee to Chest, page 90	1	30 sec	30 sec

LEVEL 1

How do you know when you're ready to start this level? If the Introduction to Kettlebells workout seems too easy, then you're ready. However, if you're experiencing some soreness or awkwardness with the movements, don't progress until you're more comfortable.

Always perform a thermal warm-up for at least 10 minutes to prepare your body for the workout. Then try out all kettlebell motions without a kettlebell until you're familiar with the movements. After your kettlebell routine, perform the post-workout stretches that have been included to facilitate flexibility and reduce injury. In this program, start to challenge yourself by increasing the load or extending the time you perform the movements.

LEVEL 1

Warm up for at least 10 minutes.

EXERCISE	SETS	REPS/TIME	REST
Double-Bell Squats, page 322	1–2	5–15	30 sec
Deadlifts, page 326	1–2	5–15	30 sec
Bent-Over Rows, page 334	1–2	5–15	30 sec
Curl-Ups (Kettlebells), page 340	1–2	5–15	30 sec
Gunslinger Curls, page 347	1–2	5–15	30 sec
Picture Frame, page 70	1	30 sec	--
Soup Can Pours, page 65	1	30 sec	--
Double Wood Chops, page 64	1	30 sec	--
Standing Wrist Stretch, page 77	1	30 sec	--
Inward/Outward Wrist Stretch, page 76	1	30 sec	--

LEVEL 2

By the time you move to this level, you should feel confident with the kettlebell movements. Your level of fitness should also be increasing, and you should be ready to start challenging yourself. Only you will know when you're ready. If you overdo it, your body will tell you; back off a little or downsize some of the exercises in this workout to best match your current level. Treat this fitness routine as a living document that can be amended as needed. Nothing is written in stone.

Always perform a thermal warm-up for at least 10 minutes to prepare your body for the workout. Then try out all kettlebell motions with a lighter kettlebell until you're familiar with the movements. Finally, challenge yourself by pushing up the reps or load. Since you'll be including a second set, consider doing the first set lighter with more reps and the second set heavier with fewer reps. Post-workout stretches have been included to facilitate flexibility and reduce injury.

LEVEL 2

Warm up for at least 10 minutes.

EXERCISE	SETS	REPS/TIME	REST
Double-Bell Squats, page 322	2	5–15	30 sec
Side-Step Squats, page 324	2	5–15	30 sec
Overhead Presses, page 331	2	5–15	30 sec
Bent-Over Rows, page 334	2	5–15	30 sec
Bent-Over Triceps Extensions, page 335	2	5–15	30 sec
Double-Bell Kneeling Get-Ups, page 341	2	5–15	30 sec
Curl-Ups (Kettlebells), page 340	2	5–15	30 sec
Plank, page 167	2	1 min max	30 sec
Lateral Arm Raise & Squats, page 345	2	5–15	30 sec
Rear Calf Stretch, page 116	2	30 sec	15 sec
The Zipper, page 71	2	30 sec	15 sec
V Stretch, page 101	2	30 sec	15 sec
Mad Cat Stretch, page 122	2	30 sec	15 sec

LEVEL 3

If Level 2 seems too easy and you feel no discomfort, you're ready to try Level 3. Your body will tell you when to proceed and when to back off. If some portions of this workout are too difficult, you can keep some of your favorites from Level 2 if you wish.

In this workout, the rest time has been shortened and you should be pushing to increase the load. Consider challenging yourself by progressively increasing the load and reps. This workout is really the beginning of a solid fitness routine. Treat it as a living document that can be amended as needed. Nothing is written in stone.

Always perform a thermal warm-up for at least 10 minutes to prepare your body for the workout. Then try out all kettlebell motions with a lighter kettlebell until you're familiar with the movements. Since you'll be including a second set, consider doing the first set lighter with more reps and the second set heavier with less reps. The third set should lie somewhere in between. Post-workout stretches have been included to facilitate flexibility and reduce injury.

LEVEL 3

Warm up for at least 10 minutes.

EXERCISE	SETS	REPS/TIME	REST
Single-Bell Squats, page 321	3	5–15	15 sec
Deadlifts, page 326	3	5–15	15 sec
Lunges (Kettlebells), page 328	3	5–15	15 sec
Lunges with Overhead Lockout, page 330	3	5–15	15 sec
Plank Rotations with Arm Extension, page 339	3	5–15	15 sec
Rocking Horse, page 343	3	5–15	15 sec
Double-Bell Kneeling Get-Ups, page 341	3	5–15	15 sec
Arm & Leg Curls, page 344	3	5–15	15 sec
Diagonal Knee to Chest, page 87	2	30 sec	10 sec
Side-to-Side Neck Stretch, page 57	2	30 sec	10 sec
Skyscraper, page 58	2	30 sec	10 sec
The Butterfly, page 96	2	30 sec	10 sec
Standing Wrist Stretch, page 77	2	30 sec	10 sec
Inward/Outward Wrist Stretch, page 76	2	30 sec	10 sec

POWERHOUSE

This advanced-level workout, designed to foster greater levels of power, is for elite 50+ athletes who are highly trained and can perform or have performed heavy resistance training in the past. Your doctor has cleared you in the past for high-intensity training—your blood pressure is within acceptable limits and you're pain-free.

This workout can be hard on joints and should only be done one to two times a week for no more than four weeks. After you've performed this workout for four weeks, back off for a period. This routine will push you to your limits—don't overdo it. Most people won't do this routine nor need to. Treat this routine as a living document that can be amended as needed. Nothing is written in stone.

Always perform a thermal warm-up for at least 10 minutes to prepare your body for the workout. Note that since this workout encourages heavy lifting, greater recovery time between sets and fewer reps are necessary. Since you'll be including a second set, consider doing the first set lighter with more reps and the second set heavier with fewer reps. The third set should lie somewhere in between. Post-workout stretches have been included to facilitate flexibility and reduce injury.

POWERHOUSE

Warm up for at least 10 minutes.

EXERCISE	SETS	REPS/TIME	REST
Double-Bell Squats, page 322	1–3	3–5	60 sec
Lunges with Overhead Lockout, page 330	1–3	3–5	60 sec
Overhead Presses, page 331	1–3	3–5	60 sec
Bent-Over Rows, page 334	1–3	3–5	60 sec
Kneeling Get-Ups & Presses, page 342	1–3	3–5	60 sec
V Stretch, page 101	1–3	30–60 sec	30 sec
Quad Stretch, page 108	1–3	30–60 sec	30 sec
Rear Calf Stretch, page 116	1–3	30–60 sec	30 sec
Standing Wrist Stretch, page 77	1–3	30–60 sec	30 sec
Inward/Outward Wrist Stretch, page 76	1–3	30–60 sec	30 sec
The Zipper, page 71	1–3	30–60 sec	30 sec

SUPER-ADVANCED FITNESS AND COORDINATION

This routine is designed for motivated and fit individuals who are highly trained and can perform or have performed heavy resistance training. Your doctor has cleared you in the past for high-intensity training—your blood pressure is within acceptable limits and you're pain-free. Don't perform this routine unless you're in super shape and are prepared for a little muscle soreness. Since it includes swings and releases, this workout requires good hand-eye coordination. It should only be done one to two times a week for no more than four weeks. After you've performed this workout for four weeks, back off for a period. Treat this routine as a living document that can be amended as needed. Always perform a thermal warm-up for at least 10 minutes to prepare your body for the workout. Since you'll be including a second set, consider doing the first set lighter with more reps and the second set heavier with fewer reps. The third set should lie somewhere in between. If you're super-fit, try four sets. Post-workout stretches have been included to facilitate flexibility and reduce injury.

SUPER-ADVANCED FITNESS AND COORDINATION

Warm up for at least 10 minutes.

EXERCISE	SETS	REPS/TIME	REST
Sword Fighters, page 336	2–3	8–15	20 sec
Alternating Overhead Presses, page 332	2–3	8–15	20 sec
Plank Row Rotations, page 338	2–3	8–15	20 sec
Rocking Horse with Press, page 343	2–3	8–15	20 sec
Kneeling Get-Ups & Presses, page 342	2–3	8–15	20 sec
Lateral Arm Raise & Squats, page 345	2–3	8–15	20 sec
Figure 8, page 351	2–3	8–15	20 sec
Double-Arm Swings, page 349	2–3	8–15	20 sec
Single-Arm Swings, page 350	2–3	8–15	20 sec
Alternating Swing & Catch, page 352	2–3	8–15	20 sec
Piriformis Stretch, page 92	2	45 sec	20 sec
Pec Stretch, page 75	2	45 sec	20 sec
Pec Stretch Variation, page 75	2	45 sec	20 sec
Rotator Cuff, page 66	2	45 sec	20 sec
V Stretch, page 101	2	45 sec	20 sec
The Butterfly, page 96	2	45 sec	20 sec
Rear Calf Stretch, page 116	2	45 sec	20 sec
Mad Cat Stretch, page 122	2	45 sec	20 sec
Standing Wrist Stretch, page 77	2	45 sec	20 sec
Inward/Outward Wrist Stretch, page 76	2	45 sec	20 sec

BASEBALL/SOFTBALL

This hurry-up-and-wait sport has a great deal of standing or sitting around and then calls upon its players to quickly react to a situation or ball. A middle infielder will have a different workout from a catcher or an outfielder, so speak to your coach about the specific needs of your position and adapt this routine accordingly. As you become more fit, decrease the recovery time and increase the load. The intensity of your training depends on your level of play. If you're a tournament player, use this routine to prepare yourself for the season.

BASEBALL/SOFTBALL

Warm up for at least 10 minutes.

EXERCISE	SETS	REPS/TIME	REST
Forward Lunges (Kettlebells), page 328	1–2	10–15	30 sec
Backward Lunges (Kettlebells), page 328	1–2	10–15	30 sec
Side-Step Squats, page 324	1–2	10–15	30 sec
Sword Fighters, page 336	1–2	10–15	30 sec
Bent-Over Rows, page 334	1–2	10–15	30 sec
Plank Row Rotations, page 338	1–2	10–15	30 sec
Double-Bell Kneeling Get-Ups, page 341	1–2	10–15	30 sec
Curl-Ups (Kettlebells), page 340	1–2	10–15	30 sec
Figure 8, page 351	1–2	10–15	30 sec
Alternating Swing & Catch, page 352	1–2	10–15	30 sec
Mad Cat Stretch, page 122	1–2	60 sec	30 sec
Standing Wrist Stretch, page 77	1–2	60 sec	30 sec
Inward/Outward Wrist Stretch, page 76	1–2	60 sec	30 sec
The Butterfly, page 96	1–2	60 sec	30 sec
Rotator Cuff, page 66	1–2	60 sec	30 sec
Soup Can Pours, page 65	1–2	60 sec	30 sec
Picture Frame, page 70	1–2	60 sec	30 sec
The Zipper, page 71	1–2	60 sec	30 sec

BASKETBALL

Basketball requires an excellent aerobic baseline to accommodate bouts of explosive speed and jumps. If you're practicing and playing a couple of games a week, you might just do this workout in the off-season to reduce your risk of overtraining or use it as a pre-season conditioning routine. Train to play, not the other way around! As you become more fit, decrease rest time.

BASKETBALL

Warm up for at least 10 minutes.

EXERCISE	SETS	REPS/TIME	REST
Single-Bell Racked Squats, page 323	2–3	10–15	15–30 sec
Side-Step Squats, page 324	2–3	10–15	15–30 sec
Deadlifts, page 326	2–3	10–15	30 sec
Plank Rows, page 337	2	10–15	15–30 sec
Gunslinger Curls, page 347	2	10–15	15–30 sec
Double-Arm Swings, page 349	2	10–15	15–30 sec
V Stretch, page 101	2	60 sec	10 sec
Piriformis Stretch, page 92	2	60 sec	10 sec
Double Knee to Chest, page 90	2	60 sec	10 sec
Pec Stretch, page 75	2	60 sec	15–30 sec
Pec Stretch Variation, page 75	2	60 sec	15–30 sec
Double Wood Chops, page 64	2	60 sec	15–30 sec
Quad Stretch, page 108	2	60 sec	30 sec
Side-to-Side Neck Stretch, page 57	2	60 sec	30 sec
Skyscraper, page 58	2	60 sec	30 sec
The Butterfly, page 96	2	60 sec	30 sec

GOLF

When designing a golf program, check with your golf pro to see which kettlebell moves best serve your particular needs and think about which muscles are involved in golf. Since golf is an asymmetrical sport, you'll need to make sure to train both sides in order to balance out your body. The level of your training is dependent on you—the recreational player has a different agenda from a tournament player. Be careful with lower back moves since many golfers have a bad back. My recommendation is to perform kettlebell workouts in the off-season.

GOLF

Warm up for at least 10 minutes.

EXERCISE	SETS	REPS/TIME	REST
Deadlifts, page 326	1–2	8–10	30 sec
Side-Step Squats, page 324	1–2	8–10	30 sec
Plank Row Rotations, page 338	1–2	8–10	30 sec
Curl-Ups (Kettlebells), page 340	1–2	8–10	30 sec
One-Legged Deadlifts, page 327	1–2	8–10	30 sec
Single-Bell Squats, page 321	1–2	8–10	30 sec
Side-to-Side Neck Stretch, page 57	1–2	30 sec	30 sec
Double Knee to Chest, page 90	1–2	30 sec	30 sec
Pec Stretch Variation, page 75	1–2	30 sec	30 sec
Piriformis Stretch, page 92	1–2	30 sec	30 sec
Rear Calf Stretch, page 116	1–2	30 sec	30 sec
Double Wood Chops, page 64	1–2	30 sec	30 sec

KAYAKING

Kayaking can be a recreational hobby done paddling around a lagoon or an intense sport when performed in rivers or the open sea. Kayaking demands upper-body endurance along with strength and power to place the kayak on top of the car or to carry it down to the beach. Some level of lower-body strength is needed as well, not to mention excellent core stability. Kayaking requires strength and endurance on both sides of the body. The intensity of your kettlebell program is dependent on the level of fitness you need. It's also wise to add an aerobic component to your routine.

KAYAKING

Warm up for at least 10 minutes.

EXERCISE	SETS	REPS/TIME	REST
Sumo Squats, page 320	2	8–10	60 sec
Single-Bell Squats, page 321	2	8–10	60 sec
Single-Bell Racked Squats, page 323	2	8–10	60 sec
Racked Lunges, page 329	2	10–15	30 sec
Overhead Presses, page 331	2	10–15	30 sec
Upright Rows (Kettlebells), page 333	2	10–15	30 sec
Bent-Over Rows, page 334	3	10–15	30 sec
Sword Fighters, page 336	3	10–15	30 sec
Plank Rows, page 337	3	30 sec	30 sec
Curl-Ups (Kettlebells), page 340	3	60 sec	30 sec
Lateral Arm Raise & Squats, page 345	3	10–15	30 sec
Double-Arm Swings, page 349	1	8–10	60 sec
Single-Arm Swings, page 350	2	8–10	60 sec
Clean & Press, page 356	1	6-8	--
Lunges (Weights), page 236	1	30 sec	--
Deadlifts, page 326	1	30 sec	--
Arm Swings with Neck Turn, page 67	1	60 sec	--
Skyscraper, page 58	1	30 sec	--
Pec Stretch, page 75	1	30 sec	--

SKIING

Downhill skiing can be a fun recreational hobby done on the bunny slopes or an extreme sport that tackles the black diamonds of the mountains. The intensity of your kettlebell routine is dependent upon your expectations. The ability to enjoy a full day of skiing is dependent on the strength and endurance of your legs and core.

SKIING

Warm up for at least 10 minutes.

EXERCISE	SETS	REPS/TIME	REST
Sumo Squats, page 320	3	10–15	60 sec
Side-Step Squats, page 324	3	10–15	60 sec
Lunges (Kettlebells), page 328	3	10–15	60 sec
Sword Fighters, page 336	2	8–10	30 sec
Plank Rows, page 337	2	5-7	60 sec
Curl-Ups (Kettlebells), page 340	2	10–15	60 sec
Double-Bell Kneeling Get-Ups, page 341	2	10–15	30 sec
Arm & Leg Curls, page 344	2	8–10	30 sec
Double-Arm Swings, page 349	2	10–15	30 sec
Lunges (Weights), page 236	1	30 sec	--
Deadlifts, page 326	1	10	--
Plank, page 167	2	30 sec	--
Quad Stretch, page 108	2	30 sec	15 sec
The Butterfly, page 96	2	30 sec	15 sec
Rear Calf Stretch, page 116	2	30 sec	15 sec

SOCCER

This sport requires cardiovascular endurance, muscular endurance, agility, and explosive speed, among other physical qualities. As you're well aware, each position has its own subset of physical requirements, so design the kettlebell workout to best suit your positional needs. Speak with your coach as to how best to include kettlebells in your existing training routine. If you're playing soccer several times a week and playing on the weekends, this kettlebell workout is best done in the off-season to avoid overtraining injuries. It can be performed as a pre-season conditioning program to complement your existing programs. As your fitness increases, decrease recovery time and increase reps and intensity.

SOCCER

Warm up for at least 10 minutes.

EXERCISE	SETS	REPS/TIME	REST
Deadlifts, page 326	2	8–10	20 sec
Side-Step Squats, page 324	2	8–10	20 sec
Forward Lunges (Kettlebells), page 328	2	8–10	20 sec
Backward Lunges (Kettlebells), page 328	2	8–10	20 sec
Plank Rows, page 337	2	8–10	20 sec
Plank Row Rotations, page 338	2	8–10	20 sec
Plank Rotations with Arm Extension, page 339	2	8–10	20 sec
Double-Bell Kneeling Get-Ups, page 341	2	8–10	20 sec
Arm & Leg Curls, page 344	2	8–10	20 sec
Double-Arm Swings (light), page 349	2	8–10	20 sec
Double Knee to Chest, page 90	2	60 sec	10 sec
Diagonal Knee to Chest, page 87	2	60 sec	10 sec
V Stretch, page 101	2	60 sec	10 sec
The Butterfly, page 96	2	60 sec	10 sec
Side-to-Side Neck Stretch, page 57	2	60 sec	10 sec

SURFING

Surfing can be a fun recreational hobby done in the lapping waves of Honolulu or an intense sport done in major waves in chilly water. Surfing requires upper-body endurance to paddle out to the waves and explosive power to stand up quickly. It also demands excellent balance and agility. The intensity of your kettlebell routine should be done according to your intentions.

SURFING

Warm up for at least 10 minutes.

EXERCISE	SETS	REPS/TIME	REST
Lunges with Overhead Lockout, page 330	2	10–15	30 sec
Bent-Over Triceps Extensions, page 335	3	10–15	30 sec
Sword Fighters, page 336	3	10–15	30 sec
Plank Row Rotations, page 338	2	5–10	30 sec
Kneeling Get-Ups & Presses, page 342	3	10–15	30 sec
Double-Arm Swings, page 349	3	10–15	30 sec
Single-Arm Swings, page 350	3	10–15	30 sec
Figure 8, page 351	2	5–10	60 sec
Alternating Swing & Catch, page 352	3	10–15	30 sec
Arm Swings with Neck Turn, page 67	1	45 sec	--
Pec Stretch Variation, page 75	2	30 sec	15 sec
Double Wood Chops, page 64	2	45 sec	15 sec
Soup Can Pours, page 65	1	10–15	--
Rotator Cuff, page 66	1	10–15	--
Mad Cat Stretch, page 122	1	10–15	--

SWIMMING

Swimming is an excellent method to develop overall fitness. However, since it's not weight bearing, all swimmers should do some level of weight training. Therefore, a regular dose of kettlebell training two to three times week is an excellent idea. Swimming involves many types of strokes, from freestyle to butterfly, so if you're a competitive swimmer, speak with your coach about what the most important muscles are for you. Keep in mind that many swimmers have shoulder issues so be careful not to overdo the shoulder motions or use excessively heavy kettlebells.

SWIMMING

Warm up for at least 10 minutes.

EXERCISE	SETS	REPS/TIME	REST
Lunges (Kettlebells), page 328	2	10–15	30 sec
Upright Rows (Kettlebells), page 333	2	10–15	30 sec
Bent-Over Triceps Extensions, page 335	2	10–15	30 sec
Sword Fighters, page 336	3	10–15	30 sec
Kneeling Get-Ups & Presses, page 342	2	8–10	30 sec
Arm & Leg Curls, page 344	2	8–10	30 sec
Overhead Press & Squats, page 346	2	8–10	30 sec
Gunslinger Curls, page 347	2	8–10	30 sec
Double-Arm Swings, page 349	3	10–15	30 sec
Sumo Squats, page 320	2	10–15	30 sec
Lunges (Weights), page 236	1	10–15	--
Arm Circles, page 67	1	10–15	--
Plank, page 167	2	30 sec	15 sec
Pec Stretch Variation, page 75	2	30 sec	15 sec
Double Wood Chops, page 64	1	60 sec	15 sec
Soup Can Pours, page 65	1	10	--
Rotator Cuff, page 66	1	10	--
The Zipper, page 71	2	30 sec	15 sec
Mad Cat Stretch, page 122	1	10	15 sec

TENNIS/PICKLEBALL

Tennis and pickleball are sports that can be played well into later life and at all levels. As you know, tennis and pickleball involve quick starts and stops and prolonged matches. If you're not doing two-handed backhands, it can be a somewhat one-sided sport, which means upper body imbalances. Thus your kettlebell routine should be designed for your level of play and fitness level. Ask your tennis or pickleball pro to review your workout to match your level of play. Try to design one that equalizes the development on both sides of the body. This kettlebell workout should complement your existing training schedule. Use caution when doing kettlebell moves that include the knee and shoulders.

TENNIS/PICKLEBALL

Warm up for at least 10 minutes.

EXERCISE	SETS	REPS/TIME	REST
Side-Step Squats, page 324	2	10–15	30–45 sec
Overhead Presses, page 331	2	10–15	30–45 sec
Sword Fighters, page 336	2	10–15	30 sec
Plank Row Rotations, page 338	2	10–15	45 sec
Curl-Ups (Kettlebells), page 340	2	10–15	30 sec
Gunslinger Curls, page 347	2	10–15	30 sec
Double-Arm Swings, page 349	2	10–15	45 sec
Figure 8, page 351	2	10–15	30 sec
Mad Cat Stretch, page 122	2	45 sec	10 sec
Standing Wrist Stretch, page 77	2	45 sec	10 sec
Inward/Outward Wrist Stretch, page 76	2	45 sec	10 sec
Quad Stretch, page 108	2	45 sec	20 sec
The Butterfly, page 96	2	45 sec	30 sec
Rotator Cuff, page 66	2	45 sec	30 sec
Soup Can Pours, page 65	2	45 sec	30 sec
Double Wood Chops, page 64	2	45 sec	20 sec
The Zipper, page 71	2	45 sec	30 sec
Piriformis Stretch, page 92	2	45 sec	30 sec
Side-to-Side Neck Stretch, page 57	2	45 sec	30 sec

KETTLEBELL EXERCISES

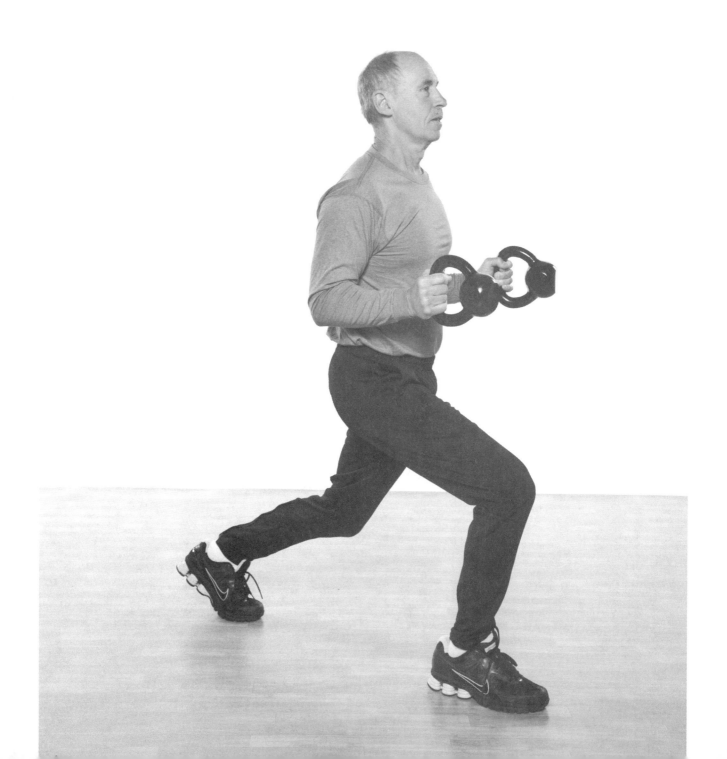

SQUAT SERIES

The squat series is designed to enhance the power and strength of the legs as well as tone the torso. The legs are the foundation of independence for 50+ folks. For all squats, keep your back in neutral position, your head up, and your legs a comfortable distance apart. Engage your core, and try to keep your heels down. Lower yourself down until your thighs are parallel with the floor. Make sure your knees point in the same direction as your feet throughout the movement; to protect your knees, don't allow them to extend past your toes. As you get stronger, you may move on to heavier bells.

If you need to modify any of these squats, feel free to either squat into a chair or place the kettlebell on a table or block so you don't need to lower yourself down as much.

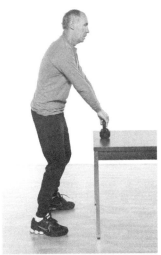
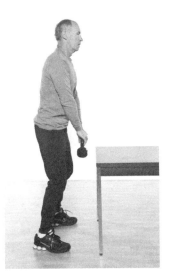
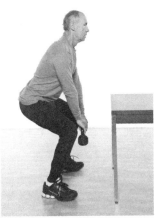

Table modification

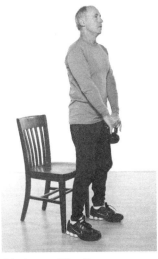
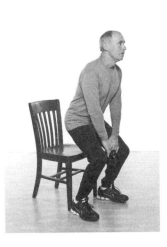
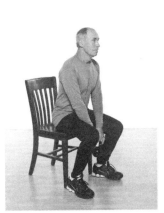

Chair modification

Sumo Squats

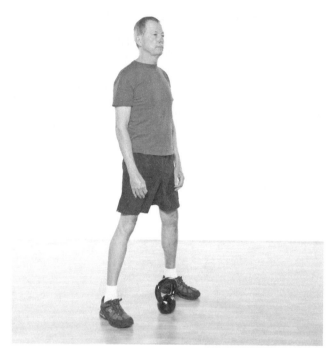

1. Assume a regular stance that's comfortably wide with a kettlebell placed between your feet. You may angle your toes slightly outward if this is more comfortable for your knees.

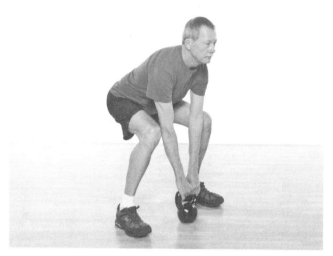

2. Keeping your back straight and your head high, squat down and grab the handle with a side-to-side grip.

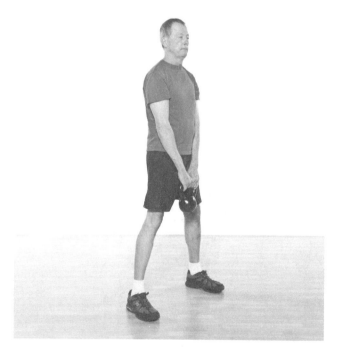

3. Squeezing your butt and thigh muscles, stand up tall.

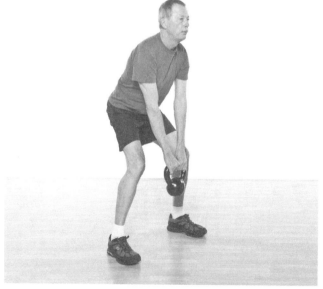

4. Lower into a squat. Use the power of your thighs, not your back.

Single-Bell Squats

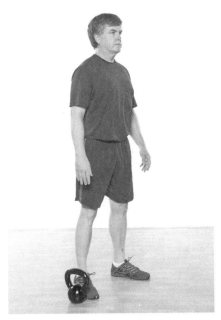

1. Assume a regular stance that's comfortably wide with the kettlebell placed just outside your right foot. You may angle your toes slightly outward if this is more comfortable for your knees

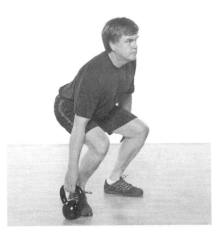

2. Lower your rear end into a squat until your thighs are parallel with the floor, and grab the bell using a right overhand grip.

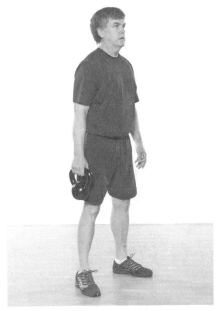

3. Stand up, keeping your arm at your side. Do not hold your breath.

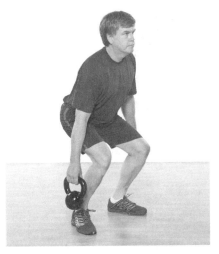

4. Lower into a squat. Use the power of your thighs, not your back.

Repeat, then switch sides

Double-Bell Squats

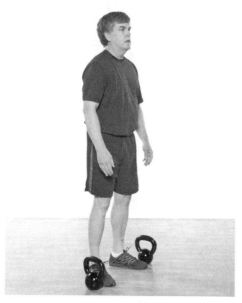

1. Assume a regular stance that's comfortably wide with a kettlebell placed just outside each foot. You may angle your toes slightly outward if this is more comfortable for your knees.

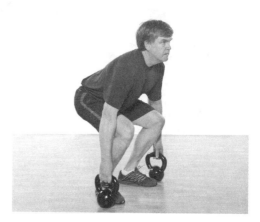

2. Lower your rear end into a squat until your thighs are parallel with the floor, and grab a bell in each hand using an overhand grip.

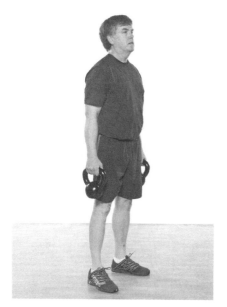

3. Stand up, keeping your arms by your sides.

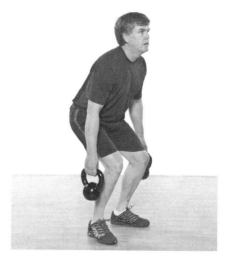

4. Take a deep breath and exhale as you lower into a squat. Use the power of your thighs, not your back.

Return to the upright position.

Single-Bell Racked Squats

Target: glutes, thighs, upper torso

Before you can do a racked squat, you need to know how to rack your bell (see page 298).

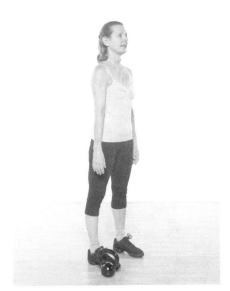 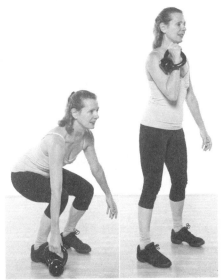 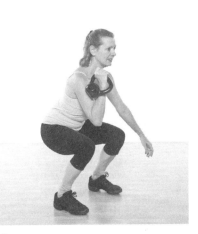

1. Assume a regular stance that's comfortably wide with the kettlebell placed just outside your right foot. You may angle your toes slightly outward if this is more comfortable for your knees.

2–3. Lower your rear end into a squat until your thighs are parallel with the floor, and grab the bell in your right hand. Stand up, keeping your arm at your side, and move the bell to rack position at your right shoulder. Protect your wrist by maintaining neutral wrist position; your grip should be relaxed.

Repeat, then switch sides.

4. Lower into a squat.

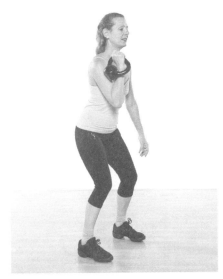 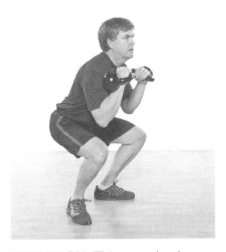

5. Use the power of your legs to stand up.

VARIATION: This can also be done with two bells.

Side-Step Squats

You can start with a heavier bell in this squat.

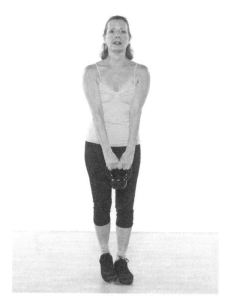 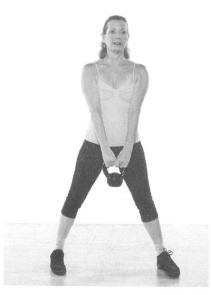 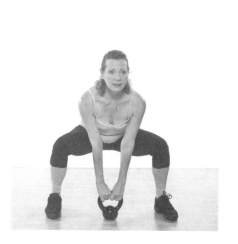

1. Stand with your feet together and hold a kettlebell in both hands using a side-by-side grip.

2–3. Step sideways to the left with your left foot, keep everything facing forward, and squat down, getting your thighs parallel and touching the kettlebell to the floor if possible.

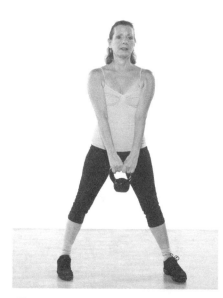 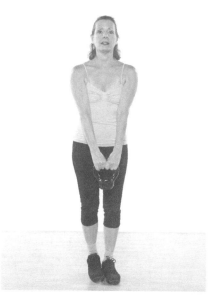

4. Use the power of your legs to stand up.

5. Step your left foot back to starting position.

Step to the right with your right foot and perform a squat.

Continue alternating sides.

DEADLIFT SERIES

Avoid this series if you have lower back issues. To make sure you can do this safely, practice this move without a kettlebell first, or place the kettlebell on a table or block so you don't have to extend back so much. Don't bounce or overstretch, and don't jerk the bell off the floor.

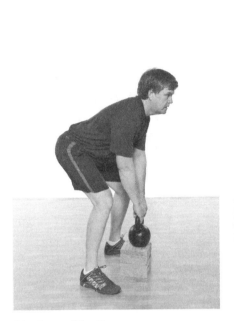 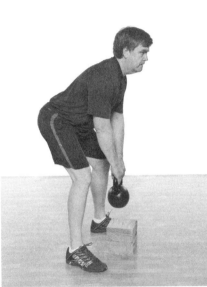 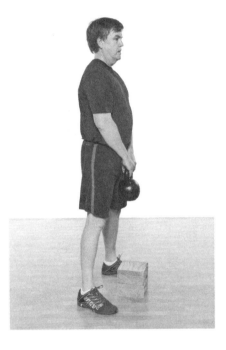

Block modification

Deadlifts

Target: glutes, thighs, core

Traditionally this move is performed with heavy weights. I don't recommend that until you know how your body responds. Instead, perform this slowly a few times without a kettlebell until you know your body can handle the move. The deadlift is done from the hip hinge joint, not by the rounding of the back. CAUTION: This is a controversial move so if you decide to perform it, be careful and do so slowly.

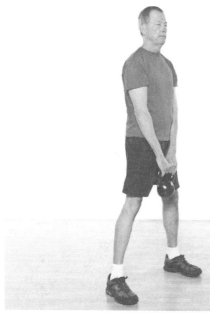 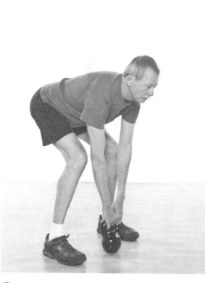 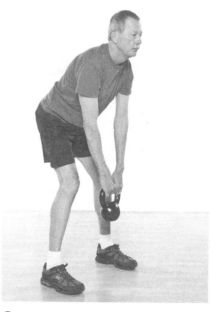

1. Assume a regular stance with your feet a little wider apart than normal.

2. Keeping your back straight from the base of your skull to the base of your tailbone (a yardstick should be able to rest flat on your back), bend at the hip hinge joint, only going as far as your hamstrings will allow. Don't bounce or overstretch.

3. Engage your gluteal muscles—not your back—to slowly return to standing.

One-Legged Deadlifts

Start with a lighter kettlebell, watch your form in a mirror, and avoid rounding your back.

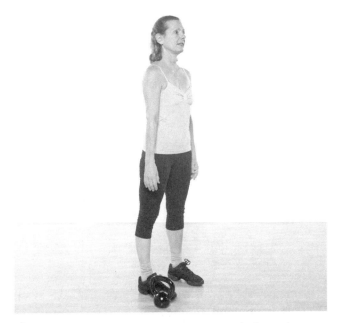

1. Stand with your feet together and place the kettlebell just outside your right foot.

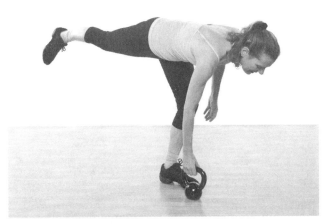

2. Bending over from the hip hinge joint, grab the handle using a right thumb-up or overhand grip. Extend your right leg straight back to counter-balance. Keep your hips level to the floor.

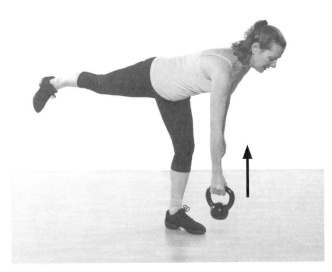

3. Engaging your torso and gluteal muscles, slowly return to starting position.

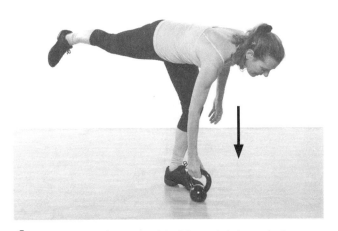

4. Bend over from the hip hinge joint again to return the bell to the floor.

Repeat, then switch sides.

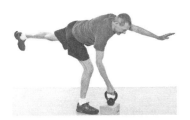

MODIFICATION: To reduce the distance, raise the bell's height by placing it on blocks or a stack of thick books.

Lunges (Kettlebells)

Target: thighs, core

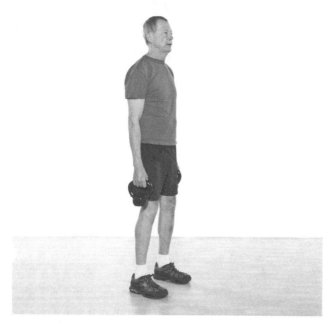

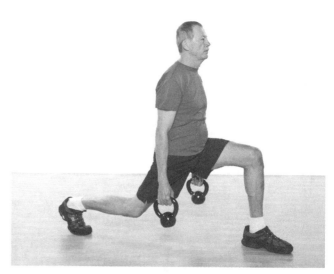

1. Assume a regular stance and hold a kettlebell in each hand, arms along your sides.

2. Lunge a comfortable distance forward with your left leg. Bend your right knee toward the floor, allowing your heel to come off the floor. Keep your front knee pointed in the same direction as your foot, but don't let it extend over your toes. Pay attention to your lower back posture.

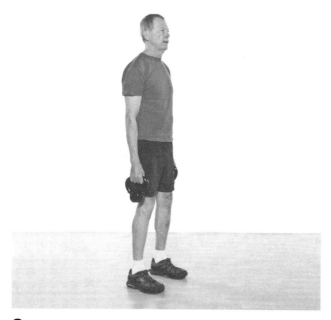

3. Return to starting position.

Perform with your other leg and continue alternating legs.

VARIATION: This can also be done by stepping backward into a lunge.

Racked Lunges

Target: thighs, core

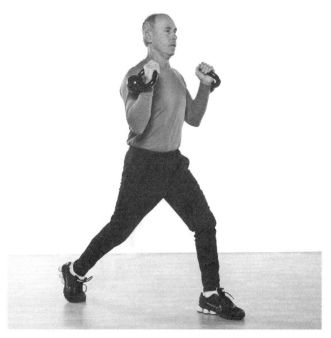

1. Assume a staggered stance with a bell held in rack position at each shoulder. Allow your rear heel to lift off the ground.

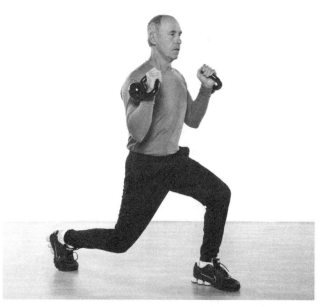

2. Slowly bend both knees, bringing your rear knee toward the floor. Keep your front knee pointed in the same direction as your foot, but don't let it extend over your toes. Pay attention to your lower back posture.

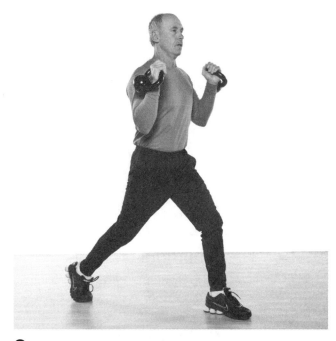

3. Return to starting position.

Repeat, then switch sides.

Lunges with Overhead Lockout

Target: thighs, core, shoulders, triceps

Caution: If you have high blood pressure or heart issues, holding a kettlebell overhead might be ill-advised.

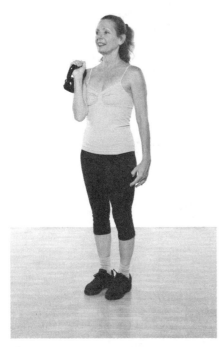 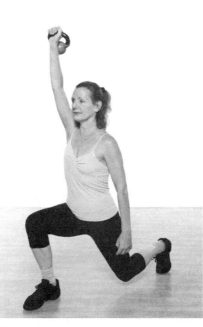 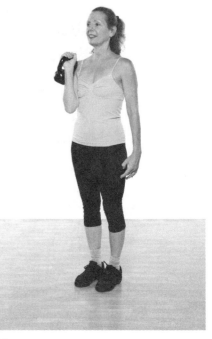

1. Assume a regular stance and hold the kettlebell with your right hand in rack position.

2. Press the bell overhead to lockout position, keeping your wrist in proper position, and lunge a comfortable distance forward with your right leg. Keep your knees, hips, and torso pointed in the same direction as your feet throughout the movement. Bend your left knee toward the floor, allowing your heel to come off the floor.

3. Return to starting position. Repeat, then switch sides.

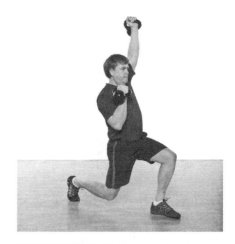

VARIATION: This can also be done by stepping backward into a lunge.

ADVANCED: Hold a kettlebell in each hand and alternate the overhead press with each lunge.

Overhead Presses

Target: thighs, glutes, core, shoulders, triceps

Because you'll be generating extra power with your legs, you can use a heavier bell if your joints can tolerate it. Remember to breathe properly with each rep, exhaling when pressing upward.

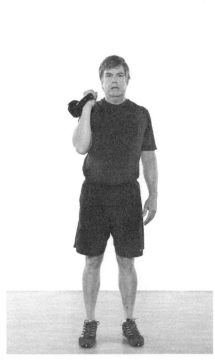

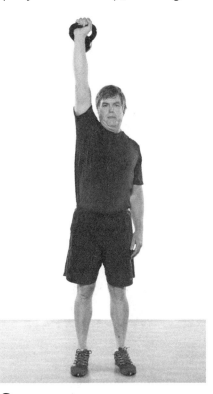

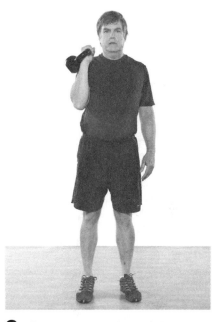

1. Assume a regular stance and hold the kettlebell with your right hand in rack position.

2. Slightly bend your knees then use your legs to transfer the power up through your hips and pelvis and into your shoulder and arm to press the bell up while turning your palm forward. Hold for a moment, keeping your arm above your head and your elbow straight.

3. Return to starting position.

Repeat, then switch sides.

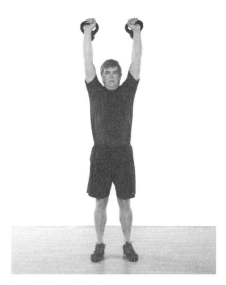

VARIATION: This can also be done with two bells.

Alternating Overhead Presses

Target: thighs, glutes, core, shoulders, triceps

Because you'll be generating extra power with your legs, you can use heavier bells if your joints can tolerate it. Remember to breathe properly with each rep, exhaling when pressing upward.

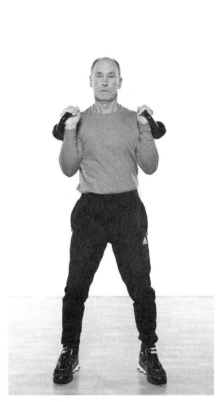

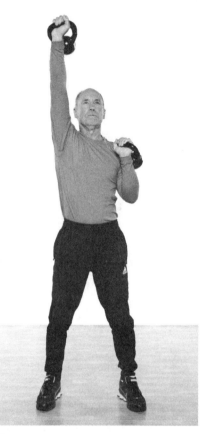

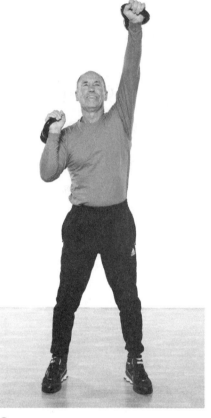

1. Assume a regular stance with a slight bend in your knees and hold a bell in rack position in each hand.

2. Press the right bell overhead while turning your palm forward (you may bend your knees slightly to assist in powering up the bell). Hold for a moment.

3. Return to starting position then press the left bell overhead while turning your palm forward. Hold for a moment.

Continue alternating arms.

Upright Rows (Kettlebells)

Target: shoulders, arms, upper back, core

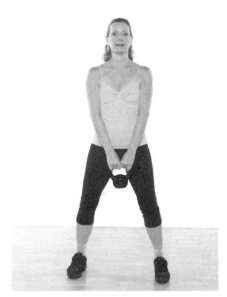
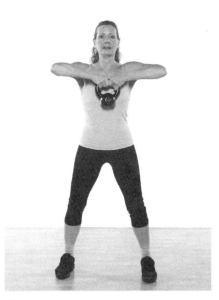
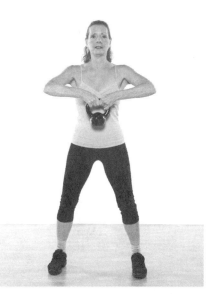

1. Assume a wide stance and hold a kettlebell in both hands using a side-by-side grip. Keep your arms extended in front of your hips.

2. Keeping the bell close to your body, pull it up to chest height. Your elbows will come out to the sides.

3. Lower the bell to starting position.

Shrugs (Kettlebells)

Target: shoulders, upper back

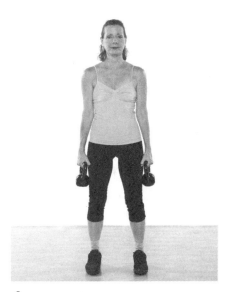
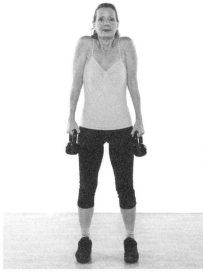
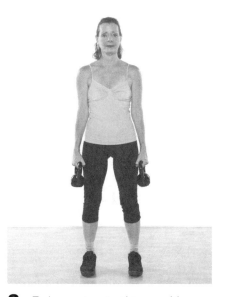

1. Assume a regular stance and hold a bell in each hand, arms by your sides.

2. Shrug your shoulders up to your ears and hold for a moment.

3. Release to starting position.

Bent-Over Rows

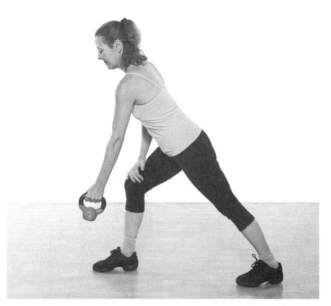

1. Assume a staggered stance with your right leg forward. Bending at the waist about 45 degrees, place your right hand on your right thigh for support and grasp the handle with your left hand. Keeping your arm extended, bring the bell off the ground.

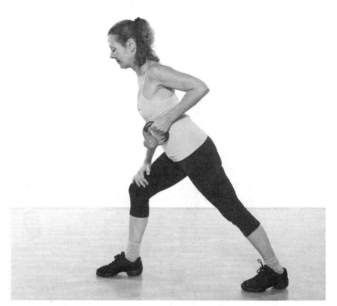

2. Squeezing your shoulder blades together, pull the bell up toward your waist.

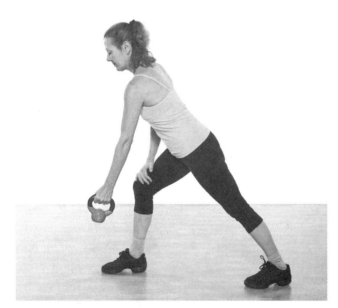

3. Extend your arm toward the floor.

Repeat, then switch sides.

Bent-Over Triceps Extensions

Target: triceps, upper back

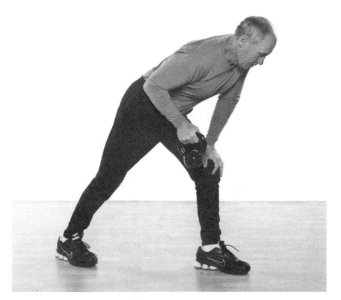 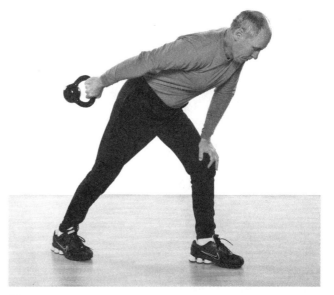

1. Assume a staggered stance with your left leg forward. Bending at the waist about 45 degrees, place your left hand on your left thigh for support and grasp the handle with your right hand, thumb up. Squeezing your shoulder blades together, pull the bell up toward your chest until your arm makes a 90-degree angle and your elbow is next to your ribs.

2. Keeping your right elbow next to your ribs, extend your arm straight back.

Return to starting position.

Repeat, then switch sides.

Sword Fighters

Target: shoulders, upper back, rotator cuff

Use this movement to learn how to control and stop a moving weight.

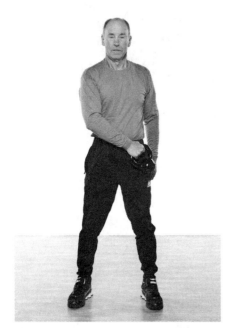

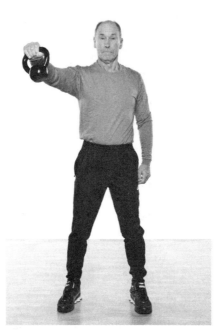

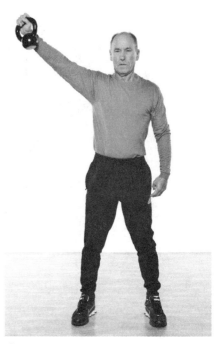

1. Assume a regular stance and hold the kettlebell with a right overhand grip, positioning the bell at your left hip.

2. Keeping your arm straight but not locked, swing the bell diagonally up and across your body to full extension.

3. Hold momentarily.

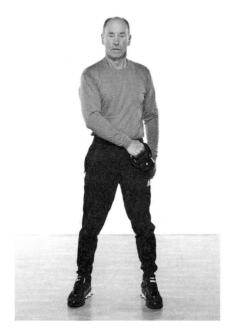

4. Return to starting position.

Repeat, then switch arms.

VARIATION: You can also perform this by rotating your torso, moving your hips and shoulders as a unit with a pivoting motion of your feet.

Plank Rows

Target: full body

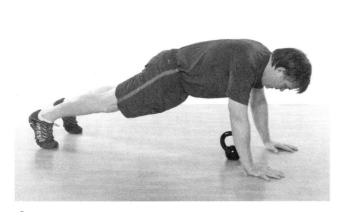

1. Assume a plank (high push-up) position with your hands beneath your shoulders and your legs extended straight back behind you. Position the kettlebell under your sternum.

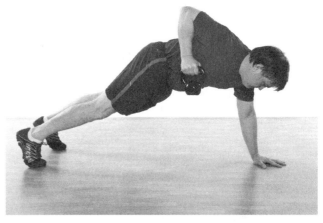

2. Balancing on your left hand and keeping your body as parallel to the floor as possible, grab the bell with your right hand and pull it to your waist. Focus on not rotating your torso by engaging your abs and glutes.

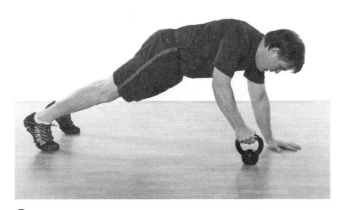

3. Return the bell to the floor.

Repeat, then switch sides.

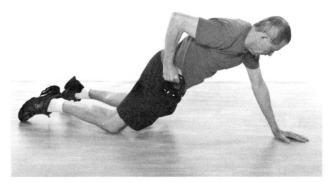

MODIFICATION: This can also be done from your knees.

Plank Row Rotations

Target: full body

This advanced exercise challenges the total kinetic chain and, when done correctly, recruits total-body engagement from the calf muscles to the neck in addition to the core.

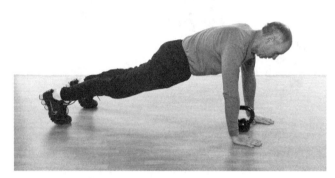

1. Assume a plank (high push-up) position with your hands beneath your shoulders and your legs extended straight back behind you. Place the kettlebell under your sternum.

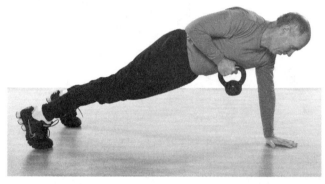

2. Balancing on your left hand and keeping your body as parallel to the floor as possible, grab the bell with your right hand and pull it to your chest.

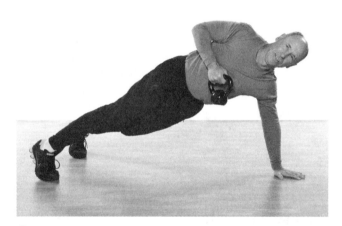

3. Rotate your body to the right, keeping the bell in front of your sternum, until your shoulders are stacked.

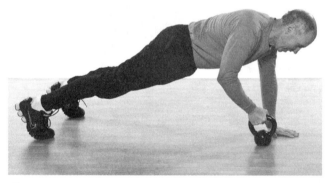

4. Return the bell to the floor.

Now grab the bell with your left hand and perform the same move in the opposite direction. Continue alternating between left and right hands.

Plank Rotations with Arm Extension

Target: full body

This advanced exercise challenges the total kinetic chain and, when done correctly, recruits total-body engagement from the calf muscles to the neck, with special emphasis on the arm and shoulders as well as the core and upper back muscles, which are used as stabilizers. Practice this move without a bell first or with a very light kettlebell. Form is critical!

Caution: Avoid this exercise if you have back or shoulder concerns.

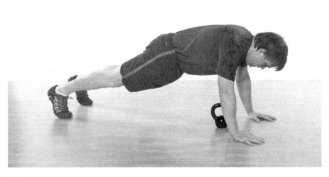

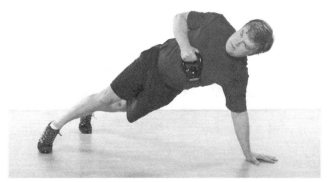

1. Assume a plank (high push-up) position with your hands beneath your shoulders and your legs extended straight back behind you. Place the kettlebell under your sternum.

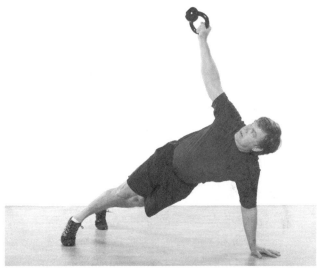

2–3. Grab the bell with your right hand and rotate your body to the right as the bell moves up and over your right shoulder. Your body should nearly be at right angles to the floor.

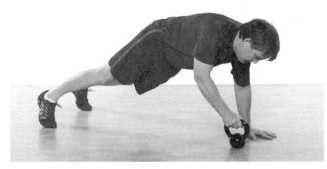

4. Return the bell to the floor and switch sides.

Continue alternating between left and right hands.

Curl-Ups (Kettlebells)

You may want to do this on an exercise mat to provide some cushioning for your back.

Caution: Avoid this exercise if you have back or neck issues.

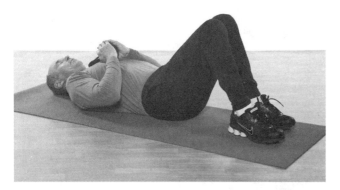

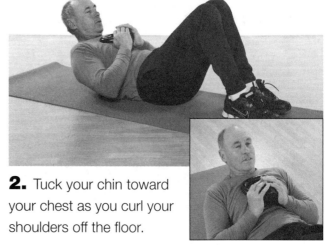

1. Lie on your back with your knees bent and feet flat on the floor. Grasp the ball of the bell firmly with both hands and rest it on your chest.

2. Tuck your chin toward your chest as you curl your shoulders off the floor.

Slowly return to starting position.

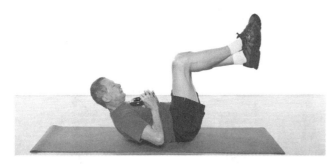

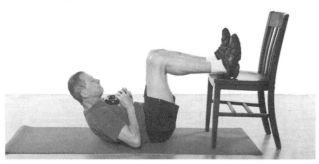

VARIATION: You can also do this with your feet off the ground or placed on a chair.

Double-Bell Kneeling Get-Ups

If you have sensitive knees, place a mat under your kneeling knee.

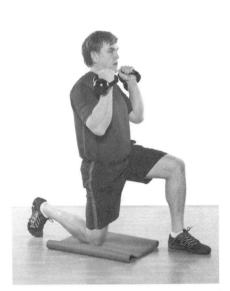 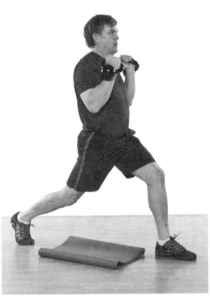 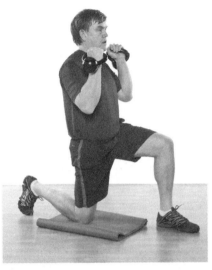

1. Kneel on your right knee and place your left foot in front of you on the floor. Hold a bell in rack position in front of each shoulder.

2. Stand up, staying mindful of the mechanics of your lower back and knees.

3. Return to kneeling position.

Repeat, then switch sides.

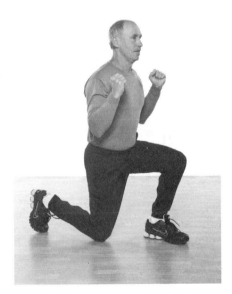

MODIFICATION: You can also try this with a light kettlebell or no weight at all.

Kneeling Get-Ups & Presses

Target: full body

If you have sensitive knees, place a mat under your kneeling knee. Do not do this advanced move until you can do the Double-Bell Kneeling Get-Ups (page 341).

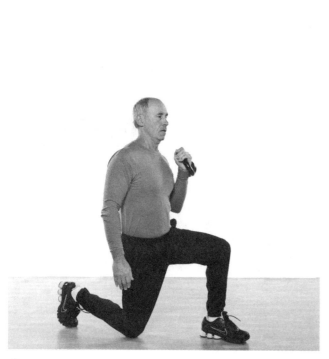 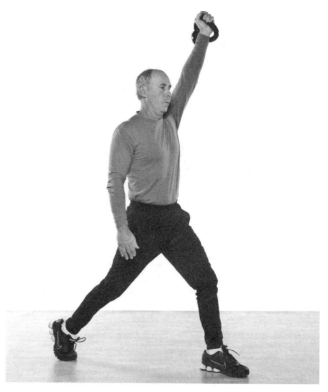

1. Kneel on your right knee and place your left foot in front of you on the floor. Hold the bell in rack position in front of your left shoulder.

2. Stand up and press the bell overhead, rotating your hand forward.

Return to kneeling position.

Repeat, then switch sides.

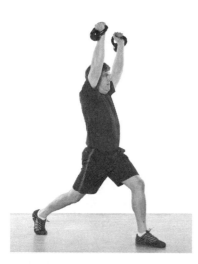

DOUBLE-BELL VARIATION: This can also be performed with two bells held in rack position.

Rocking Horse

This is an advanced exercise. You may want to do this on an exercise mat to provide some cushioning for your back and tailbone.

Caution: Avoid this exercise if you have back or neck issues.

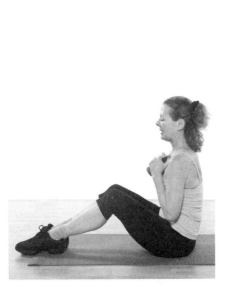 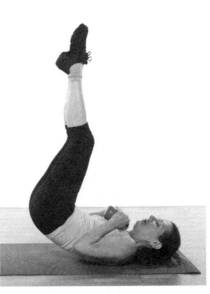 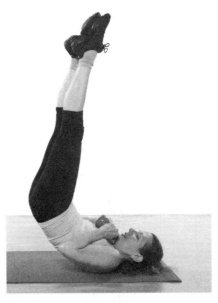

1. Sit on the floor with your knees bent and feet flat on the floor. Hold the handle of the bell with both hands at your chest.

2. Keeping the bell next to your chest and engaging your core, roll back, allowing your hips to lift off the floor.

3. As your hips come off the floor, extend your feet toward the ceiling, pointing your toes and keeping your legs as straight as possible.

Roll back to starting position.

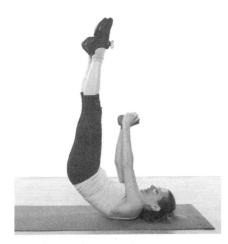

ROCKING HORSE WITH PRESS: For an advanced challenge, press the bell toward the ceiling as you roll back, keeping the bell over your chest.

COMPOUND SERIES

The exercises in this series are more complex and are often called "compound exercises" because they include multiple movements and target several muscles. Make sure you can perform the individual components with correct form before combining the movements or introducing heavier bells.

Arm & Leg Curls

Target: biceps, hamstrings, core

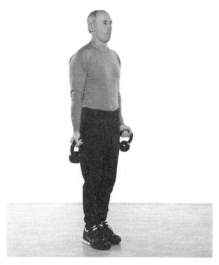 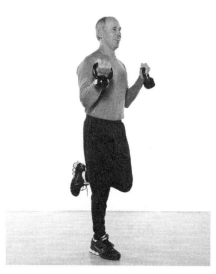 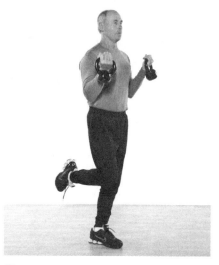

1. Stand with your feet together and hold a bell in each hand in front of your body with an overhand grip, arms straight yet relaxed. Your palms should face forward.

SINGLE-BELL VARIATION:
This can also be performed with one bell. Remember to switch the bell to the other hand at some point.

2. Inhale and curl the bells to rack position as you simultaneously curl your left leg toward your left buttock.

3. Exhale and return to starting position.

Perform the arm curl, this time curling the opposite leg.

Lateral Arm Raise & Squats

Target: shoulders, upper back, thighs, core

Since this is primarily a shoulder/arm exercise, use a lighter bell.

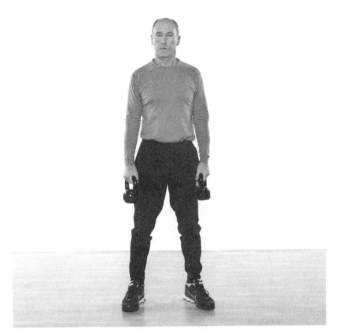

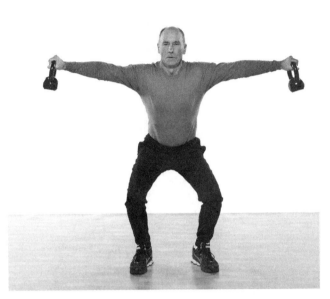

1. Assume a regular stance, or slightly wider stance if need be. Hold a kettlebell in each hand using an overhand grip, keeping your arms alongside your body.

2. Perform a half squat and lift the bells out to the sides, no higher than shoulder level. Hold momentarily.

Return to starting position.

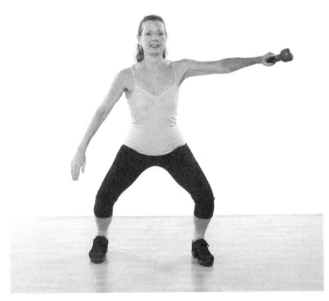

VARIATION: You can also hold the kettlebell in one hand and pass the bell from hand to hand as you stand up.

Overhead Press & Squats

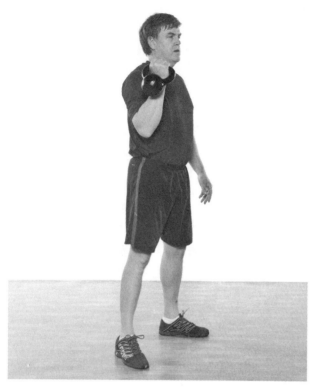

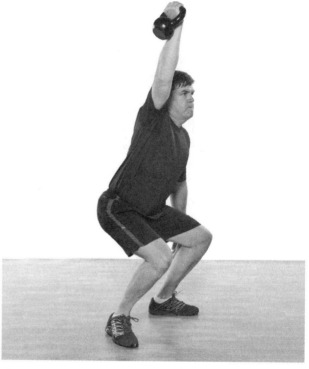

1. Assume a regular stance and hold the bell in rack position at your right shoulder.

2. Inhale as you squat down halfway and press the bell directly overhead, turning your palm forward as you press. Hold momentarily.

Exhale as you return to starting position.

Repeat, then switch sides.

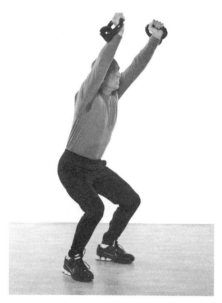

VARIATION: This can also be done with two bells.

Gunslinger Curls

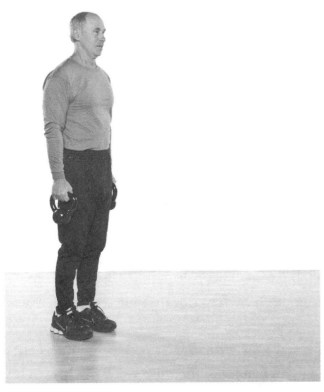

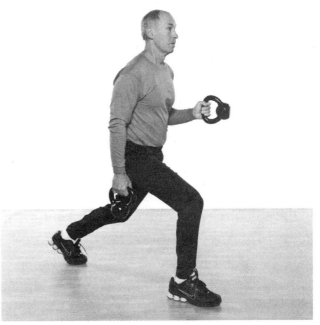

1. Assume a regular stance and grab a kettlebell in each hand using an overhand grip, keeping your arms at your sides, palms facing in.

2. Lunge forward with your right leg, bending your rear knee to the floor, if possible. At the same time, bend your left elbow 90 degrees—you'll look like an old-time gunslinger.

Return to starting position.

Repeat, then switch legs.

VARIATION: You can also lunge backward.

SWING SERIES

Swing movements are unique to kettlebell training in that they engage the total-body kinetic chain. Most conventional weight-training exercises focus on controlled concentric and eccentric contractions while working through the full range of motion. A kettlebell workout is much like performing Olympic lifts—dynamic and explosive. Swings are where the momentum concept comes into play. When you do a swing, you'll engage your legs, butt, and hips, as well as your torso; your arms really only serve as a fulcrum. The beauty of swing moves is that they engage prime mover muscles as well as deep-lying stabilizers. The advantage of kettlebell swings for 50+ folks is that very often as we get older, not only do we lose muscle mass and strength, we lose what's called fast-twitch muscle fibers even more. Swings, when performed safely, foster development of fast-twitch muscle fiber development, which will slow down the decline of your reaction time.

Keep in mind that a body in motion tends to stay in motion, and if you can't maintain control of the kinetic chain, pain will invade your body. Often the reason people get hurt while performing kettlebell swings is because the weaker deep-lying muscles have never been trained prior to a kettlebell workout.

Swings will help you improve power, but learning and practicing the correct technique is critical. It's also important to learn how to slow down a kettlebell too; otherwise you'll be thrown off balance or your joints will be taken past a safe range of motion, injuring the supporting joints and muscles. If you don't believe this, imagine trying to catch yourself while falling.

Swings are very advanced moves. I strongly believe you need to have a solid foundation of muscular endurance, strength, and coordination before you should engage in them since they allow you to lift more weight than you could without momentum. Don't overdo it! Ironically, in traditional weight training, a good trainer never allows you to swing the weights (this is called cheating), but using momentum in certain kettlebell movements is okay. Start slowly and with a light weight.

Double-Arm Swings

Make sure you have a firm grip on the bell and that the area around you is free of things and people. You may use gloves or chalk to secure the kettlebell.

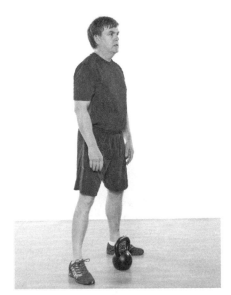

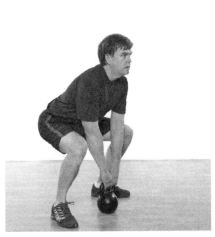

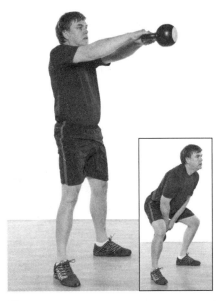

1. Assume a regular stance. Place the kettlebell with its handle angled 45 degrees between your legs.

2. Lower your hips back and down to squat and grasp the handle with both hands using an overhand grip. Your arms and torso should move as a unit.

3. Hike the bell back between your legs and then contract the muscles of your hips and legs simultaneously while you stand up straight and allow the bell to swing forward to chest or head height. Keep your arms extended.

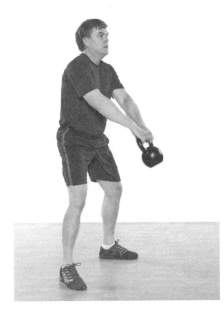

4. Allow gravity to bring the bell back between your legs but control its downward motion.

Quickly reverse the direction upward again.

Single-Arm Swings

You may use gloves or chalk to secure the kettlebell. Some people like to place the free arm out to the side, on the hip, or behind the back; experiment to see which provides the most control and counterbalance for you.

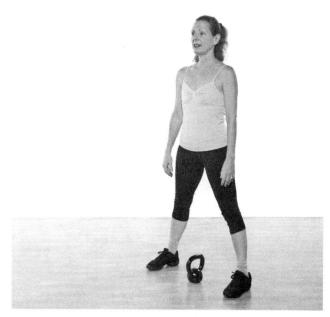

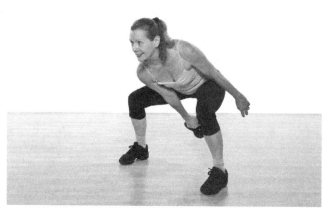

1. Place the kettlebell with its handle angled 45 degrees between your legs.

2. Lower your hips back and down to squat. Grasp the handle with your right hand using an overhand grip, then hike the bell between your legs. Your arm and torso should move as a unit.

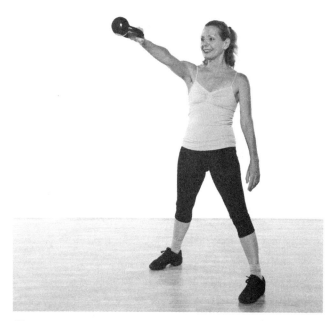

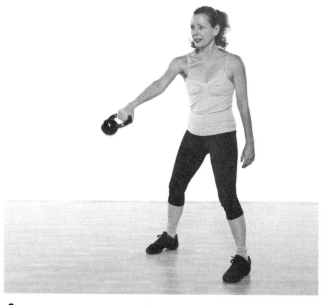

3. Contract the muscles of your hips and legs simultaneously while you stand up straight and allow the bell to swing forward to chest or head height. Keep your arm extended.

4. Allow gravity to bring the bell back between your legs but control its downward motion.

Quickly reverse the direction upward again. Repeat, then switch arms.

Figure 8

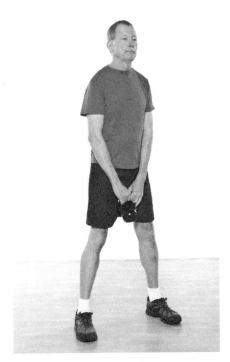

1. Assume an athletic stance and hold the kettlebell in both hands using a side-by-side grip.

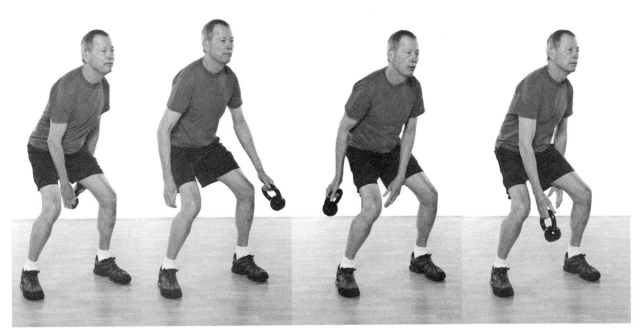

2–5. Squat slightly to pass the kettlebell under, around, and through your legs several times. Make the transition slowly at first and progress to a quicker transfer from hand to hand. Be careful not to drop the bell!

Once you've done this several times, reverse direction. When you're done, stand up straight to stretch your back muscles (the Double Wood Chops stretch, page 64, works well).

Alternating Swing & Catch

This very challenging advanced kettlebell exercise emphasizes hand-eye coordination. Make sure you've mastered the basic swings before trying this—swings should be done without any shoulder or lower back discomfort. Start with a light bell—this exercise can be dangerous if you drop the bell. In addition, you must control the motion at all times—don't let the bell take you into unsafe zones. This exercise demands good grip strength; gloves are highly recommended.

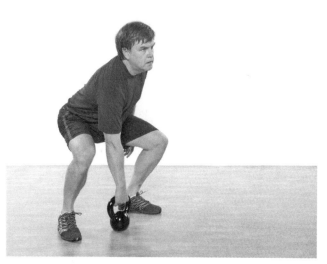 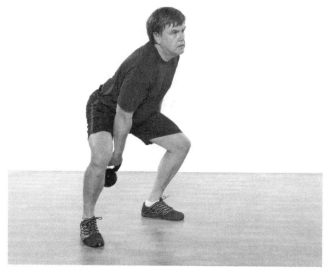

1. Straddle the bell with your feet slightly wider than your shoulders, squat slightly, and grasp the handle with a right overhand grip. Keep your arm straight but not locked throughout the movement.

2. Gently swing the bell several times to prepare the body and generate some momentum.

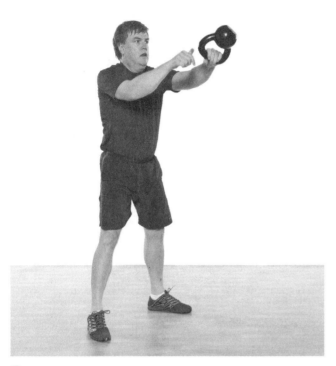

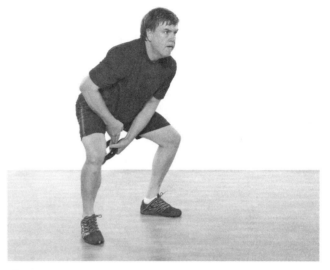

3. As the bell reaches its apex (between shoulder and eye height), quickly release the bell and re-grab the handle with your left hand. The height at which you release the bell is based upon your vision and reaction time.

4. As the kettlebell comes back down, decelerate the motion by squatting down and bending slightly at your hips and knees, allowing the bell to go between your legs.

Continue swinging the bell back up while coming to an upright posture, engaging your core and leg muscles and switching hands at the apex of each upward swing.

CLEAN SERIES

Often as a person get older, explosive power declines. If you're healthy, this series is an excellent way to maintain your explosive power; in some cases it'll improve. The clean is an advanced movement that takes the kettlebell off the floor and to the shoulder using a light upward swing. Learn the motion with a light weight first. You may want to do only one rep at a time and rest and re-group between reps. Some people complain that the kettlebell hitting the forearm bothers them. If you're banging the bell on your forearms, you're probably swinging the bell too far. Pay attention to your form and body mechanics. If this continues to bother you, avoid this exercise or wear something to protect your forearms.

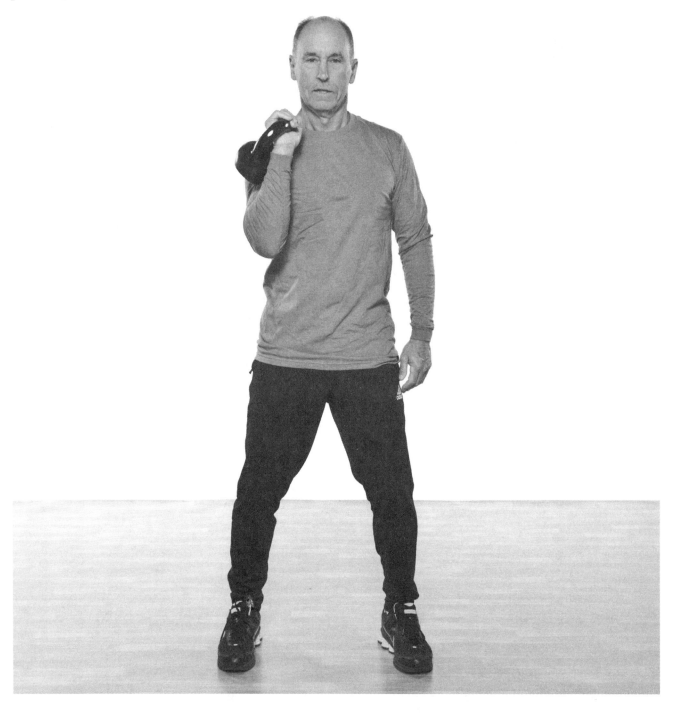

Basic Clean

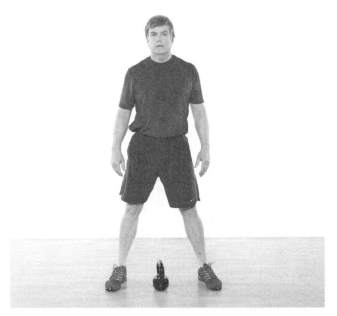

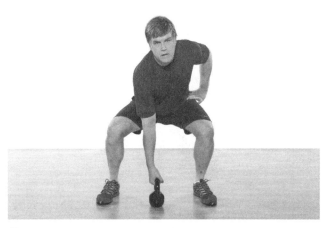

1. Assume a regular or wide stance with the kettlebell slightly out in front of your body and between your legs, handle angled 45 degrees.

2. Lower your hips backward and down and grasp the handle with an overhand grip.

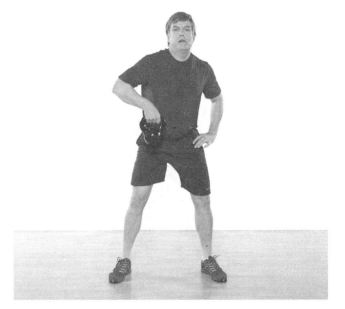

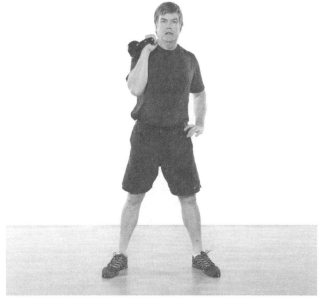

3–4. Perform a light upward swing, moving the arm and torso as a single unit; when the bell reaches waist height, bend your elbow to bring your hand to your shoulder and loosen your grip to allow the bell to flip over. The bell should end up in rack position.

Push the bell off your forearm, flip the handle, and return to starting position.

Clean & Press

The goal of this exercise is to teach the body to work as a team by recruiting your whole body in a systematic fashion to generate power.

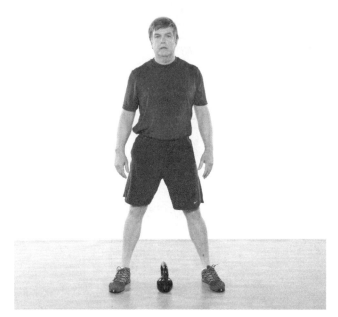

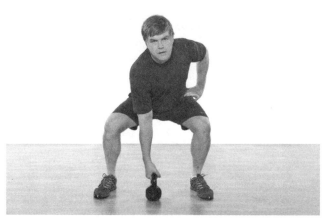

1. Assume a regular or wide stance with the kettlebell slightly out in front of your body and between your legs, handle angled 45 degrees.

2. Lower your hips backward and down and grasp the handle with an overhand grip.

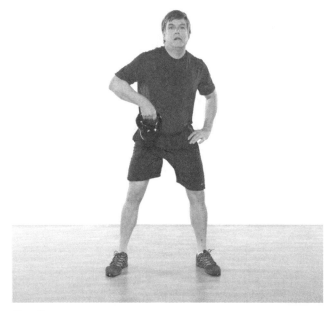

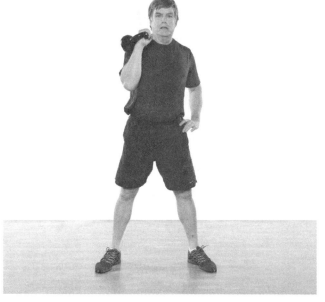

3–4. Perform a light upward swing, moving the arm and torso as a single unit; when the bell reaches waist height, bend your elbow to bring your hand to your shoulder and loosen your grip to allow the bell to flip over. The bell should end up in rack position for a short moment.

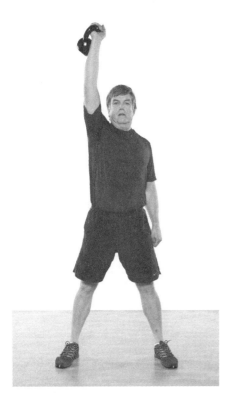

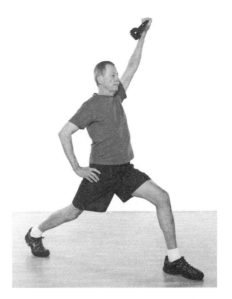

5. Bend your knees to "drop" under the bell and then drive up through your feet, extending your legs and pressing the kettlebell upward.

Return to starting position with control.

ADVANCED VARIATION: When you're comfortable with this movement, you can step backward/forward as you press the bell upward.

SUGGESTED STRETCHES FOLLOWING A KETTEBELL WORKOUT

APPENDIX

EXERCISE AND AGING TO PERFECTION

Many people, when they think of aging, imagine becoming more and more disabled. But previous surgeons general have estimated that close to 85 percent of our most dreaded diseases could be prevented with appropriate lifestyle changes such as good diet and regular exercise. Proper healthy behaviors and sensible exercise prevent disease and untimely death and improve quality of life. Exercise allows people not only to survive but to thrive! Age is no excuse for infirmity! Unhealthy aging is not what our bodies are programmed for, but rather for longevity.

Research supports the conclusion that we can control many aspects of our own aging. Many scientists believe that with a healthy lifestyle, we may be able to turn back the biological clock 10 to 20 years, or at least slow it down. A healthy, active person ages approximately half a percent a year, compared to an inactive person with poor health habits, who ages at approximately 2 percent a year. If you do the math, you can see how an unhealthy lifestyle can make a significant difference over a period of a lifetime. That is why many older people find chairs to be too low and steps too high. But fortunately for all of us, aging to perfection can be found in a daily dose of prudent exercise that includes strength training.

Unfortunately, I had a client come up to me and say, "If I knew I was going to live this long, I would have taken better care of myself." Don't let that person be you. The good news is that this person joined my resistance band strength-training class and now no longer uses his walker and is enjoying a more vibrant life. Research shows that it is never too late to feel great, and a sensible exercise strength-training program is the way to begin.

The average life expectancy of females born in 1930 was 62 years and for males it was 58 years. By 2050 the expected lifespan in the United States will be 82 years of age. In 1980 there were more than 25 million people over the age of 65. By the year 2030, predictions are there will be more than 63 million people over the age of 65 and more than 160 million Americans who are 50+. The 85+ age group is swelling, but the centenarians are the fastest growing age cohort. Today, there are almost double the number of people over the age of 100 than there were in 1980.

While aging is inevitable and extremely desirable when compared to the alternative, being frail is not desirable. Unsuccessful aging is the result of abuse, neglect, and misuse of the human machine. This is much like the old grandfather clock in the living room that does not work. Does it not function fully because the springs have lost their ability to recoil or because they are over-worn, or is it because somebody forgot to wind it up?

For decades we've seen shriveled and non-energetic people among the older segment of the population and have considered this the norm in our society. Now, in studies of older athletes, researchers are finding that fit older people don't slow down like their sedentary counterparts. When such deterioration does occur, it's not the result of old age but, again, of disuse.

The expectation of a slow, steady decline with progressing years is not true for those individuals who prioritize fitness and healthy lifestyles. We now know that a fit person (someone on a regular exercise program) of 90 can be compared to a moderately fit person (someone who exercises occasionally) of 50, if there are no underlying medical disorders. As remarkable as that may seem, more and more evidence supports the fact that chronological age has very little to do with aging and is nothing to worry about. Even mental sharpness is retained at a higher level when the older person stays physically engaged. *The real purpose of exercise is not to add years to one's life but rather life to one's years!*

The mantra of today's older adult needs to be "Life begins at 50." Most of today's older adults are better educated and are wealthier than any previous middle-age generation. The 50+ age group of today is much different than previous 50+ generations. Nowadays most 50+ folks don't consider themselves "seniors." They go by many names—"Baby Boomer," "Gen Xer," "older American," "mature adult," "retiree"—while some prefer to be called "vintage athlete."

In the United States, people are living longer than ever before, and most desire to engage in an active lifestyle. With improved antibiotics, water quality, and sanitation, life expectancy has improved significantly within the USA over the past 100 years. The Centers for Disease Control attributes the increased longevity to the reduction of six of the fifteen leading causes of death: heart disease, cancer, stroke (also known as a cerebrovascular accident or CVA), the flu, liver disease, and falls.

Yet, the CDC found in a study that only 1 in 16 Americans manages to address the five important factors that ward off chronic health issues: smoking, not exercising regularly, drinking to excess, being overweight, and not getting adequate sleep. Today, research indicates that if a person rests too much and eats too much, there is a good chance they will rust out before their expiration date.

Longevity is in our hands: 30 percent of it lies in our genes, leaving the other 70 percent up to how we behave. While there is still much to learn about the aging process, one thing is known for sure: everybody ages differently. Factors that influence the human lifespan include gender, genetics, habits, health care, levels of stress, nutrition, exposure to pollutants, socialization, adherence to safe practices, zest for life, and sometimes just plain luck.

Experts are continually discovering that health-related issues ranging from childbirth to heart disease can be improved by the intervention of exercise. Study after study demonstrates that proper exercise, in addition to making us look and feel better, actually lengthens and improves the quality of our lives. Aging affects the function of all body systems. In the book *We Live Too Short and Die Too Long,* Dr. Walter Bortz writes, "Almost everything we've been taught about aging is wrong. We now know that a very fit body of seventy can be the same as a moderately fit body of forty." We are now entering an exciting time, when medical doctors, exercise physiologists, and gerontologists are all redefining what aging is. No longer should we expect to get sick, get heart disease, get Alzheimer's disease, or any of the other maladies commonly associated with the passage of time.

COMMON BIOMARKERS OF NORMAL AGING

There are generally agreed-upon physical changes that occur during the normal aging process:

- Metabolism slows. Calorie requirements drop by 2 to 10 percent each decade over age 30.

- Muscle mass decreases.

- Nerve cells degenerate, resulting in slower reaction and movements.

- Blood cholesterol levels and body fat levels may increase, likely due to decreased activity.

- Bone mass decreases, vertebral discs degenerate, and osteoporosis may set in.

- Muscular strength decreases.

- Skin becomes darker, more pigmented, and more vulnerable to bruises and skin sores. It also loses elasticity.

- Joints stiffen and bone density decreases, often resulting in stooped posture and a loss of height. Breathing, urination, and defecation can be impaired.

- The heart muscle loses strength, and cardiac output (the amount of blood pumped with each beat) declines. The hardening and shrinking of the arteries (arteriosclerosis) makes it more difficult for blood to flow freely throughout the body. The body may compensate with an increase in the systolic blood pressure. Increased workload placed on the heart and circulatory system can lead to strokes and heart attacks.

- Tendency toward hypertension increases in some individuals as a result of increased peripheral vascular resistance.

- The respiratory system weakens, and the exchange of oxygen and carbon dioxide in the lungs may become more difficult and less efficient, resulting in a decrease in vital capacity, total lung capacity, and oxygen intake.

- The gastrointestinal system can change, leading to different dietary demands.

- Bladder control may be lost, and more frequent urination may occur.

- The nervous system is altered, in part because of a loss in bulk of the brain. Brain weight in a 75-year-old is about 92 percent of that of a 30-year-old.

- Kidney filtration declines with age. The kidney filtration rate of a 75-year-old is 60 percent of the rate of a 30-year-old.

- The sensations of touch and pain are reduced with age.

- Visual acuity diminishes. Less light reaches the retina in an aging eye, and the lens often acquires a yellow cast. Cataracts are increasingly found.

- Taste and smell become less sensitive.

- Reflexes and reaction time are slowed.

CHANGING THE PARADIGM OF AGING

Most of us know what "lifespan" is, but most people are not familiar with the term "health span." Health span includes being more energetic, being more flexible, and being able to enjoy life more fully. Simply put, it's being fit for life and for the challenges and demands presented by it.

Today's group of 50+ clients are not satisfied by living on past achievements. They are looking for new challenges physically, intellectually, and socially.

The bad news is that we all are aging. The good news is that we all are aging—definitely better than the alternative. Technically, we all begin to age from the moment of conception. When we are 15 years of age, we can't wait to be 16 and drive. At 20 we can't wait to be 21, whereas at 49 years of age some fear being over the hill. Unfortunately, by middle age, if the body is not well cared for, the effects of "normal" aging, such as heart disease, hypertension, joint disorders, and changes in our skin, manifest themselves. While we can see the visual effects of aging on the outside, things are also occurring internally, such as glucose intolerance, a loss of bone density, and vascular changes, to mention a few. That is the bad news!

The good news is that how we age is, to a large extent, determined by the choices we make daily. What we do today determines our tomorrows. Age is just a number! What is more important is how a person feels, performs, and behaves. Most older adults don't want to live long only to survive in the back room of a nursing home—they want to thrive and enjoy a fulfilling quality of life. Age is no excuse for being sedentary and weak.

Not all aging is "normal" aging, though. Dr. Bortz maintains that aging can often be attributed to:

- **Abuse:** smoking, excessive eating, recreational drugs, or drinking.
- **Disuse:** engaging in a zoo-like existence of sedentary living.
- **Misuse:** beating oneself up with overtraining or performing activities biomechanically incorrectly, resulting in joint disorders.

If a person does not maintain fitness, they will lose adequate function to perform activities of daily living and become frail. A major culprit is extended periods of sitting, which can increase the risk of metabolic diseases, cardiovascular diseases, and a decreased lifespan. Getting up and moving around every 30 minutes or so is at least as important as getting enough exercise overall. "Move it or lose it" has real meaning to the 50+ generation!

For decades we have accepted getting weak, stiff, frail, and non-energetic as normal aging. Those expectations are beginning to shift. Exercise physiologists who are involved in exercise programming for older adults strongly believe that stooped shoulders, halting steps, and other so-called age-related conditions can be prevented or even corrected with proper exercise. Study after study bears out that older athletes' metabolism does not slow down as much as first thought. When older people stay engaged in a moderate strength-conditioning program, their muscle mass does not decrease as much as that of a sedentary person of the same age. We now have evidence that a fountain of youth does exist! It exists in the form of your local fitness center, pool, or exercise class.

THEORIES ON AGING

Theories about the causes of aging abound. Dr. Frank Schneider, while at the University of Southern California Andrus Gerontology Center, said, "If you think cancer is complex, look at aging." Today most experts agree that the effects of the aging process may arise from a multitude of parallel and interconnecting factors. Aging is a complex and multidimensional process.

One current group of theories holds that aging follows a biological timetable, one that regulates both childhood growth and development and also adult aging, such when one gets gray hair. Another major theory suggests that environmental assaults on the body gradually cause things to go wrong. Many researchers believe that these factors may occur in combination. It is also suggested that many factors, both intrinsic and extrinsic, are yet to be discovered. Because these theories of aging are not mutually exclusive, it seems unlikely that one theory will ever be able to describe the process of aging in its entirety.

The following provides a brief and very simplified explanation of some of the major theories being proposed.

Extrinsic and Error Theories

Many things we associate with aging, such as brittle bones, forgetfulness, and loss of strength, are brought on due partially to extrinsic factors, such as mental or physical inactivity. Failure to use our muscles and other bodily systems regularly can result in premature aging, either from disuse or from development of disease. Each of us ages at our own pace. Many of the changes we expect with the passage of time can be positively influenced by the inclusion of sensible lifestyle behaviors and regular exercise.

Intrinsic Theory

In 1961 scientists at Vistar Institute of Anatomy and Biology found that human cells have a finite capacity to duplicate or divide. When cells from older adults were compared to those of younger adults, the younger cells had a greater capacity to divide. Interesting fact: scientists discovered that people with Werner's Syndrome (a disease that results in premature aging and ultimately death) show a reduced capability to replicate their cells when compared to those of the same age without the disease.

Lifespan/Metabolic Theory

The lifespan, or metabolic, theory of aging suggests that the organism has a theoretical metabolic time limit. The premise is that the metabolic time limit is pre-set and is passed from one generation to the next. For years researchers have known that certain species have fairly predictable lifespans. Elephants usually live approximately 70 years; horses about 40 years, and mice survive two to three years.

Human mortality is characterized by the longer you live, the longer you are expected to live. If a baby can avoid infant mortality and stay well the first few years of life, their chances to live a long life increase significantly. If a young person can avoid accidents, drugs, chronic and acute illness, etc., in the middle years of life, their chances of living a long life increase. Quality of life depends on how you live—how you eat, sleep, manage stress, avoid toxins, and get proper physical activity. The earlier you start, the better, but it is never too late to feel great.

Quality of life and health span is more important than quantity of life. Most people don't want to live to be 100 in the back rooms of a nursing home. They would rather live fully until they die, without severe mental and physical limitations. It is important to note that life expectancy, lifespan, and healthy lifespan are all uniquely different, yet often confused.

The process of aging still remains an enigma, yet the following factors are generally accepted:

- **Programmed senescence.** Aging is the result of the sequential switching on and off of certain genes, with senescence being defined as the time when age-associated deficits are manifested.

- **Endocrine theory.** Biological clocks act through hormones to control the pace of aging.

- **Immunological theory.** A programmed decline in immune system functions leads to an increased vulnerability to infectious disease, resulting in greater age-related characteristics that influence death.

- **Error theory.** One theory suggests that our cells (specifically, our telomeres) are designed to multiply a limited number of times. There appears to be a relationship between this "programmed death of the cell" and the rate at which we age and the length of the human lifespan.

- **Catastrophe theory.** Damage to mechanisms that synthesize protein results in faulty proteins, which accumulate to a level that causes catastrophic damage to cells, tissues, and organs.

- **Wear and tear.** Cells and tissues have vital parts that wear out.

- **Rate of living.** The greater the rate of oxygen metabolism, the shorter the lifespan.

- **Cross-linking.** The accumulation of cross-linked proteins damages cells and tissues, thereby slowing down bodily processes.

- **Free radicals.** Accumulated damage caused by oxygen radicals causes cells, and eventually organs, to stop functioning.

- **Somatic mutation.** Genetic mutations occur and accumulate with increasing age, causing cells to deteriorate and malfunction.

How to circumvent aging is a topic that has fascinated people since the beginning of time. Even the most respected scientists and gerontologists do not fully understand the mechanisms of aging, but they recognize that no one ages exactly the same. Thus, they speak in terms of each person having several ages: chronological, biological, and social.

CHRONOLOGICAL AGE

Chronological age is simply the number of times your body has circled the sun, the number that a liquor store clerk or a traffic cop can calculate by looking at your driver's license. Chronological age has relevance in the context of studies that address demographics and statistics—and, of course, in studies on aging. We all know that some people age faster than others: the number of years someone has lived does not always reflect their functional ability. We often see 70-year-olds running 10K races, but we also see 70-year-olds in nursing homes.

BIOLOGICAL AGE

Biological age, also called physiological age or functional age, reflects a person's physical condition and how well they have maintained function. The interesting thing about aging is there can be a large discrepancy between chronological and biological age. Even within our own bodies, some of our parts wear out faster than other of our body parts.

SOCIAL AGE

Social age, also called behavioral age, has to do with how a person acts and feels about themselves and their age. It also relates to how old they perceive themselves to be and the manner in which they are able to function independently. Many commercials imply that wrinkles are bad, and that people should cover up their age. Too many stereotypes exist about aging. Two people with the identical age can be radically different in how they function; one may be functioning quite well with very few limitations while the other may be severely impaired. A person's ability to function normally, rather than a diagnosis of a disease or old age, is what is most important for older adults. But in spite of age-related changes, adhering to a healthy lifestyle and having a positive attitude can give us a better chance of independent functioning. Growing older should not reduce the quality of life. Evidence suggests that a dose of daily action and positive attitude have a more profound effect on positive aging than does genetics. Having a positive attitude toward the aging process will enhance your experience of it. When we lose motivation, we need to encourage ourselves with a simple motto: *When challenges and changes come, strive to overcome.*

EXERCISE AND LONGEVITY

We are the first generation that have the opportunity and knowledge to dictate how we age. More and more research suggests that lifestyle has a significant influence on how a person ages, maybe even more than genetics. Alex Lief, MD, and Harvard Medical School professor of gerontology, has said that exercise is the closest thing we have to an anti-aging pill. Dr. Walter Bortz said, "Our aging is in our own hands. It is no one else's responsibility. If we depend on our doctors, our families, our government, we risk compromising the quality of our lives." If we take charge of our lives, we have a better chance of ensuring that our future years are creative and radiantly alive. Science confirms that exercise can slow down the aging process.

The purpose of exercise is not to make senior athletes out of all older adults or even to extend their lifespan, but rather to afford older adults the opportunity and capability to do whatever they wish to perform—whether it be to have adequate strength to get out of a chair and go for a walk, or to play catch with their grandchildren, or even go on a vacation that they always wanted to take. I have an older friend at the gym who told me the only reason she exercises is so that she is fit enough to take advantage of the over-75-years ski free program!

Dr. Herbert DeVries, a well-respected professor and exercise physiologist at the University of Southern California, is convinced that men and women in their 70s and 80s can achieve levels of vigor usually associated with people 30 years younger. A study conducted by Dr. Steven Blair of the Cooper Institute for Aerobics Research in Dallas found that the data plainly indicates that as much as one and one-half of all functional decline typically associated with aging is the result of disease syndrome and can be reversed with proper exercise. It has been implied that preparation for a healthy and fit old age should begin as a young person. How many times have we heard our friends say, "If I knew I was going to live this long, I'd have taken better care of myself!" Fortunately, we now know that it is *never too late* to start taking better care of ourselves and one of the first steps is to begin with a sensible exercise program.

A few years ago, we knew exercise was good for you and it would put zest in your step. But now we're finding it may *add years to your life* and *life to your years*! What would you estimate is the maximum lifespan for humans? Most researchers believe that the maximum lifespan is slightly over 110 years. Scientists are suggesting that we should not have a steady decline starting in our 30s, but rather live successfully until our 80s before body systems start to slow down and break down.

A study conducted jointly by the American College of Sports Medicine and the Center for Disease Control found that 12 percent of deaths in Americans are *indirectly* related to lack of exercise, or what we call hypokinetic disease, or what might be better known as "couch potato syndrome." With all of the attention exercise is receiving, it is depressing that only one in four Americans get adequate exercise.

Living a long and healthy life is dependent upon many factors, including a healthy and active lifestyle, strong genes, and plain good luck. The *Journal of the American Medical Association* stated that even a minimal amount of exercise, such as a 30-minute brisk walk two times a week, has a protective effect against cardiovascular disease and cancer. Another exciting study shows that unfit men who exercised their way to physical fitness cut their overall death rate by nearly half (after adjusting for age, health status, and other risk factors for premature death) when compared to those who stayed out of shape. The more physically fit the men became, the more they cut their risk.

Current research does show an increase in lifespan for those who exercise regularly and follow a prudent and healthy lifestyle. Older adults must come to realize that "use it or lose it" has real meaning to them if they want to age successfully and remain independent. Unfortunately, many older adults believe it is too late to start exercising and that their past abilities and present disabilities are predictors on how fit or healthy they can become. This is false! A motto for today's older adult: *I want to grow strong and capable, not old and frail!*

AGING AND THE BODY

Aging affects all the systems of the body. We now know that a person does not grow too old to exercise but grows old from lack of exercise. In the 1970s, when the effects of space travel were first explored, some researchers found that 21 days of total bed rest shows the same effects that are seen in 30 years of normal aging. Exercise physiologists have proven that a trained and fit 60-year-old person is equivalent in their oxygen carrying capacity as an untrained, unfit sedentary 30-year-old person. We also understand that although various medical interventions can improve the body's ability to transport oxygen, that is only a fraction of what can be accomplished through exercise and improved cardiopulmonary fitness. Studies have shown that improved fitness may extend life, and it is indisputable that exercise improves quality of life.

We all know changes occur as we age; however, the amount of effect is different for every individual. Today, medical doctors, along with exercise physiologists and gerontologists, are redefining the aging process. We know that normal aging, healthy aging, and sickness as seen in older people are not the same. Few people die strictly of old age, but rather from the repercussions of diseases such as cancer and heart disease so often found in older, unhealthy people. Shoring up one's functional reserves through a healthy lifestyle can delay a functional decline often seen in aging.

In normal aging, people decline about 2 percent a year while active and fit people age at about half a percent. Multiply 2 percent versus half a percent over 30 years and that decline can be the difference between remaining independent or being confined to a nursing home. As we age, we lose about 6 to 8 percent in relative power. Power declines to a greater degree than strength over time, and it accelerates even faster after the age of 60. Flexibility declines about 5 percent each decade, which can lead to impaired balance and difficulty in doing simple things like tying your shoes. After 70, we can experience a significant loss of aerobic ability.

COMMON CHANGES SEEN WITH NORMAL AGING

Heart

Maximal oxygen consumption during exercise declines in men by about 10 percent with each decade of adult life; in women VO_2 max drops by about 7.5 percent per decade. Cardiac output is the product of stroke volume and heart rate. All three have been shown to decrease with age, though exercise can reverse or lessen this decline.

Brain

With age, the brain loses some cells (neurons) and others become damaged. However, it adapts by increasing the number of connections (synapses) between cells and by regrowing the branch-like extensions (dendrites and axons) that carry messages in the brain. Physical exercise has been shown to improve motor skills and cognitive skills.

Kidneys

The kidneys gradually become less efficient at extracting wastes from the blood. This decrease in efficiency is partially attributed to the general decrease in the size of the kidneys that occurs with age, and also the decrease in blood or plasma flow to the kidneys. Bladder capacity declines and tissues atrophy, sometimes resulting in urinary incontinence, which can often be managed with exercise and behavioral techniques.

Body Fat

Body fat increases with age, commonly from a combination of acquiring more storage fat from sedentary living and redistribution of existing stored fat. Women are more likely to store it in the lower body—hips and thighs. Men will tend to carry their stored fat in the abdominal area. An unhealthy change in body composition has many health risks associated with it, but these risks can be reduced with physical activity.

Muscle

Lean muscle mass is the amount of muscular tissue that you have, in relation to total body mass. The average decline in muscle mass between the ages of 30 and 70 has been measured at 22 percent for women and 23 percent for men. Type II fibers, the muscle fibers responsible for high levels of strength, have been shown in some studies to decrease as much as 50 percent in men by the age of 80. Strength training can prevent loss of muscle mass and help in regaining the lean mass you may have already lost. Leg strength is critical to independent living.

***

Can we slow down the aging process? Many of these so-called effects of aging can be reversed or slowed down with the intervention of a proper and regular exercise routine. However, no matter how well we maintain ourselves, the physiological process of aging will eventually take its toll. However, proper exercise is an important ingredient in maximizing physiological capacity and slowing down the effects. Exercise training does not stop the biological clock, but at the present time it is the only means available of slowing it down.

EXERCISE AND THE CIRCULATORY SYSTEM

The circulatory system, which includes the cardiovascular system and the respiratory system, many times limits the functional abilities of older people. With normal aging some structural, anatomical changes take place within our bodies that affect our ability to function fully. Some unfit older adults fatigue easily or experience shortness of breath when participating in simple activities. Specifically, with normal aging we see the size of the heart decrease and the ability of the heart to pump blood efficiently decrease. It is not uncommon to see heart valves and the vascular system become more rigid and thicker with age.

One of the most common effects of aging seen in the vascular system is an increase in blood pressure. I remember when I was in college many years ago, the common belief was that a systolic blood pressure (the top number in the blood pressure fraction which measures the amount of force used to push blood through the arteries) was acceptable if it was 100 plus your age. The new theory is that a consistent blood pressure of 150/90 is reason for concern. The belief is that the artery walls lose their elasticity with age and become hardened (thus the term hardening of the arteries), which affects the ability of the blood to flow freely. Some researchers contend that the greater difference between the upper number and lower number of the blood pressure represents an increased risk of myocardial infarction, which literally means death of the heart muscle, more commonly referred to as a heart attack.

Today we know that age alone does not wear out the heart; it is disuse, misuse, and disease that does that. In two comprehensive studies involving women with heart disease and exercise, researchers found that moderate exercise, such as brisk walking several times a week, cut heart attack risk by up to 50 percent. The other study, which analyzed 73,000 women enrolled in the Boston-based Nurses' Health Study, found that physical activity can reduce the risk of stroke by more than 40 percent. This was one of the first strong suggestions that exercise works as well for women as it does for men.

A landmark study completed by Dr. DeVries found that when he followed a group of older men through 42 weeks of vigorous conditioning, they improved in the way their bodies consumed oxygen and how their lungs took in air and how effectively they used it. That is because the body's ability to use oxygen efficiently is a sign of fitness. Another landmark study, which revealed that older adults can improve cardiovascular fitness as they age, was performed by Dr. Kasch at San Diego State University. Dr. Kasch carefully observed 15 men, aged 45 to 65, for over 20 years. What he found should be reassuring to all of us. These men maintained a healthy body weight, and their oxygen carrying ability decreased by only 12 percent rather than the 40 to 50 percent expected to occur with aging. This demonstrates that getting slower and tiring easily is not inevitable with age. The next time there is an older adult foot race, look at the times of these older men and women. They will be faster than you might expect. Numerous studies support these findings.

Cardiovascular training will increase maximum ventilation, and the improvements parallel those of cardiac output (the heart's ability to pump blood). Although the breathing muscles can be strengthened through exercise, most previous damage as a result of disease or smoking is irreversible. While that is discouraging, a progressive aerobic fitness program as seen in hospital-based "better breather programs" can improve function. The nurses who operate better breather programs surmise that this is possible because of the large reserve capacity of the lungs. These changes can be tolerated quite well.

Older adults can demonstrate improvements in maximal oxygen consumption similar to that of their younger counterparts, but it may take longer to achieve such enhanced function. An older adult participating in an aerobics program may enjoy some or all of the following improvements in cardiorespiratory fitness: a decrease in submaximal heart rate at a similar workload, a faster recovery heart rate, and a decreased systolic blood pressure at rest and during exercise. Most older adults who exercise will show improvement slowly and will not progress as far as younger exercisers.

EXERCISE AND THE SKELETAL SYSTEM

The skeletal issues that are seen in older adults range in severity from mild arthritis to severe osteoporosis. Arthritis is a major crippler of Americans. The severity of degenerative joint disease ranges from mild to severe. In severe cases of degenerative joint disease, it is common to have a person consider a joint replacement. Osteoporosis is another serious problem seen in older people, particularly in women.

Osteoporosis versus Osteoarthritis

Many people confuse osteoporosis and osteoarthritis since they sound very similar, yet they are very different. Osteoporosis is a reduction of bone mass, whereas osteoarthritis is a degenerative joint disease that usually affects the weight-bearing joints (as opposed to *rheumatoid* arthritis, which is a systemic autoimmune disorder).

Osteoporosis is Latin for "porous bone." It's a silent condition with no outward symptoms that causes the bones to become weak, brittle, and easily breakable. Osteoporosis is when a person's bone mass density (BMD) is low compared to normal peak BMD. Osteopenia is the term that refers to a decrease in bone density that, while too low to be called normal, isn't low enough to be considered osteoporotic. Having osteopenia means there's a greater risk that you may develop osteoporosis.

In people with osteoporosis, bones can break from a minor fall, or even a simple cough can fracture a rib. In older men and women, osteoporosis can sometimes be an indirect cause of death, but more often it's a cause of a decreased quality of life. The good news is that today treatments for osteoporosis, as well as methods to prevent it, are available. And one of the easiest, least expensive treatments is weight-bearing exercise.

Just about everyone gets osteoporosis. It's an equal-opportunity disease. Most people think that osteoporosis is only a concern for women, but did you know that one out of four men over the age of 50 could develop a fracture in his lifetime? While osteoporosis can lead to an increased risk of fractures of the hip, spine, and wrist in women, men are susceptible to the same effects as women from a less-than-ideal lifestyle, including poor diet choices over a lifetime, smoking, drinking too much, and lack of weight-bearing exercise. Unfortunately, men never seem to discuss this topic with their health professional. Men generally have a higher bone mass than do females overall and don't experience the rapid loss that women do as a result of menopause. Unfortunately, for men osteoporosis goes undetected until much later in life, often after preventive measures could have been employed. Men's bones like the same things that women's bones do: a healthy diet including calcium and vitamin D, along with a sensible dose of weight-bearing exercise and resistance training. Both men and women should consult their health professional about the proper intake of calcium and vitamin D, which often depends upon age and health history.

While osteoporosis is often thought of as an older person's disease, it can strike at any age. Osteoporosis is a major public health threat for an estimated 44 million Americans, or 55 percent of the people 50 years of age and older. Of the 10 million Americans estimated to have osteoporosis, 8 million are women and 2 million are men. Osteoporosis is underrecognized and undertreated not only in Caucasian women, but in African-American women as well. Significant risk has been reported in people of all ethnic backgrounds.

After people reach maturity, they often forget about their bones. But in order to understand osteoporosis, it's important to think about bones and understand what they really are. Bone is living, growing tissue. Throughout our lives, our bodies are continually breaking down old bone and rebuilding new bone. When we're young, we gain more bone than we lose. Bones then progressively increase in density until a maximum level is reached, usually around age 30. But after about age 35, things change and we start to lose more bone than we make. Over time, this causes bone density to slowly decrease, and bones become more brittle. In a lifetime, a woman may lose up to 38 percent of peak bone mass, whereas a man may lose only 23 percent.

Bone density is much like a honeycomb. A person with good bone strength will have a tightly woven bone matrix, whereas someone with osteoporosis will have big gaps in the honeycomb that make it weak. Everybody gets weaker bones as they age. The causes of osteoporosis are multifactorial and therefore are difficult to isolate. Genetic and environmental factors interact to affect the rate of bone loss and the integrity of the remaining structure. Metabolic disorders involving the digestive system, renal function, diabetes, or hormonal levels increase the rate of bone loss. Poor lifestyle habits such as insufficient calcium intake, physical inactivity, and smoking can further accelerate bone loss. Physical activity is necessary for maintaining bone material content and serves as a stimulus for increasing bone mass. Studies have shown that immobility leads to bone loss and that the stress of weight-bearing exercise builds up mineral mass.

Osteoarthritis, which is the inflammation and swelling of the cartilage and lining of a joint, is sometimes called "wear-and-tear" arthritis because it's often caused by the misuse and abuse we put our bodies through. It's also called degenerative joint disease, or simply arthritis. The most common form of arthritis in the United States, osteoarthritis causes the cartilage to break down, commonly producing pain and stiffness. Osteoarthritis is often found in weight-bearing joints such as the ankle, hips, and knees. It also occurs in the hands, lower back, and any other joint. The causes of arthritis are multifactorial, including biomechanical as well as biochemical issues. Genetics, dietary issues, and bone density, along with joint looseness, obesity, and lack of muscle all contribute to arthritis. Once osteoarthritis has occurred, it's irreversible. It is difficult to separate deterioration caused by aging from that caused by accumulated wear and tear. Trauma to joint cartilage results in the formation of scar tissue that causes the connective tissue to become stiffer and less responsive. This build-up can result in a thickened joint capsule that often contains debris, which in turn impairs range of motion. Decreased range of motion in joints affects posture, gait, balance, and skeletal flexibility, thus increasing the potential for falls and injury. The kyphosis that occurs with aging leads to diminished stature and poor use of respiratory muscles, which predisposes older people to respiratory infection. Breakdown of the joint cartilage leads to osteoarthritis and pain, reduced mobility, and a diminished ability to accomplish activities of daily living.

POSSIBLE EXERCISE BENEFITS FOR BONES OF AN OLDER ADULT

- Improve bone density
- Improve flexibility
- Improve range of motion

THE EFFECTS OF EXERCISE ON MUSCLE MASS AND STRENGTH IN OLDER ADULTS

By adolescence we are equipped with all the muscle cells we will have; therefore, after that time, a muscle can get either bigger or smaller. When we build muscles, hypertrophy, we enlarge the muscle cell. The opposite is the shrinking of the muscle cell, or atrophy. By the time most people are 70 years of age, they have lost about 25 percent of their muscle mass due to disuse atrophy. In some cases, the loss of strength is so severe that a person cannot climb or descend stairs or rise from a chair without pushing up with their hands.

The loss of mean muscle mass, strength, and muscle endurance are universal changes found in normal aging muscles. The reduction of muscle mass is critical in many older adults, who lose about three to five ounces of muscle mass per year. According to one respected researcher, when we strip away the fat and skin in an autopsy, we find very skinny old people with regard to muscle mass. Among the physical changes that occur with age, the loss of lean muscle mass is one of the most noteworthy. Strength in men is maximal between the ages of 30 and 35 years and remains relatively constant until around 50 years of age, after which time it declines. The rate of decline in muscular strength with age appears to be slightly less in the upper extremities (small muscle groups) than in the back and legs (large muscle groups). Leg and back muscle strength decline by 40 percent. Men 80 years old may exhibit a 40 percent lower lean muscle mass than men 30 years old. Between the middle-aged and older men, overall body weight drops 10 percent and is attributed to a decline in lean muscle mass.

The classic study performed by DeVries in 1986 found that strength-training exercise has a tremendous impact on the maintenance and development of muscle mass in the aging adult. The reductions in the musculoskeletal system result in reductions of muscle tone and size, which usually leads to an avoidance of heavy physical activity, which leads to less strength—and thus, the vicious circle of decline in function and strength. Research has found that the major declines seen in muscle strength are not an expected outcome of age. In a landmark study that took 10 frail men and women as old as 96 years and had them work out with free weights, within two months participants had already boosted thigh muscle strength by an average of 174 percent and muscle mass had increased by 9 percent. What does this mean in real life terms? Five volunteers who originally could walk only one quarter of a mile doubled their walking distance. Two other volunteers who had previously needed canes to walk, no longer needed them at all. (I personally have a 94-year-old woman who couldn't get up out of a chair without the use of her hands. After two weeks of instruction, she is now "popping" out of the chair.)

The well-respected scientist Mime Nelson, PhD, maintains that "our muscles have the ability to grow and get stronger from birth until we die." By making a lifelong habit of even minimal weight-bearing exercise and resistance training (for 15 minutes a day, two times per week) we can maintain as much as 94 percent of our muscle mass well into old age. Recent research suggests that increased strength leads to improved balance and functional mobility among older people. Myths about the inability of older people to increase their strength are just that. Nearly every senior patient can benefit from basic resistance and strength-training programs.

In decades past, the cry from most exercise physiologists was that aerobic exercise was critical. Unfortunately, in their enthusiasm to make that point, they didn't remind the public that a totally fit person needs strength training along with stretching exercises combined with cardiovascular conditioning. To be truly "physically fit," a person must incorporate all components of exercise.

According to the experts at Tufts University in Boston, strength training is the single most critical step a person can take to retard the aging process. "...if older people can maintain muscle mass and functional strength, many of these things we call 'biomarkers' of aging might actually be 'biomarkers' of inactivity," according to Dr. Evans. Physical therapists and fitness trainers who work with older adults on a daily basis have observed firsthand that older adults can increase their strength, power, and functional performance. Personally, I have seen older women who initially came to my exercise classes frail and using walkers and canes improve their strength to the extent that they no longer rely on their canes and walkers. Recent research shows that improvements in strength lead to functional improvements in the ability to perform normal, daily activities more easily. Strength training improves balance and mobility. A total fitness program includes flexibility, aerobic exercise, and strength training.

BENEFITS DERIVED FROM STRENGTH TRAINING FOR THE OLDER ADULT

- Increase in muscle tone, muscle size, and muscle strength and strong bones
- Improvement in bone density
- Reduction of the risk of colon cancer and diabetes
- Improvement in muscle coordination
- Improvement in functional independence

EFFECTS OF EXERCISE ON THE BRAIN AND NEUROLOGICAL SYSTEM

As years pass, the brain may decrease in weight, and the interconnections among neurons may be reduced. Biologically, the brain actually continues to develop throughout our lives. Dr. Marian Diamond of the University of California, Berkeley, contends there is mounting evidence that so long as disease does not intervene, the brain retains its capacity to grow new anatomical connections, to learn, and to function at high levels. As a person ages, mental capacity does not necessarily deteriorate, especially in people who continue to learn and think, who are well nourished, and who exercise their bodies throughout their lives. Studies show that intellectual challenge can enhance this growth. As our bodies change, so do our brains change, either positively or negativity depending upon numerous factors, some genetic, some behavioral, some health related. Note that there is a significant difference between normal forgetting and Alzheimer's disease. The best example of that was told to me by Dr. Dean Edell: normal forgetting is when you forget where you put your glasses; a reason to be concerned is not knowing that you wear glasses.

From the age of 30 onward there is a slight mental slowdown, such as in reaction time, which determines how quickly you can step on the brake while driving or how fast you come up with the answers while watching *Jeopardy!* But other functions, such as vocabulary, get better through your 50s and 60s. It is true that some mental skills do begin to decline around age 70, but this varies greatly.

The Baltimore Longitudinal Study of Aging, which followed volunteers over the age of 70 for over 20 years, found no significant decline in memory. Some participants continued to perform well on the cognitive tasks well into their 80s. The brain, like the heart, may do more adapting and less declining with age than previously thought. One example the researchers cited was problem-solving skills: when faced with a task, the older volunteers drew on different capacities to complete the task. At least up to age 70, there is little or no decline in problem solving.

Research has demonstrated that there is a strong association between regular, vigorous exercise and successful aging. Some preliminary research even indicates that exercising can improve brain function in older people. The tests measured response time, memory, and mental flexibility. More and more research confirms that older adults who are physically active have been reported to have faster movement times than their younger, inactive counterparts. Physical exercise can help brain functions, too. Robert Dustman, chief of the Neuropsychology Laboratory at the Salt Lake City VA Hospital, found that aerobically fit individuals in their 50s did as well as those in their 20s. These active people had more mental flexibility and adjusted more quickly to changing tasks than did people their same age who were "couch potatoes." Dr. Dustman postulates that the improved circulation produces the effect. Another study analyzed women aged 57 to 85 who started exercising regularly, and showed they were able to gain back some of the mental speed they had previously lost. As older people become fit, all the predictable good things happen to the bones, muscles, arteries, and so forth, but the most exciting finding is that exercise increases an older person's IQ. Exercise can be responsible for a quicker and more alert brain.

Exercise helps to maintain the integrity of the central nervous system and psycho-motor control, possibly due to increases in regional cerebral blood flow or elevated cerebral metabolism from increased sensory stimulation and arousal. Hence, age-related decreases in reaction and movement times are minimized. What does the brain need to function? It needs oxygen. How does it obtain oxygen? Via the blood. And the best way to move oxygen-rich blood to the brain is through exercise.

THE EFFECTS OF EXERCISE ON BODY FAT IN OLDER ADULTS

For decades, we've seen shriveled and non-energetic older people and have accepted that as the norm. We have also seen substantially fat older people and have accepted that, too, as the norm. The old excuse was, "Oh, my metabolism has just slowed down." Scientists looking at metabolic rates in senior athletes found that the metabolism doesn't really slow down that much if the person stays active and if their muscle mass is similar to when they were younger. The key factor to remember is that fit people use more calories at rest than do sedentary people.

That's because exercise not only increases metabolism during exercise but keeps it revved up for some time after exercise. Also, muscle burns more calories at rest than fat does, so the more muscle you have, the more calories you are burning.

Increased body fat that occurs with age is a concern because of its relationship with heart disease and diabetes, which often lead to premature mortality. It is not uncommon for people to gain significant fat during their mid-life, especially women. Contrary to the belief that women were insulated against heart disease no matter what, a study conducted at Harvard University School of Public Health found that weight gains of even 11 to 18 pounds in mid-life increased a woman's chance of having a heart attack by 25 percent. Remember, heart disease is a major killer in both men and women!

EFFECTS OF EXERCISE ON JOINT MOBILITY

A common issue seen by fitness trainers are sprains, which are a partial or complete tear of a ligament, which attach bone to bone. Ankle sprains, often the result of landing incorrectly and the joint moving in an abnormal direction, are reportedly the most common sports injury.

Bursitis is pain and swelling of the bursae, small fluid-filled sacs located in or near the joints. These sacs help cushion any tissues that rub against or slide over hard bone. Repetitive motions can result in bursitis, with shoulders, elbows, hips, and knees being commonly affected areas. Healing time varies due to the severity of the condition.

Strains, commonly called "pulled muscles," are injuries involving the muscle-tendon connection. They're most often caused by using a muscle in a way that it's not trained for. Essentially, a strain is the overstretching or overstressing of a muscle. Strains have three classifications. A first-degree strain is mild and doesn't cause disability. A second-degree strain involves significant tearing of the fibers, and recovery time can last several weeks. A severe, third-degree strain is the complete destruction of the muscle-tendon unit.

RESEARCH TO PRACTICE

Arthur Kramer, psychologist at the University of Illinois, measured how quickly 40 sedentary adults between the ages of 63 and 82 responded simultaneously to two differently pitched tones by hitting buttons. Half the adults went through a 10-week water aerobics course, three times a week for 45 minutes of exercise, while the others all remained sedentary. The regular exercisers responded more quickly upon hearing a tone than did sedentary adults, even when the non-exercisers were younger by 20 to 50 years. (Normally, reaction time hits its peak when people are in their 20s, begins a subtle decline in the 30s, and is on a downhill roll in our 60s). Roberta Rikli, PhD, at Cal State Fullerton believes that the decline seen in reaction time that begins in the mid-30s is not related to aging so much as to fitness level.

Tendinitis is the inflammation of a tendon, connective tissue that attaches a muscle to a bone. The most obvious example is perhaps the Achilles tendon (feel the back of your heel and follow it up to your calf muscle). As the muscle turns into a tendon it becomes denser. The purpose of the tendon is to transmit force and help provide stability to the joint area. Tendinitis can be caused by irritation seen in overuse syndromes (think tennis elbow) or by poor technique.

EXERCISE AND AGING

The research on physical activity and aging has taught us:

- Exercise doesn't have to be hard or vigorous to make improvements. In fact, Dr. William Haskell at the Stanford Prevention Research Center has said that four bouts of exercise, such as walking for 5 minutes each time, will improve cardiovascular fitness.

- Exercise programs for older adults must include flexibility, strength, and cardiovascular exercise in addition to balance and coordination.
- Fit people have an increased metabolism.
- A regular dose of mild to moderate exercise along with proper diet can have a positive influence on the incidence of type II diabetes.
- Exercise makes the brain better and improves psychosocial aspects such as increased self-esteem, better socialization, and less anxiety.
- Exercise improves insulin efficiency and increases blood plasma volume.
- There is a strong association between regular exercise, improved sleep patterns, and decreased fatigue levels.
- Fit people have increased lean body mass, which contributes to reduced risk of heart disease, stroke, diabetes, and much more.
- Fit older people take less medication and have fewer doctor and hospital visits than sedentary older people, as well as living longer and fuller lives!
- How you live is more important than the genes you were born with.

Growing older should not mean losing the sense of joy and dignity, or the ability to function fully. Rather, masterful aging means maintaining a sense of humor and having a strong foundation of hope, health, and gratitude for every stage of life. Remember, as you embrace the fitness challenge, you will add years to your life and life to your years!

GLOSSARY

Atrophy: a decrease in size of a muscle resulting from de-conditioning or immobilization.

Cardiovascular endurance: the capacity to continue physical performance over an extended period of time.

Circuit training: a series of different exercises done with no significant rest in between each set.

Concentric contraction: an isotonic contraction in which muscle shortens; e.g., bringing a glass of water to your mouth.

Contraction: muscles utilizing energy and expending heat to exert a force.

Cross-training: a method of training in which a variety of exercises or sports are employed to stimulate a training effect without increasing the risk of injury. A positive example of cross-training is when a runner takes one to two land workouts into the pool to perform deep water running; their cardiovascular system stays conditioned but the lower-impact water workout allows for other parts of the body to avoid repetitive stress.

Eccentric movement: a movement in which the muscle lengthens while resisting the load; e.g., bringing down the glass of water slowly from your mouth.

Extension: making the joint angle larger.

Flexibility: the ability of the joint to move freely and comfortably through a complete range of motion.

Flexion: making the joint angle smaller.

Hypertrophy: an increase in muscles size as a result of progressive resistive exercise training.

Isokinetic contraction: where the resistance stays constant through a full range of motion. A basic example of isokinetic exercise is moving your arms through the water, or expensive hydraulic resistance equipment.

Isometric contraction: when no movement occurs because the resistance is constant. A common example is pushing your hands together in front of the chest.

Isotonic contraction: when the muscle lengthens and shortens. Types of isotonic contractions:

> **Concentric contraction:** an isotonic contraction in which the muscle shortens. When you drink a glass of water you are performing a concentric contraction of the bicep.

> **Eccentric contraction:** an isotonic contraction in which the muscle lengthens. When you lower a glass of water to the table you are performing an eccentric contraction the bicep.

Muscular endurance: the ability of a muscle to contract for a prolonged time.

Muscular strength: the amount of weight/force a muscle can exert.

Overtraining: when a training routine exceeds the capabilities of the athlete, creating deleterious outcomes to the trainee. Overtraining takes many shapes, from injuries to personality changes to extreme weight loss. The key is to train not strain.

Periodization: a systematic approach of changing your training routine at a regularly scheduled interval. Periodization optimizes results and prevents the athlete from overtraining or getting stale. The goal of periodization is for the athlete to "peak" in time for season competition. This approach allows for year-round training without causing overuse syndrome. A common example is when swimmers go from swimming long course to short course.

Plyometrics: exercises that maximize the stretch reflex to teach muscles to produce maximum force. Plyometrics usually include sport-specific movements such as hopping and jumping. These high-impact exercises are very traumatic to the body and can cause overuse injuries in some athletes. Plyometric routines should be spread out and used cautiously to avoid putting too much stress on the body.

Power: a combination of strength applied over a short period of time. Plyometric exercise is an example of power. Most sport skills rely on power.

Progression: the process of changing the challenges placed upon the body to stimulate the desired gains. The progression can be adapted by changes to the intensity, volume, or frequency to the training routine.

Progressive resistance exercise: commonly referred to as strength training; as the muscle gets stronger you increase the load to further challenge the muscle.

Recovery: the rest interval in place for the energy system to recover. Recovery can be the time between sets, or the time between workouts. The critical question with recovery is how much time is needed for the body to recover and repair itself before it starts to de-condition.

Reps (or Repetitions): the number of times a movement is repeated.

Set: a grouping of repetitions.

Specificity of training: matching the physical training program to the specific demands required for the sport.

Training variables: customization to be considered when designing a fitness routine. A training session is much like a "grandma's recipe." It can be modified by tweaking the ingredients that go into the training session. The major ingredients that most trainers tweak are called FITT or:

F = Frequency—how often the exercise should be performed. For most individuals three to five times a week is ideal. For competitive athletes the frequency will increase. It is important to note that with increased frequency the risk of injury increases.

I = Intensity—the overload necessary to promote the desired outcome. An example of intensity is how heavy you lift a weight or how hard you sprint a quarter-mile. Overload is loading the muscles beyond normal capacity to promote increase in muscular strength and/or endurance.

T = Type—the mode of exercise. For example, there are several options to increase aerobic fitness, such as biking, walking, or swimming, to name just a few. Cross-training is a good way to foster fitness and prevent overuse syndrome.

T = Time—time on task, or duration, is the length of each training section.

EXERCISE INDEX

ACKNOWLEDGMENTS

A sincere thanks goes out to Keith Riegert, Brian McLendon, and Kierra Sondereker for their vision and conceiving of this book concept. I would also like to express my appreciation to all those talented people behind the scenes that made this book possible—especially Claire Chun and Mary Calvez—as well as those who contributed to my previous books from which much of the information in this book was gleaned.

A special recognition goes out to my wife Margaret and my children Chris and Kevin.

May this book assist you in growing strong, not old and frail. Recent research has shown that a modest amount of regular exercise can contribute to an improved quality and quantity of life. Note that most chronic conditions can be positively influenced with a regular dose of physical activity.

Always remember and never forget you are never too old to engage in a prudent exercise program, and it is the elixir of youth and vitality.

ABOUT THE AUTHOR

Dr. Karl Knopf (or Dr. Karl, as his students called him) has been involved with the health and fitness industry in numerous capacities for more than four decades. He started teaching older adult fitness classes in the 1970s when little was known about the relationship between exercise and seniors. He also taught adaptive PE classes at Foothill College for 40 years. In addition to his full-time job as a college professor, Dr. Knopf was the president of the Fitness Educators of Older Adults Association for 20 years and the former director of fitness therapy and senior fitness for the International Sports Science Association (ISSA) until 2021. He is currently an advisor to public television's *Sit and Be Fit* show.

Dr. Knopf was involved in many professional activities outside of his teaching duties. He has been a consultant to Time Life Medical's video series, the State of California, Stanford University, and the University of California, and served as an expert witness in several lawsuits pertaining to controversial exercises. He has been interviewed for and featured in many print media publications, including the *Wall Street Journal, San Jose Mercury News, Los Angeles Times, Washington Post,* and most recently, *Bottom Line.* In the past, he was a frequent guest on Joanie Greggains's KGO radio show and briefly served as an advisor to the Santa Clara County Public Health advisory board.

Since his retirement in 2013, Dr. Knopf has provided numerous wellness and aging workshops to local community and nonprofit organizations. In 2018, he received a Global Award from the aquatic exercise association for his lifetime contributions to the aquatic fitness industry.